D0187996

Moritz Kaposi

(1837–1902)

Professor of Dermatology, University of Vienna

Courtesy of Professor Klaus Wolff,
Department of Dermatology, University of Vienna, Austria

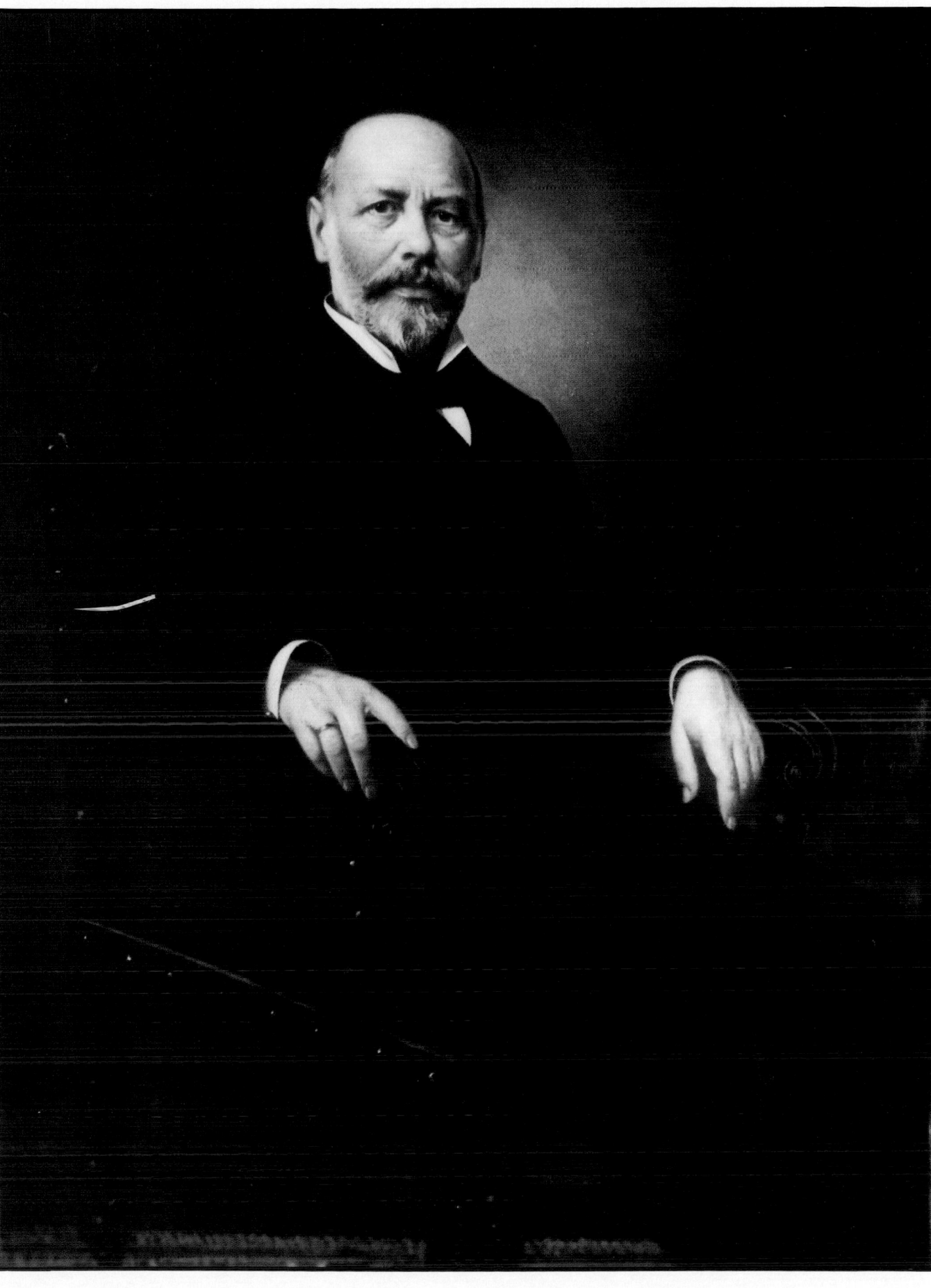

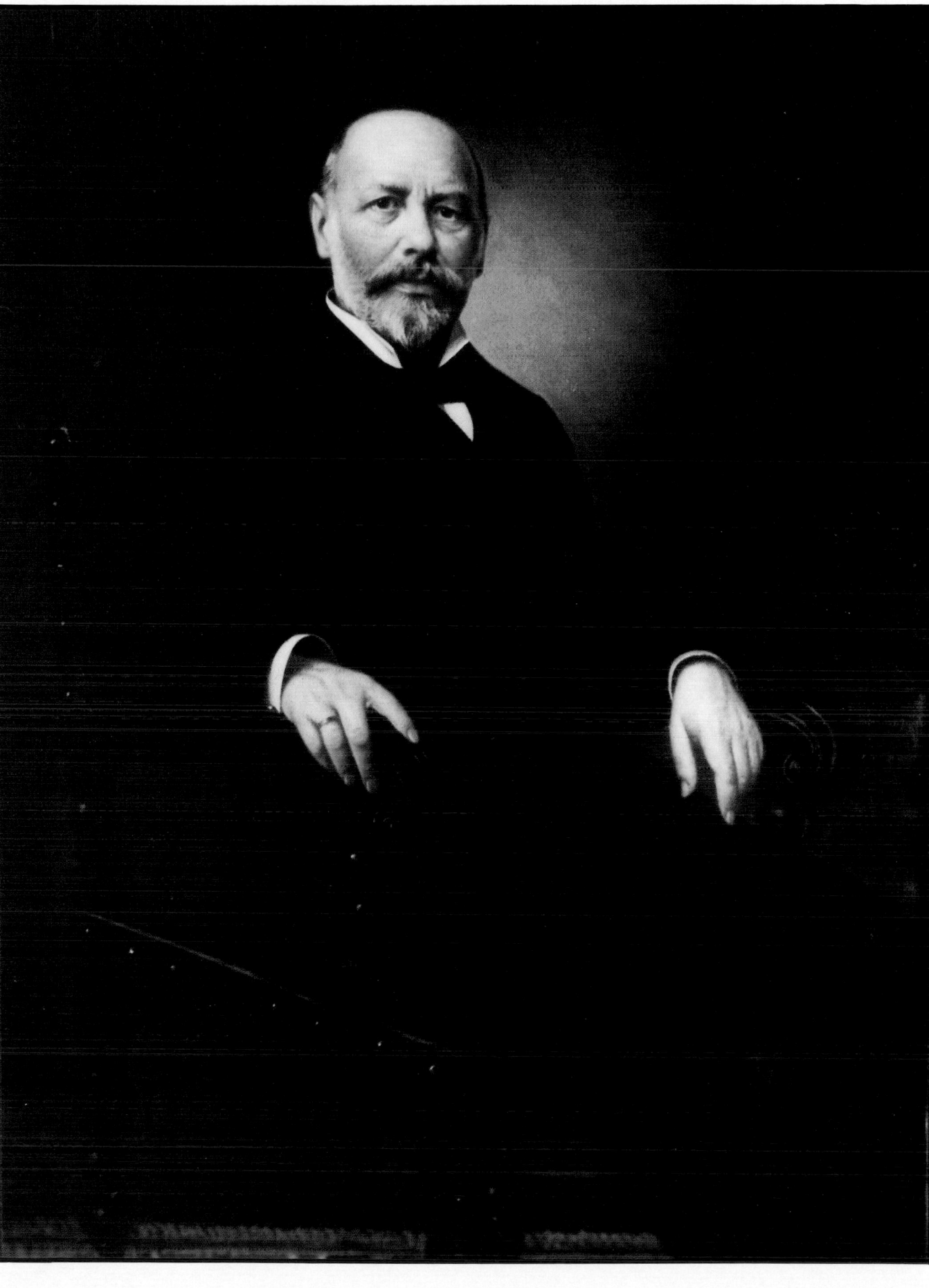

Color Atlas of AIDS

Alvin E. Friedman-Kien, M.D.

Professor of Dermatology and Microbiology
Departments of Dermatology and Microbiology
New York University Medical Center
New York, New York

1989

W.B. SAUNDERS COMPANY
Harcourt Brace Jovanovich, Inc.
Philadelphia London Toronto Montreal Sydney Tokyo

W. B. SAUNDERS COMPANY
Harcourt Brace Jovanovich, Inc.

The Curtis Center
Independence Square West
Philadelphia, PA 19106

Library of Congress Cataloging-in-Publication Data

Color atlas of AIDS.

1. AIDS (Disease)—Atlases.   I. Friedman-Kien,
   Alvin E. [DNLM: 1. Acquired Immunodeficiency
   Syndrome—atlases.   WD 308 C7192]

RC607.A26C654   1989   616.97′92075   88–24013

ISBN 0–7216–2759–5

Cover art: *Top,* Herpes zoster; *center,* Pneumocystis carinii cysts; *bottom,* Epidemic Kaposi's sarcoma.

Editor: Tracy Tucker
Designer: Patti Maddaloni
Production Manager: Peter Faber
Manuscript Editor: Lee Walters
Illustration Coordinator: Brett MacNaughton
Page Layout Artist: Patti Maddaloni
Indexer: Ruth Low

Color Atlas of AIDS   ISBN 0–7216–2759–5

© 1989 by W. B. Saunders Company. Copyright under the Uniform Copyright Convention. Simultaneously published in Canada. All rights reserved. This book is protected by copyright. No part of it may be reproduced, stored in a retrieval system, or transmitted in any form or by any means, electronic, mechanical, photocopying, recording, or otherwise, without written permission from the publisher. Made in the United States of America. Library of Congress catalog card number 88–24013.

Last digit is the print number: 9   8   7   6   5   4   3   2   1

*This book is dedicated to Howard Gilman,
who has provided continued support for AIDS research
since the beginning of the epidemic.
We are grateful to him for making the publication of this book possible.*

Contributors

Clay J. Cockerell, M.D.
Assistant Professor in Dermatology
Associate in Dermatopathology
New York University Medical Center
New York, New York

Vincent T. DeVita, Jr., M.D.
Clinical Director
National Institutes of Health
National Cancer Institute
Bethesda, Maryland

Alvin E. Friedman-Kien, M.D.
Professor of Dermatology and Microbiology
New York University Medical Center
New York, New York

N. Patrick Hennessey, M.D.
Clinical Instructor
Department of Dermatology
New York University Medical Center
New York, New York

Kenneth H. Mayer, M.D.
Associate Professor of Medicine
Brown University
Chief, Infectious Disease Division
Memorial Hospital
Pawtucket, Rhode Island

Steven M. Opal, M.D.
Assistant Professor of Medicine
Brown University
Director, Traveler's Clinic
Memorial Hospital
Pawtucket, Rhode Island

Richard Ostreicher, M.D.
Department of Dermatology
Yale University Medical School
New Haven, Connecticut

Brian Saltzman, M.D.
Department of Medicine
New York University Medical Center
New York, New York

David N. Silvers, M.D.
Associate Clinical Professor
Departments of Dermatology and Pathology
Director, Section of Dermatopathology
College of Physicians and Surgeons
Columbia University
New York, New York

Dorothea Zucker-Franklin, M.D.
Professor of Medicine
Department of Medicine
New York University Medical Center
New York, New York

Acknowledgments

We wish to express our deepest gratitude to the Sandoz Corporation and especially to Dr. Max Link, President, Sandoz, USA, who recognized the urgent need for this Atlas and generously provided a grant that subsidized the production of all the color illustrations.

We thank Dr. Milton R. Salton, Professor and Chairman of the Department of Microbiology, and Dr. Irwin M. Freedberg, Professor and Chairman of the Department of Dermatology of New York University Medical Center, for their constant encouragement and sound advice in the conception and preparation of this atlas.

Special words of appreciation are extended to Senior Project Assistants Thomas M. Nichols and W. Dean Hiatt for their dedication, patience, and excellent help throughout the organization and preparation of the various manuscripts for this book. We also wish to thank Claudia Boak and Ellen Arntz for their superb typing assistance.

We thank Dr. Klaus Wolff, Professor of Dermatology, University of Vienna, Austria, who kindly provided us with the photograph of the fine portrait of Professor Moritz Kaposi that now hangs in the offices of the Department of Dermatology at the University of Vienna, Austria.

We are most grateful to several physicians who contributed photographs for this book, including Dr. Charles L. M. Olweny, former Director of the Uganda Cancer Institute, Kampala, Uganda; Dr. Alexander C. Templeton, St. Luke's Medical Center, Department of Pathology, Chicago; Dr. Charles L. Vogel of the Comprehensive Cancer Center of the State of Miami, Florida; and Dr. John D. Ziegler of the University of California School of Medicine, Department of Medicine, San Francisco, who all worked together in Uganda during the 1960s to study Kaposi's sarcoma seen in Africa; as well as Dr. Paul L. Gigase, Professor of Medicine, University of Antwerp, Belgium. Each of these men generously contributed several of the photographs of African patients from their own personal collections, which have been used to illustrate the various forms of endemic Kaposi's sarcoma in this atlas. We also thank Dr. Nathan Clumeck, Division of Infectious Diseases, St. Pierre Hospital, Brussels, Belgium, one of the first clinical scientists to describe AIDS among African patients, who kindly allowed us to use his photographs of some African patients with AIDS-associated Kaposi's sarcoma. Dr. John Li, Director of Pathology, North Central Bronx Hospital, Bronx, New York, generously provided the photographs used to illustrate the gross pathologic specimens of Kaposi's sarcoma involving visceral organs of patients with AIDS.

We extend our special appreciation to the Howard Gilman Foundation, Bernard Bergreen, Esq., Edward Klagsbrun, Esq., and Fred Greenman, Esq., whose concern and excellent advice were instrumental in bringing this book into fruition.

We wish to acknowledge the assistance of Dr. Mead Morgan, Director of the Statistics Branch of the AIDS Program, Centers for Disease Control, Atlanta, Georgia, who kindly provided much of the statistical data on epidemic Kaposi's sarcoma used in Chapter 2.

A special thanks is due to Dr. Harry Haverkos of the National Institutes of Health, who conscientiously reviewed some of the chapters of this book and offered many helpful suggestions.

We are enormously indebted to William Slue, Photography Division, Department of Dermatology, New York University Medical Center, New York City, who photographed most of the clinical lesions used as color illustrations in this atlas. We are very grateful to Mr. Slue and his assistant, Meryll Krolik, who were especially considerate and humane in dealing with our patients.

It is my pleasure to acknowledge the personal interest, diligence, and careful consideration this book has received in the capable hands of many people at W. B. Saunders Company, who made the process of publishing this atlas a gratifying experience. These include Vice President and Editor-In-Chief Thomas E. Mackey, Jr., our Editor, Tracy Tucker, as well as Patti Maddaloni, Peter Faber, Lee Walters, Evelyn Weiman, Brett MacNaughton, Jack Farrell, Stephen Zellers, and Ruth Low. To these individuals with whom we worked directly, and to all the others at Saunders who labored "behind the scenes" to make this atlas a reality, we offer our deepest appreciation.

Most of all, on behalf of the physicians and other health care workers who will use this atlas as a reference, we wish to express our profound appreciation to each of the patients who willingly agreed to be photographed and granted us permission to use their pictures for publication in this book. They did so with the knowledge and hope that their participation would benefit other patients by providing the medical community with a heightened awareness, better recognition, and deeper understanding of both the subtle and more overt visual diagnostic signs and symptoms associated with human immunodeficiency virus infection and AIDS.

Contents

6
Cutaneous Signs of AIDS Other Than Kaposi's Sarcoma
Clay J. Cockerell

7
Opportunistic Infections in Patients
with Human Immunodeficiency Virus Infection
Kenneth H. Mayer
Steven M. Opal

Index

Introduction

It is a rare patient with AIDS who does not present with or develop a cutaneous manifestation of the disease. As with some of the opportunistic infections that complicate AIDS, the cutaneous manifestations of the disease overlap with similar manifestations that occur in illnesses quite different from AIDS. Drawing the distinction between a benign condition and a dermatologic presenting sign of AIDS is, therefore, becoming increasingly important to the general physician as the AIDS epidemic spreads.

This color atlas of the cutaneous manifestations of AIDS is the most extensive collection of photographs of these skin conditions available. It is edited by one of the world's foremost authorities on these problems, Dr. Alvin Friedman-Kien. In 1981, Dr. Friedman-Kien and his colleagues were astute enough to detect an unusual frequency of a variant of Kaposi's sarcoma in young homosexual men. This observation, and the detection of an epidemic of *Pneumocystis carinii* pneumonia in the same population, marked the beginning of what we have come to know as the AIDS epidemic. In the scant six years since then, the causative agent, a retrovirus, has been discovered; its molecular biology characterized; its site of attack on the immune system described; diagnostic tests developed; new, albeit primitive, treatments developed; and candidate vaccines prepared for clinical trials. This sequence of events began at the bedside and, once again, illustrates the important role observations made by discerning physicians play in the history of research and medicine.

A large portion of this atlas is appropriately enough devoted to Kaposi's sarcoma. Kaposi's sarcoma is truly one of mother nature's puzzle games. For those of us interested in the cancer problem, the unraveling of the puzzle of Kaposi's sarcoma offers to clarify many more general mechanisms of the development of malignancy and, hence, its importance. It is hard to escape the conclusion, for example, that Kaposi's sarcoma is somehow associated with disorders of the immune system. In the classic indolent form, it is linked to an unusually high incidence of HLA DR5 antigens, and affected patients have an extraordinarily high increase of lymphomas, malignancies of the immune system. It also appears with a markedly increased frequency in immunosuppressed transplant patients, as do lymphomas, where it has a tendency to wax and wane with the degree of immunosuppression. Its occurrence in African blacks who reside near the equator in areas endemic for Burkitt's lymphoma and its failure to occur with any frequency in American blacks add to the speculation that it shares a common mechanism, or etiologic agent, with lymphomas. Of course, it appears in about one third of patients with AIDS, and lymphomas are also appearing with greater frequency in this disease. Its frequency in homosexual men with AIDS is now mysteriously decreasing.

AIDS is not yet a common disease, and many physicians have a limited personal experience with it. The rapidly increasing incidence and spread to the heterosexual population will soon present the general physician with many diagnostic problems. This text will provide a valuable visual course on the cutaneous manifestations of AIDS.

Vincent T. DeVita Jr., M.D.

1

An Overview of the Acquired Immune Deficiency Syndrome

Alvin E. Friedman-Kien
Kenneth H. Mayer

Historical Perspective

In June and July of 1981, cases of an extremely uncommon opportunistic infection, *Pneumocystis carinii* pneumonia, and a very rare skin tumor of endothelial cell origin, Kaposi's sarcoma, were first reported in New York and California in epidemic proportions among previously healthy young homosexual and bisexual men who were not previously known to be predisposed to these diseases.[1, 2] With the rapidly increasing number of cases, it was soon recognized that other life-threatening infections and neoplastic diseases were also observed and found to be associated with an unexplained defect in cell-mediated immunity, common to each of these patients.[3]

In the early days of this epidemic, when these hitherto unusual diseases appeared to be limited to homosexual men, the acronym "GRID" was briefly used, an abbreviation for gay-related immunodeficiency diseases. However, within a few months further epidemiologic observations proved this term to be incorrect when several intravenous drug users, recent Haitian immigrants, and eventually hemophiliacs and recipients of blood transfusions were also found to have an unexplained immunodeficiency and similar opportunistic infections.[4] By early 1982 this group of disease entities, associated with a specific pattern of immunodeficiency, was renamed the acquired immune deficiency syndrome (AIDS) by the Centers for Disease Control (CDC).[3] The term "syndrome" has been used because AIDS does not constitute a single illness, but rather encompasses a wide range of clinical diseases including specific life-threatening infections and neoplasms associated with a profound and irreversible unexplained acquired disorder of cell-mediated immunity. At the outset, there was no etiologic agent identified which could explain the underlying immunodeficiency and its protean manifestations.

AIDS was originally defined by the CDC for epidemiologic surveillance purposes as "the presence of a reliably diagnosed disease at least moderately predictive of an underlying defect in cell-mediated immunity in the absence of known causes of such diminished host resistance (e.g., immunosuppressive therapy, or Hodgkin's disease)."[3] The original CDC case definition has been useful in the epidemiologic surveillance of AIDS, but the delineation of the retroviral etiology and wider spectrum of associated immune disregulation has resulted in a broadened understanding of the current global epidemic (Tables 1–1 and 1–2). The initial definition was appropriately restructured so that overreporting of non-AIDS-related cases did not occur and a true picture of the epidemic curve emerged, but the spread of the virus associated with AIDS, the human immunodeficiency virus (HIV), and its varied clinical manifestations could not be encompassed by the initial definition. Thus, the CDC case definition of AIDS has been subsequently updated and modified to include the growing list of infectious and neoplastic complications of the syndrome (Table 1–3).[5–9] The most recent revision of the case definition occurred on September 1, 1987, when severe HIV-related neurologic disease and constitutional symptoms were formally classified as AIDS (CDC class IV, subgroups A and B).[10] Patients at increased risk for AIDS may have other serious infections and malignancies that do not ipso facto fit in the more restrictive case definition (Table 1–4).

Although in retrospect clinical cases of AIDS-associated illness can be traced back to the late 1970s, epidemiologic evidence strongly supports the fact that AIDS appears to be a new illness previously not seen in the United States. Both Kaposi's sarcoma and *Pneumocystis carinii* pneumonia were very unusual diseases before the current AIDS epidemic. Regarding the sudden increased incidence of Kaposi's sarcoma, the registry data from the

Table 1–1. Opportunistic Infections Indicative of a Defect in Cellular Immune Function Associated with AIDS

A. *Helminthic infection*
 1. Strongyloidiasis (disseminated beyond the gastrointestinal tract)*

B. *Protozoan infection*
 1. *Pneumocystis cariniii* pneumonia
 2. Disseminated toxoplasmosis, or *Toxoplasma* encephalitis, excluding congenital infection
 3. Chronic *Cryptosporidium* enteritis (>1 month)
 4. Chronic *Isospora belli* enteritis (>1 month)

C. *Fungal infection*
 1. *Candida* esophagitis, bronchopulmonary candidiasis*
 2. Cryptococcal meningitis, or disseminated infection
 3. Disseminated histoplasmosis*

D. *Bacterial infection*
 1. Disseminated (not just pulmonary or lymphatic) *M. avium-intracellulare* or *M. kansasii*

E. *Noncongenital viral infection*
 1. Chronic (>1 month) mucocutaneous herpes simplex
 2. Histologically evident cytomegalovirus infection including liver or lymph node
 3. Progressive multifocal leukoencephalopathy

*Not listed in original CDC definition of AIDS, but subsequently added.

New York State Department of Health, Bureau of Cancer Control, included only 19 reported cases of Kaposi's sarcoma in young men between the ages of 15 and 49 in all of New York State from 1971 to 1979, supporting the view that the occurrence of this rare neoplasm was uncommonly seen in this group before 1980. In retrospect, none of these reported cases were found to be related to AIDS.[11]

Pneumocystis carinii pneumonia is usually treated with trimethoprim-sulfamethoxasole (Bactrim, Septra, Co-trimoxazole) or pentamidine isoethionate.[12] Pentamidine was not initially commercially available and could only be obtained from the CDC at the onset of the epidemic, and thereby enabled this agency to monitor the incidence of *Pneumocystis carinii* pneumonia by the number of requests received for the drug to treat this infection. The sudden and marked increase in the number of such requests for pentamidine in 1981 to treat *Pneumocystis carinii* pneumonia in the absence of diseases commonly known to be associated with immunosuppression suggested that a new epidemic was occurring.

When the first cases of AIDS were reported, many hypotheses were proposed to explain the possible cause(s) of the newly recognized syndrome of diseases associated with an underlying cell-mediated immunodeficiency. The striking prevalence of the opportunistic infections and neoplastic disorders seen initially in homosexual men and soon recognized among intravenous drug users suggested that the observed immunologic disorder common to both groups might be related to the particular life styles of those affected. Most of the early cases were seen in young homosexual men who had frequent exposures to multiple sex partners,[13] and soon thereafter among male and female intravenous drug users,

Table 1–2. Opportunistic Malignancies Indicative of a Defect in Cellular Immune Function Associated with AIDS

Neoplasm	Comments
1. Kaposi's sarcoma (in a person less than 60 years old)	Most commonly presents in homosexual males with AIDS in USA; uncommon elsewhere and among other risk groups
2. High-grade, B-cell non-Hodgkin's lymphoma*	
A. Burkitt's lymphoma	Unusual in United States except in AIDS
B. Undifferentiated non-Hodgkin's lymphoma, immunoblastic sarcoma	
3. Primary brain lymphoma	Limited to brain; hard to diagnose

*Not listed in original CDC definition of AIDS, but subsequently added.

Table 1–3. Summary of Centers for Disease Control Classification System for HIV Infections

Group I	Acute infection
Group II	Asymptomatic infection*
Group III	Persistent generalized lymphadenopathy*
Group IV	Other disease
Subgroup A	Constitutional disease†
Subgroup B	Neurologic disease†
Subgroup C	Secondary infectious diseases
Category C-1	Specified secondary infectious diseases listed in the CDC surveillance definition for AIDS‡
Category C-2	Other specified secondary infectious diseases
Subgroup D	Secondary cancers‡
Subgroup E	Other conditions

*Patients in groups II and III may be subclassified on the basis of a laboratory evaluation.
‡Includes those patients whose clinical presentation fulfills the definition of AIDS used by the CDC for national reporting until 9/1/87.
†Includes those patients whose clinical presentation fulfills the definition of AIDS used by the CDC for national reporting after 9/1/87.

Table 1–4. Other Diseases Noted in Patients at Increased Risk for AIDS, But Not Considered Sufficiently Indicative of Underlying Cellular Immunodeficiency to be Classified As AIDS

Protozoan infections
  Amebiasis
  Giardiasis

Bacterial infections
  Legionellosis
  Nocardiosis
  Salmonellosis
  Shigellosis
  Tuberculosis
  Pulmonary or lymphatic atypical mycobacteriosis

Fungal infections
  Aspergillosis
  Candida oropharyngitis
  Coccidioidomycosis
  Histoplasmosis
  Zygomycosis

Viral infections
  Herpes simplex encephalitis or nonchronic mucocutaneous infections
  Herpes zoster
  Cytomegalovirus mononucleosis
  Epstein-Barr virus mononucleosis

Malignancies
  Squamous cell carcinoma of the anus, rectum, mouth, tongue
  Hodgkin's lymphoma
  Carcinoid tumor

known to share unsterilized needles and syringes. Most of the patients from both of these identified high-risk populations had clinical and serologic evidence of prior exposure to multiple viral and other microbial pathogens, such as cytomegalovirus, hepatitis B virus, Epstein-Barr virus, and enteric parasites.[14] Among the early postulated causes or contributing factors to the irreversible immune disorder characteristic of AIDS was the concept of an "immunologic overload," possibly due to prior, and often repeated, exposure to multiple infectious agents which were known to be common infections in both sexually active homosexual men and intravenous drug users.

Frequent exposure to allogeneic semen resulting in the development of autoantibodies to semen that has been reported to also cross-react with lymphocytes was also suggested as a possible cofactor in the development of the immune defect occurring in the homosexual cohort of AIDS patients.[15] The repeated systemic insults of injected foreign substances (drugs) by intravenous drug abusers was also suggested as a likely factor contributing to the development of the immunodeficiency seen in these individuals.

Epidemiologic evidence strongly supported the hypothesis that AIDS was due to a specific viral agent with a pattern of infectivity similar to hepatitis B virus, which may be either sexually transmitted or blood-borne. The common cell-mediated immune dysfunction was characterized by the specific depletion of the T-helper lymphocytes in the peripheral blood. Because bacterial, fungal, and parasitic pathogens have not been known to have a predilection for infecting and replicating within a particular subset of lymphocytes, a virus with a particular tropism for T-helper lymphocytes seemed the most likely etio-

logic agent causing the immunologic disorder seen with AIDS.[16] It is now widely accepted that AIDS is caused by a previously unknown human retrovirus, which was initially discovered and isolated in 1983 from patients with persistent generalized lymphadenopathy at the Institut Pasteur in Paris by Luc Montagnier and his colleagues, and named lymphadenopathy-associated virus (LAV).[17] Several months later in 1984, a nearly identical retrovirus was cultured from AIDS patients in the United States by Robert Gallo and his associates at the National Cancer Institute, who called their viral isolate the human T-cell lymphotropic virus type III (HTLV-III).[14, 18, 19] They believed that it was related to the two previously identified human retroviruses, HTLV-I and HTLV-II. At about the same time, Jay Levy and his coworkers isolated a similar virus from AIDS patients in San Francisco which they called the AIDS-related virus (ARV).[20] For the sake of uniformity, the virus has been renamed the human immunodeficiency virus (HIV) by the International Committee on the Taxonomy of Viruses in 1986.[21]

Virology and Immunology of HIV Infection

For two years after HIV was isolated it was incorrectly classified as an oncornavirus, which is a subfamily of retroviruses which have been closely associated with maligant diseases, such as HTLV-I and HTLV-II, which are believed to cause cutaneous T-cell lymphoma and "hairy" cell leukemia in humans, and other species of these viruses which are related to neoplastic diseases in animals.[22] HIV has now been reclassified as a member of a distinct subfamily of retroviruses known as *lentiviruses*, of which only three other, nonhuman,

species were known, the maedivisna virus in sheep, the encephalitis-arthritis virus in goats, and the equine anemia virus in horses.[23]

The lentiviruses generally had been neglected because no species known to cause diseases in humans had been identified prior to AIDS. No antiviral therapies for any of the lentivirus infections in domestic animals have been found to be effective, and the resulting diseases are ultimately fatal. Vaccines against lentiviruses have not yet been successfully developed, as opposed to the oncovirinae (e.g., feline leukemia virus).

The human immunodeficiency virus has been found to have a particular affinity to infect, and replicate within, a small number of mature thymic-derived T-helper lymphocytes. Infection of other cells, including B-cells, Langerhans cells of the skin, macrophages, and oligodendricytes, as well as cells in the central nervous system, have also been reported.[24–28] After infecting the T-helper lymphocyte, the virus may remain latent for long periods and suddenly become reactivated and then replicate, causing dysfunction and eventually destruction of the infected lymphocytes.[29] The virus can spread from cell to cell by fusion with the formation of syncytia of giant cells similar to that observed with the herpes simplex virus.[30] This *intra*cellular spread of infection could protect the virus from serum neutralizing antibodies, resulting in a depletion of the T-helper lymphocyte population in the infected host, ultimately creating a deficiency which may develop insidiously. Other cytopathic effects of HIV-infected lymphocytes have been studied.[31–33]

A second human member of the lentivirus subfamily of retroviruses, closely related to HIV, was isolated in 1985 and is known as HIV-II.[34]

The significance of this new human lentivirus isolated from patients from areas of Central and West Africa, its relationship to HIV-I, and its relative pathogenicity has not yet been fully determined.[35, 36] More detailed immunologic and epidemiologic studies are under way to better determine the relative pathogenicity of this newly described retrovirus.

All the known retroviruses are capable of establishing long-term latent infections within their target host cells during which time the virus can be detected as both unintegrated and proviral DNA integrated into the host cell genome; however, the virus may be periodically reactivated, inducing a viral specific enzyme, reverse transcriptase, and may become expressed as complete RNA virions.[29] Viremia may occur intermittently or may persist in infected animals and humans, even in the presence of specific humoral antibodies, which do not effectively neutralize lentiviruses in vivo.[37] Because of the apparently prolonged latency period that may ensue after infection, the ultimate morbidity and mortality rates of HIV for the millions already affected is not yet known and probably will not be known for several decades.

Several strains of HIV have been isolated from different patients in different locations as well as from the same patient. These different viral isolates have been shown to have significant variations in their env gene, which codes for the virus envelope glycoproteins, which serve as a major antigenic stimulus for specific HIV antibody production by the infected host.[38] The phenomenon, known as "antigenic variation," is characteristic of all the known lentiviruses and is believed to be responsible for the production of a variety of slightly different antigenic strains of these viruses

throughout the life of an infected animal.[39] Combined with the apparent inability of existing antibodies produced by the infected hosts to neutralize, and therefore eliminate, these viruses from their circulation, the antigenic variability of retroviruses has made previous efforts to produce effective specific vaccines extremely difficult with the available technology.

Human immunodeficiency virus has also been found to infect and become integrated in the genome of cells within the nervous system, including the brain. The cytopathic effects result in progressive clinical neurologic disorders, including aseptic meningitis, peripheral neuropathy, myelopathy, and dementia, which may gradually develop over a period of several years.[27, 40] The cells of the blood and nervous system of the animals infected with the other known lentiviruses are found to remain infected for life. In contrast to HIV, the maedi-visna virus only causes a neurologic disease in sheep and has not been found to be cytopathic for peripheral blood lymphocytes. Infection apparently results in progressive brain disease without causing an immunodeficiency.[41] In humans, HIV-induced progressive encephalopathy has been reported in the absence of severe immunodeficiency in patients who have not developed either opportunistic infections or systemic neoplasms such as Kaposi's sarcoma or lymphomas.[42]

Epidemiology and Clinical Spectrum of HIV Infection

Although the majority of the U.S. patients with AIDS are homosexual and bisexual men, AIDS is now recognized as a pandemic, global disease affecting men, women, and children. The heterosexual transmission of HIV infection and AIDS has steadily increased in the United States and has been found through-

out the world, especially in Africa, where AIDS is seen equally among sexually active men and women and also in children born to HIV-infected mothers.[43]

In 1987 homosexual and bisexual men accounted for almost 73 per cent of the total number of persons with AIDS in the United States (8 per cent of persons with AIDS were both homosexually active men and intravenous drug users). Other populations have also been found to be at increased risk, including heterosexual male and female intravenous drug users (17 per cent), hemophiliacs (1 per cent), recipients of HIV-contaminated blood transfusions or blood products (2 per cent), heterosexual partners of HIV-infected individuals (3 per cent), and infants born to HIV-infected mothers (1 per cent). For the remaining 3 per cent of reported cases of AIDS in the United States, none of the known risk factors have been determined.[44]

As the epidemic has progressed, the spectrum of clinical manifestations recognized to be associated with HIV infection has become far broader than that initially covered by the original CDC case definition of AIDS. Although the acute infection with HIV may be totally asymptomatic, a few weeks after infection HIV can cause a transient, febrile illness associated with malaise resembling influenza or mononucleosis.[45, 46] Seroconversion is usually followed by an asymptomatic latent period lasting from several months to at least seven years (the current duration of observation).[47] Up to 35 per cent of homosexual men infected over a three- to five-year period have been reported to develop AIDS.[48] HIV infection may remain latent for years in asymptomatic individuals and still be transmitted to others. Some patients have developed a generalized lymphadenopathy that may persist for years.[49, 50] Other HIV-infected individuals may eventually develop one or more constitutional symptoms, including unexplained weight loss, low-grade fevers, malaise, diarrhea, night sweats, "hairy" leukoplakia of the tongue, and oral candidiasis, commonly called "thrush."[51] Unofficially, the term AIDS-related complex (ARC) has been widely used in a nonstandardized fashion to describe the condition of patients who have developed three or more of these HIV-related constitutional symptoms, and laboratory evidence of a defect in cell-mediated immunity especially, including significantly decreased absolute numbers of peripheral blood T-lymphocytes.

The patients with CDC-defined AIDS who manifest the more severe clinical complications of HIV infection may develop Kaposi's sarcoma or one or more life-threatening opportunistic infections including *Pneumocystis carinii* pneumonia,[52] disseminated systemic *Mycobacterium avium-intracellulare*,[53, 54] cytomegalovirus disease,[55] toxoplasmosis,[56] cryptococcosis,[57] and cryptosporidiodis[58] (see Table 1–1). These patients are also prone to develop lymphoreticular neoplasms such as non-Hodgkin's lymphoma[59] (see Table 1–2).

By 1985, reliable diagnostic serologic tests involving ELISA and Western Blot methods were introduced for detecting the presence of serum antibodies to HIV and have been used worldwide to screen potential HIV-infected blood donors, thereby preventing transmission of the disease by transfusions.[60] The test has also been used extensively for epidemiologic surveillance of HIV infection. The HIV antibody test has been made available to physicians and the public for diagnostic purposes for individuals who are concerned about possible infection. In addition, all blood-clotting

products such as Factor VIII preparation, used in the treatment of hemophilia, are heat-treated, for this effectively inactivates any possible HIV contamination. Newer diagnostic tests are being developed which can test for HIV antibodies via immunofluorescence assays[61] or antibodies to recombinant antigens,[62] or can detect free HIV serum antigen.[63]

Future Prospects

As of mid 1988, more than 60,000 diagnosed cases of AIDS in the United States have been reported to the CDC; over half of them have died. New cases continue to be diagnosed at an alarming rate. As many as two million asymptomatic Americans and more than 20 million other individuals worldwide have been estimated to have already been infected with HIV.[43] Recent projections by the U.S. Public Health Service estimate that by the end of the year 1991, the total number of AIDS cases in the United States is expected to rise to at least 270,000, with 179,000 associated deaths.[64] It is estimated that 74,000 new cases will be diagnosed and 54,000 AIDS-related deaths will occur during 1991 alone. For the sake of comparative perspective, consider the fact that 47,000 American lives were lost during the entire course of the Viet Nam War.

In Central Africa, where HIV infection and AIDS are found equally in men and women, the disease is believed to be primarily transmitted by sexual contact.[65, 66] As of July, 1987, more than 10 million Africans were believed to be infected with HIV, and there were at least 50,000 cases of AIDS in Africa, often associated with a severe wasting syndrome, referred to as "slim disease." The opportunistic infections associated with HIV infection in Africa are frequently different from those commonly seen in American and European AIDS patients.

However, as in North America and Europe, Kaposi's sarcoma and other neoplasms occur in great frequency among HIV-infected individuals in Africa.

In the United States it was initially believed that the heterosexual transmission of HIV was essentially from male to female; however, epidemiologic evidence suggests that female to male sexual transmission of this virus may occur at an effective rate to spread HIV heterosexually.[67, 68] The transmission of HIV appears to be limited to direct exposure to particular infected body fluids, including blood and semen, and cervical secretions.[44, 69] Possible female-to-female sexual transmission of HIV infection also has been reported.[70, 71]

Epidemiologic studies evaluating the potential risk of HIV infection of heterosexual partners of AIDS patients by sexual contact have demonstrated that 58 per cent of both the male and female spouses of AIDS patients (including intravenous drug users, hemophiliacs, and transfusion recipients) were found to be seropositive for HIV.[67] However, it may be difficult to be sure that spouses of former addicts themselves were not IV drug users. Prospective epidemiologic data suggest that the prophylactic use of condoms appears to reduce significantly the risk of sexual transmission of HIV infection.[72]

HIV infection has not been shown to be transmitted by nonsexual but intimate household contacts. In one large study, the risk of household transmission of HIV infection via sharing of utensils, common bathroom facilities, and sleeping in the same bed, was not demonstrable.[73]

Although the virus has been detected in very low titers in tears, saliva, and urine from a few randomly selected HIV-infected patients, to date there is no conclusive evidence that these body fluids serve as significant vehicles for the transmission of HIV infection.[74]

Considering the large number of research personnel and health care workers who care for or are involved with research concerning AIDS or HIV, the chance of actual infection appears to be extremely minimal. Of the more than 1000 health care workers studied who experienced accidental sticks with hypodermic needles contaminated with HIV-infected blood, less than 1 per cent have developed serum antibodies to HIV. One has developed lymphadenopathy, but none have developed AIDS.[75] In health care workers who have had frequent contact with HIV-infected materials by routes other than direct parenteral exposure (e.g., direct skin or mucosal exposure to HIV-infected blood or other body fluids, or contact with open wounds), the chance of infection with HIV appears to remain very low. However, three anecdotal cases of HIV transmission occurring through nonparenteral exposure to HIV-contaminated blood among health care providers who subsequently developed HIV serum antibodies have been reported. None of them have developed clinical symptoms.[76] The occupational risk of infection by this kind of exposure is extremely low, considering the very few documented cases reported among the large number of health care workers who have been exposed to blood infected with HIV since 1981.

In order to prevent potential HIV infection it is essential that all health care workers observe the same precautions used to protect themselves against accidental infection with hepatitis B by using disposable gloves when handling all patients' blood and body fluids. Gowns, masks, and goggles are appropriate when dealing with situations in which spills are likely (e.g., emergency room) or aerosolization

may occur (e.g., centrifugation of HIV-infected blood). The same precautions should also be taken when handling *all* blood specimens and other body fluid samples in the hospital, office, or laboratory settings to avoid the risk of possible infection from any unsuspected asymptomatic carriers. The CDC has recently issued comprehensive guidelines for the management of HIV infection in the health care environment which underscore the ability of all health care workers to protect themselves while providing comprehensive care in an appropriately professional manner.[69]

Therapy and Prevention

Plagues have afflicted the human race throughout history. Had AIDS occurred in an earlier era, the course of the epidemic would have been very different. At times when intercontinental travel was much more difficult and less common, the disease might have been limited geographically.

Had AIDS appeared earlier, before the discovery of human retroviruses, the ultimate devastastation of this epidemic might have been even more ominous. Without the benefits of recent advances in medical diagnostic technology, or prior to the development of drugs that are used to treat and control some of the life-threatening opportunistic infections to which these patients are vulnerable, the survival of patients with AIDS would have been much shorter. The recent advances in the molecular virology and pathogenesis of HIV has stimulated experimental efforts to develop immunomodulators, antiviral therapeutic agents, and vaccines which may eventually lead to effective ways to treat and prevent HIV infection. In the meantime, major efforts to prevent spread of this infection are under way, including worldwide educational campaigns to inform the

world population about how this disease is transmitted and ways to protect against possible exposure.

In view of the state of urgency created by the AIDS epidemic, those at high risk and the public at large have been impatient and critical of the progress and speed with which the government and the medical community have dealt with quelling the spread of the disease and the development of prevention and cures. Although the wheels of scientific research may appear to grind slowly, an enormous amount of progress has been made in learning about AIDS and HIV infection in the relatively brief period since AIDS was first recognized in 1981. The heroic and rapid scientific accomplishments have, in fact, been unprecedented in the history of medicine. The putative agent, HIV, was discovered within two years after the disease was first recognized. Within two and a half years after the virus was discovered, reliable tests for detecting HIV antibodies were developed and have been used worldwide for the screening of blood donations to eliminate risk of HIV infection by blood transfusion. The HIV antibody tests also provide a screening test which can be used for purposes of epidemiologic surveillance to track the epidemic and to help determine the patterns of transmission. The tests have also been made available voluntarily and on an anonymous basis for individuals who wish to know if they have been infected with HIV.

By 1986, azidothymidine (AZT), the first in a series of potential therapeutic antiretroviral agents, which was found to prolong the survival of some patients with AIDS, was made more widely available to other patients with HIV infection.[77] Several other potential antiviral agents with satisfactory therapeutic-toxicity ratios are being developed. Simultaneously, a search for safe, therapeutically active immuno-modulating substances is under way. These drugs may eventually be used in conjunction with anti-viral treatment to help reconstitute the immunologic defects caused by HIV infection. In addition, tremendous efforts are being made to develop vaccines to arrest the spread of HIV infection.

The acquired immune deficiency syndrome has proved to be an unfortunate accident of nature that has provided medical science with a "window" through which to study and observe the mechanisms by which the host's immune system interacts with infectious agents and in controlling neoplastic diseases. The insights gained from the study of this disease will ultimately provide greater understanding in the fields of immunology, virology, and tumor biology that will benefit our ability to cope with many other diseases in addition to terminating this dreadful, unanticipated epidemic.

References

1. Centers for Disease Control: Pneumocystis pneumonia—Los Angeles. MMWR 30:250, 1981.
2. Centers for Disease Control: Kaposi's sarcoma, Pneumocystis pneumonia among homosexual men—New York City and California. MMWR 30:305–308, 1981.
3. Centers for Disease Control: Update on acquired immunodeficiency syndrome (AIDS)—United States. MMWR 31:507–508, 513–514, 1982.
4. Curran JW, Lawrence DN, Jaffe H, et al: Acquired immunodeficiency syndrome (AIDS) associated with transfusion. N Engl J Med 310:69–75, 1984.
5. Centers for Disease Control: Update on AIDS. MMWR 32:688–691, 1984.
6. Centers for Disease Control: Update on AIDS. MMWR 34:373–375, 1985.
7. Centers for Disease Control: Update on AIDS. MMWR 35:17–21, 1986.
8. Centers for Disease Control: Classification system for HIV infections. MMWR 35:334–339, 1986.
9. Centers for Disease Control: Update on AIDS. MMWR 35:43–46, 1986.
10. Centers for Disease Control: Revision of the CDC surveillance case definition for acquired immunodeficiency syndrome. MMWR 36(suppl 1S):3–8, 1987.
11. New York City Department of Health and Surveillance: The AIDS epidemic in New York City, 1981–1984. Am J Epidemiol 123:1013–1025, 1986.
12. Haverkos HW: Assessment of therapy for Pneumocystis carinii pneumonia. Am J Med 76:501–508, 1984.
13. Selik RM, Haverkos HW, Curran JW: Acquired immunodeficiency syndrome (AIDS) trends in the United States, 1978–1982. Am J Med 76:493–500, 1984.
14. Peterman TA, Drotman DP, Curran JW: Epidemiology of the acquired immunodeficiency syndrome (AIDS). In Szklo M, Gordis L, Gregg MB, Levine MM (eds): Epidemiologic Reviews. Vol 7. Baltimore, The Johns Hopkins University School of Hygiene and Public Health, 1986, pp 1–21.
15. Sonnabend JA: The etiology of AIDS. AIDS Res 1(1):1–12, 1983–1984.
16. Ho DD, Pomerantz RJ, Kaplan JC: Pathogenesis of infection with human immunodeficiency virus. N Engl J Med 317:278–286, 1987.
17. Barre-Sinoussi F, Chermann JC, Rey F, Nugeyre MT, Chamaret S, Gruest J, Dauguet C, Axler-Blin C, Vexinet-Brun F, Rouzioux C, Rozenbaum W, Montagnier L: Isolation of a T-lymphotropic retrovirus from a patient at risk for acquired immune deficiency syndrome (AIDS). Science 220:868–871, 1983.
18. Popovic M, Sarngadharan MG, Read E, Gallo RC: Detection, isolation, and continuous production of cytopathic retroviruses (HTLV-III) from patients with AIDS and pre-AIDS. Science 224:497–500, 1984.
19. Gallo RC, Salahuddin SZ, Popovic M, et al: Frequent detection and isolation of cytopathic retroviruses (HTLV-III) from patients with AIDS and at risk for AIDS. Science 224:500–503, 1984.
20. Levy JA, Hoffman AD, Kramer SM, Landis JA, Shimabukuro JM, Oshiro LS: Isolation of lymphocytopathic retroviruses from San Francisco patients with AIDS. Science 225:840–842, 1984.
21. Coffin J, Haase A, Levy JA, et al: Human immunodeficiency viruses (letter). Science 232:697, 1986.
22. Weiss RA: In Maby BWJ, et al: Virus Persistence. Cambridge, Cambridge University Press, 1985, pp 267–288.
23. Gonda MA, Wong-Staal F, Gallo RC, Clements JF, Narayan O, Gilden S: Sequence homology and morphologic similarity of HTLV-III and visna virus, a pathogenic lentivirus. Science 227:173–177, 1985.
24. Harper ME, Marsell LM, Gallo RC, et al: Detection of HTLV-III-infected lymphocytes in lymph nodes and peripheral blood from AIDS patients by in situ hybridization. Proc Natl Acad Sci USA 83:772–776, 1986.
25. Tschachler E, Groh V, Popovic M, Mann DL, Konrad K, Safai B, Eron L, Veronese F, Wolff K, Stingl G: Epidermal Langerhans cells—a target for HTLV-III/LAV infection. J Invest Dermatol 88:233–237, 1987.
26. Salahuddin Z, Rose RM, Groopman JE, et al: Human alveolar macrophages: One of the possible reservoirs of HTLV-III. Blood 68:281–284, 1986.
27. Gartner S, Markovits P, Markovitz DM, Betts RF, Popovic M: Virus isolation from and identification of HTLV-III/LAV-producing cells in brain tissue from a patient with AIDS. JAMA 256:2365–2371, 1986.
28. Shaw GM, Hahn B, Arya SK, Groopman JE, Gallo RC, Wong-Staal F: Molecular characterization of human T-cell leukemia (lymphotropic) virus type III in the acquired immune deficiency syndrome. Science 226:1165–1171, 1984.
29. Folks T, Powell DM, Lightfoot MM, Benn S, Martin MA, Fauci AS: Induction of HTLV-III/LAV from a nonvirus-producing T-cell line: Implications for latency. Science 231:600–602, 1986.
30. Sodroski J, Goh WC, Rosen C, Campbell K, Haseltine WA: Role of HTLV-III/LAV envelope in syncytium formation and cytopathicity. Nature 322:470–474, 1986.
31. Zagury D, Bernard J, Leonard R, Cheynier R, Feldman M, Sarin PS, et al: Immune induction of T cell death in long term culture of HTLV-III infected T cells: A cytopathogenic model for AIDS T-cell depletion. Science 231:850–853, 1986.
32. Bowen DL, Lane HC, Fauci AS: Immunopathogenesis of the acquired immunodeficiency syndrome. Ann Intern Med 103:704–709, 1985.
33. Lane HC, Depper JM, Greene WC, Whalen G, Waldmann TA, Fauci AS: Qualitative analysis of immune function in patients with the acquired immunodeficiency syndrome: Evidence for a selective defect in soluble antigen recognition. N Engl J Med 313:79–84, 1985.
34. Barin F, Denis F, Allan JS, M'Boup S, Kanki P, Lee TH, Essex M: Serological evidence for virus related to simian T-lymphotropic retrovirus III in residents of West Africa. Lancet 2:1387–1389, 1985.
35. Clavel F, Guetard D, Brun-Vezinet F, Chamaret S, Rey MA, Santos-Ferreira MO, Laurent AG, Dauget C, Katlama L, Rouzioux C, Klatzmann D, Champalimaud JL, Montagnier L: Isolation of a new human retrovirus from West African patients with AIDS. Science 233:343–346, 1986.
36. Kanki PJ, Barin F, Souleyman MB, Allan JS, Romet-Lemonne JL, Marlink R, McLane MF, Lee TH, Arbeille B, Denis F, Essex M: New human T-lymphotropic retrovirus related to simian T-lymphotropic virus type III (STLV-III_AGM). Science 232:238–243, 1986.
37. Weiss RA, Clapham PR, Cheingsong-Popov R, et al: Neutralization of human T lymphotropic virus type III by sera of AIDS and AIDS-risk patients. Nature 316:69–72, 1985.
38. Ratner I, Haseltine W, Patarca R, et al: Complete nucleotide sequence of the AIDS virus, HTLV-III. Nature 313:277–283, 1985.

39. Weiss RA: *In* Maby BWJ, et al (eds): Virus Persistence. Cambridge, Cambridge University Press, 1985, pp 267–288.

40. Shaw GM, Harper MG, Hahn BH, et al: HTLV-III infection in brains of children and adults wtih AIDS encephalopathy. Science 227:177–182, 1985.

41. Paisson PA: "Slow" virus diseases of animals and man. *In* Kimberlin RH: Amsterdam, North Holland Publishing Company, 1976, pp 17–43.

42. Price RW, Brew B, Sidtis J, Rosenblum M, Scheck AC, Cleary P: The brain in AIDS: Central nervous system HIV-I infection and AIDS dementia complex. Science 239:586, 1988.

43. Curran JW, Meade Morgan W, Hardy AM, Jaffe HW, Darrow WW, Dowdle WR: The epidemiology of AIDS: Current status and future prospects. Science 229:1352–1357, 1985.

44. Peterman TA, Curran JW: Sexual transmission of human immunodeficiency virus. JAMA 256:2222–2226, 1986.

45. Cooper DA, Gold J, Maclean P, Donovan B, Finlayson R, Barnes TG, et al: Acute AIDS retrovirus infection: Definition of a clinical illness associated with seroconversion. Lancet 1:537–540, 1985.

46. Ho DD, Sarngadharan MG, Resnick L, et al: Primary human T-lymphotropic virus type III infection. Ann Intern Med 103:880–883, 1985.

47. Francis DP, Jaffe, HW, Fultz PN, Getchell JP, McDougal JS, Feorino PM: The natural history of infection with the lymphadenopathy-associated virus human T-lymphotropic virus type III. Ann Intern Med 103:719–722, 1985.

48. Hessol N: Natural history of HIV infection in the San Francisco hepatitis B cohort. Reported at the Society for Epidemiologic Research National Meeting, June, 1987.

49. Abrams DI, Hess TP, Volberding P: Lymphadenopathy: Update of a 40-month prospective study. Presented at the International Conference on AIDS, Atlanta, GA, April 15, 1985.

50. Mathur-Wagh U, Enlow RW, Spigland I, et al: Longitudinal study of persistent generalized lymphadenopathy in homosexual men: Relation to the acquired immunodeficiency syndrome. Lancet 1:1033–1038, 1984.

51. Klein RS, Harris CA, Small CB, Moll B, Lesser M, Friedland GH: Oral candidiasis in high risk patients as the initial manifestation of the acquired immunodeficiency syndrome. N Engl J Med 311:354–358, 1984.

52. Kovacs JA, Hiemenz JW, Macher AM, Stover D, Murray HW, Shelhamer J, et al: *Pneumocystis carinii* pneumonia: A comparison between patients with acquired immunodeficiency syndrome and patients with other immunodeficiencies. Ann Intern Med 100:663–671, 1984.

53. Hawkins CC, Gold JWM, Whimbey E, Kiehn TE, Brannon P, Cammarata R, et al: *Mycobacterium avium* complex infections in patients with the acquired immunodeficiency syndrome. Ann Intern Med 105:184–188, 1986.

54. Zakowski P, Fligiel S, Berlin GW, Johnson L Jr: Disseminated *Mycobacterium avium-intracellulare* infection in homosexual men dying of acquired immunodeficiency syndrome. JAMA 248:2980–2982, 1982.

55. Laurence J: AIDS Report: CMV infections in AIDS patients. Infect Surg 5:603–610, October 1986.

56. Luft BJ, Grooks RG, Conley FK, McCabe RE, Remington JS: Toxoplasmic encephalitis in patients with acquired immune deficiency syndrome. JAMA 252:913–917, 1984.

57. Zuger A, Louie E, Holtzman RS, Simberkoff MS, Rahal JJ: Cryptococcal disease in patients with acquired immunodeficiency syndrome. Ann Intern Med 104:234–240, 1986.

58. Soave R, Danner RL, Honig CL, Ma P, Hart CC, Nash T, et al: Cryptosporidiosis in homosexual men. Ann Intern Med 100:504–511, 1984.

59. Ziegler JL, Beckstead JA, Volberding PA, Abrams DI, Levine AM, Lukes RJ, et al: Non-Hodgkin's lymphoma in 90 homosexual men. N Engl J Med 311:565–570, 1984.

60. Mortimer PP, Parry JV, Mortimer JY: Which anti-HTLV-III/LAV assays for screening and confirmatory testing? Lancet 2:873–877, 1985.

61. Sandstrom EG, Schooley RT, Ho DD, et al: Detection of human anti-HTLV-III antibodies by indirect immunofluorescence using fixed cells. Transfusion 25:308–312, 1985.

62. Lange JMA, Coutinho RA, Krone WJA, Verdonck LF, Danner SA, van der Noordaa J, et al: Distinct IgG recognition patterns during progression of subclinical and clinical infection with LAV/HTLV-III. Br Med J 292:228–230, 1985.

63. Goudsmit J, de Wolf F, Paul DA, et al: Expression of human immunodeficiency virus antigen (HIV-Ag) in serum and cerebrospinal fluid during acute and chronic infection. Lancet 2:177–180, 1986.

64. Morgan WM, Curran JW: Acquired immunodeficiency syndrome: Current and future trends. Publ Health Rep 101:459–465, 1986.

65. Mann JM, Francis H, Quinn TC, Asila PK, Bosenge N, Nzilambi N, et al: Surveillance for AIDS in a central African city: Kinshasa, Zaire. JAMA 255:3255–3259, 1986.

66. Van de Perre P, Rouvroy D, Lepage P, Bogaerts J, Kestelyn P, Kayihigi J, et al: Acquired immunodeficiency syndrome in Rwanda. Lancet 2:62–65, 1984.

67. Fischl MA, Dickinson GM, Scott GB, Klimas N, Fletcher MA, Parks W, et al: Evaluation of heterosexual partners, children, and household contacts of adults with AIDS. JAMA 257:640–644, 1987.

68. Redfield RR, Wright DC, Markham PD, Salahuddin SZ, Gallo RC, Burke DS: Frequent bidirectional heterosexual transmission of HTLV-III/LAV between spouses. Abstracts of the Second International Conference on AIDS, Paris, June 23–25, 1986, p 125.

69. Centers for Disease Control: Recommendations for prevention of HIV transmission in health-care settings. MMWR 36(suppl 2S):3–17, 1987.

70. Marmor M, Weiss LR, Lyden M, Weiss S, Saxinger WC, Spika TJ, Feorino PM: Possible female to female transmission of HIV. Ann Intern Med 105:969, December 1986.

71. Monzon OT, Capellan MB: Female-to-female transmission of HIV (letter). Lancet 2:41, July 4, 1987.

72. Conant MA, Hardy D, Sernatinger J, et al: Condoms prevent transmission of AIDS-associated retrovirus (letter). JAMA 255(13):1706, 1986.

73. Friedland GH, Saltzman B, Brian R, Rogers MF, Kahl PA, Lesser ML, Meyers MM, Klein RS: Lack of transmission of HTLV-III/LAV infection to household contacts of patients with AIDS or AIDS related candidiasis. N Engl J Med 314:344–349, 1986.

74. Groopman JE, Salahuddin SZ, Sarngadharan MG, Markham PD, Gonda M, Sliski A, Gallo RC: HTLV-III in saliva of people with AIDS-related complex and healthy homosexual men at risk for AIDS. Science 226:447–449, 1984.

75. McCray E, Cooperative Needlestick Surveillance Group: Occupational risk of the acquired immune deficiency syndrome among health care workers. N Engl J Med 314:1127–1132, 1986.

76. Centers for Disease Control: Human immunodeficiency virus infections in health care workers exposed to blood infected with HIV. MMWR Update 36:285–289, 1987.

77. Fischl MA, Richman DD, Grieco MH, Gottlieb MS, Volberding PA, Laskin OL, Leedom JM, et al: The efficacy of azidothymidine (AZT) in the treatment of patients with AIDS and AIDS-related complex. N Engl J Med 317:185–191, 1987.

2

Clinical Manifestations of Classical, Endemic African, and Epidemic AIDS-Associated Kaposi's Sarcoma

Alvin E. Friedman-Kien
Richard Ostreicher
Brian Saltzman

In 1872 Moritz Kaposi, Professor of Dermatology at the University of Vienna, published a report entitled "Idiopathic Multiple Pigmented Sarcoma of the Skin," which was the first description of multiple hyperpigmented cutaneous tumor nodules on the lower extremities in three adult males.[1] Kaposi's sarcoma, as this neoplasm became known, is a tumor of endothelial origin, arising from the cells that line the lymphatics and blood vessels of the skin and other organs.[2] The disease, its epidemiology, and clinical course, as originally described by Kaposi, is referred to as classical Kaposi's sarcoma.

Kaposi's sarcoma was once a rare and unusual neoplasm, which was considered a medical curiosity. Most of the reported cases were seen in North America and Europe primarily among elderly men of Mediterranean or Eastern European Jewish ancestry.[2–4] Variants of the tumor have also been seen in other populations as well. In the early 1950s, Kaposi's sarcoma was recognized to be a common endemic disease among young black adult males and prepubescent children in equatorial Africa.[3–5] In the 1960s, the tumor was also found to occur in renal transplant recipients, and other patients receiving immune-suppressive therapy.[6, 7] In 1981, the sudden epidemic occurrence of a fulminant and disseminated form of Kaposi's sarcoma among homosexual men in New York and California was soon recognized to be one of the most common manifestations of a new disorder, the acquired immune deficiency syndrome (AIDS).[8–13] This syndrome is believed to be caused by a newly discovered retrovirus known as the human immunodeficiency virus (HIV). We will refer to the AIDS-associated form of this disease as epidemic Kaposi's sarcoma in order to distinguish it from the classical, the endemic African, and the organ transplant–related varieties of this neoplasm. Epidemic Kaposi's sarcoma is now a global disease, with cases being reported from over 100 countries.

The histopathologic features of Kaposi's sarcoma are essentially the same as for all the variants of the tumor; however, the epidemiologic features, the clinical manifestations, and the course of the disease observed in the different populations afflicted may vary considerably.[14] The specific histopathologic characteristics of the different stages of the tumor are discussed in depth and illustrated in Chapter 3.

The lesions of Kaposi's sarcoma occur most commonly on the skin and on the oral mucosa; however, internal organs may be involved as well. These lesions vary from the earliest flat or macular *patch* lesions to thickened or indurated papules and *plaques,* which often develop into large elevated *nodules* and may occur anywhere on the body. The tumors range in color from a faint opalescent pink to red, deep blue, or purple. Lesions which have been present for several weeks or months often become hyperpigmented, and brown in color, especially in dark-complexioned individuals. They vary from a few millimeters to several centimeters in diameter, and continue to evolve and enlarge during the course of the illness. The tumors are typically asymptomatic, and in spite of their highly vascular appearance, do not bleed excessively when cut or bruised.

Unlike the typical behavior of metastatic cancers, Kaposi's sarcoma appears to be a multicentric tumor, with each lesion arising *de novo* from a localized hyperplasia of endothelial cells. With the possible exception of malignant melanoma, the tendency for the development of multiple cutaneous lesions with less frequent invasion or visceral involvement characteristic of Kaposi's sarcoma is distinct from the pattern of metastases observed with other neoplasms. In the immunocompromised host, Kaposi's sarcoma may represent a multifocal "opportunistic neoplasm" occurring in individuals who are also prone to opportunistic infections.

Classical Kaposi's Sarcoma
(Figures 2–1 to 2–22)

Although classical Kaposi's sarcoma is considered a very rare neoplastic disease, several hundred cases have been reported from around the world since 1872.[15] The classical disease as originally described by Kaposi usually runs an indolent, protracted course over several years, and those affected usually die of unrelated causes.[3, 16, 17] The vast majority of the cases have occurred in elderly men between the ages of 50 and 80 years, especially among those of Eastern European descent (e.g., Ashkenazic Jews from Russia or Poland) and individuals of Mediterranean origin.[18, 19] Infrequently, cases of the classical variety of Kaposi's sarcoma have been reported in peoples of other races.[20] The disease has been seen far less frequently in women, with a male-to-female ratio of approximately 10 or 15 to 1.[14] Although familial occurrences are unusual, cases have been reported in twins, brothers, cousins, and other members of the same family. The classical variety of the tumor has also been reported in young individuals, including children, but such cases are extremely unusual.[21] The increased prevalence of this tumor in certain ethnic groups and geographic areas suggests that there may be genetic or environmental cofactors which predispose individuals to the development of the disease.

Patients with the classical form of Kaposi's sarcoma may present with single or multiple skin lesions, which appear simultaneously or in sequence. The tumors often develop in localized clusters, most commonly found on the lower extremities, especially on the skin of the ankles and soles of the feet. However, any other mucocutaneous site may be involved at the time of presentation, or during the course of the illness.[22] With time, increasing numbers of lesions usually continue to develop. In rare instances individual lesions have been observed to totally regress spontaneously, while new lesions may appear at neighboring or distant sites.

As the disease progresses, lesions gradually increase in size, and adjacent lesions frequently coalesce. They may develop into large, painful, nodular tumors which have a tendency to ulcerate and become secondarily infected. Chronic edema of an involved lower extremity may develop owing to impairment of local lymphatic drainage and venous stasis. This may cause considerable discomfort and further complicate the course and management of the disease.[24] Infrequently, locally aggressive behavior of a skin tumor of the classical variety is observed with invasion and destruction of the underlying subcutaneous tissue and bone.

In individuals with long-standing cutaneous disease, tumors may eventually involve regional lymph nodes, the gastrointestinal tract, or other internal organs such as the liver, lungs, kidneys, or spleen. Visceral lesions are usually asymptomatic and are frequently discovered only at postmortem examination.[19, 23] Kaposi's sarcoma involving the brain or testes has only rarely been reported.[21] On occasion, the classical form of the disease has been known to take on a more aggressive, fulminant course with the rapid development of widespread mucocutaneous and visceral lesions.[16, 24] Rare cases have been observed in which single or multiple focal tumors within lymph nodes or visceral organs were detected in the absence of visible mucocutaneous involvement.

Approximately one third of the patients with classical Kaposi's sarcoma have another primary malignancy, which may antedate or follow the development of Kaposi's sarcoma. Most often these cancers are of reticuloendothelial origin, such as a non-Hodgkin's or other B-cell lymphomas.[25] This observation supports the possible role of common genetic, infectious, or environmental cofactors which may predispose certain individuals to develop these particular neoplasms in combination.[26]

Although the slow-growing, localized lesions of classical Kaposi's sarcoma usually do not require treatment, the larger chronic tumors may become cosmetically disturbing or cause local problems such as edema, pain, ulceration, or invasion of underlying soft tissues and bone, often necessitating palliative therapy. A variety of local treatment modalities are available which have proved to be effective in achieving partial to complete regression or slowing the growth of individual lesions. In those more aggressively invasive lesions, therapeutic intervention may reduce morbidity. The conventional treatment of the individual lesions of classical Kaposi's sarcoma includes local radiation or laser therapy, surgical excision, intralesional injection of chemotherapeutic agents, or electrocauterization and curettage.

In cases of widespread mucocutaneous or visceral tumor involvement, local therapeutic modalities are impractical. In these cases systemic chemotherapy, including such agents as nitrogen mustard, chlorambucil, methotrexate, 5-fluorouracil, cyclophosphamide, vinblastine, bleomycin, and etoposide (VP-16), have all been used singly or in combination, with varying success. Chemotherapy frequently provides temporary palliative effects, but there are no data to demonstrate that such therapy prolongs survival in classical Kaposi's sarcoma.[7, 24, 27]

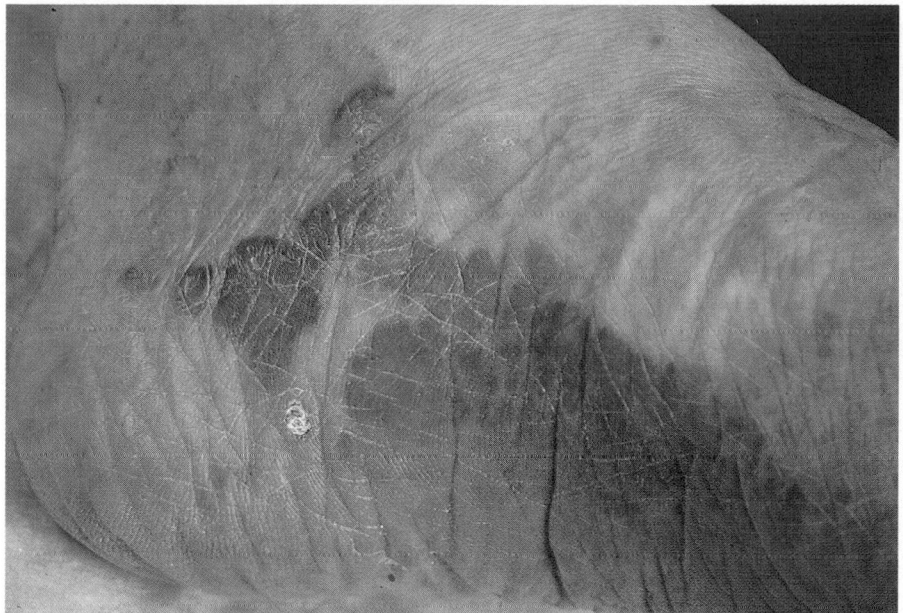

Figure 2–1. Classical Kaposi's sarcoma. Patch stage.

A 60 year old male of Eastern European origin with a large confluent pink patch-stage Kaposi's sarcoma lesion on the sole of the foot extending over the arch. This asymptomatic lesion had slowly increased in size over a five year period.

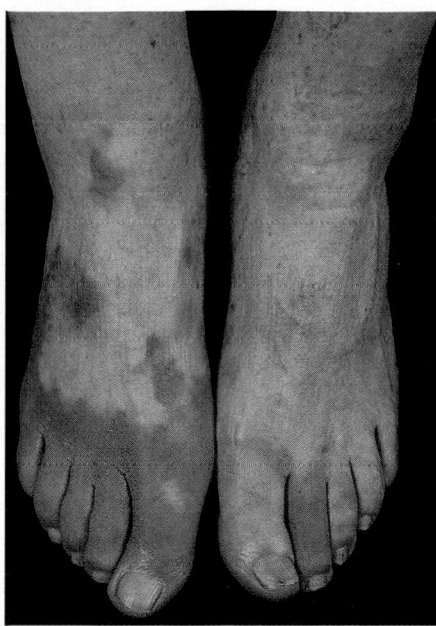

Figure 2–3. Classical Kaposi's sarcoma. Patch stage.

A large asymptomatic violaceous flat confluent lesion involving all the toes of the left foot and several other macular lesions on the dorsum of the left foot and the right second toe. The lesions had been present for four years, gradually increasing in size and number.

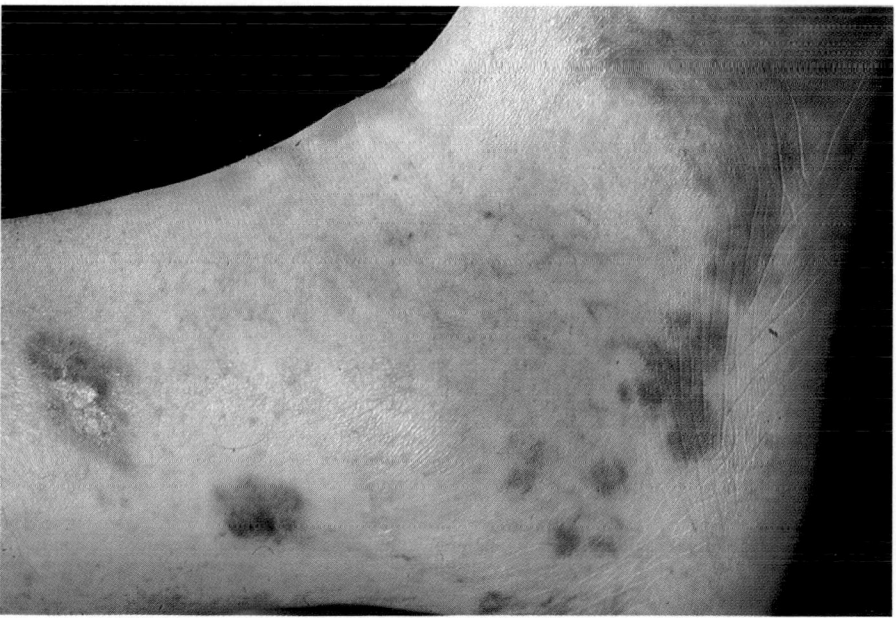

Figure 2–2. Classical Kaposi's sarcoma. Patch stage.

A 75 year old Italian male with a large red to violet confluent flat lesion on the skin over the ankle with other macular and papular lesions developing on the lateral aspect of the foot.

Figure 2–4. Classical Kaposi's sarcoma. Patch-to-plaque stage.

An 83 year old male with Kaposi's sarcoma of several years' duration, who initially presented with lesions on the feet and slowly developed lesions on the lower legs and thighs. This close-up view of the upper thigh shows multiple small papules superimposed on confluent macular patch-stage lesions.

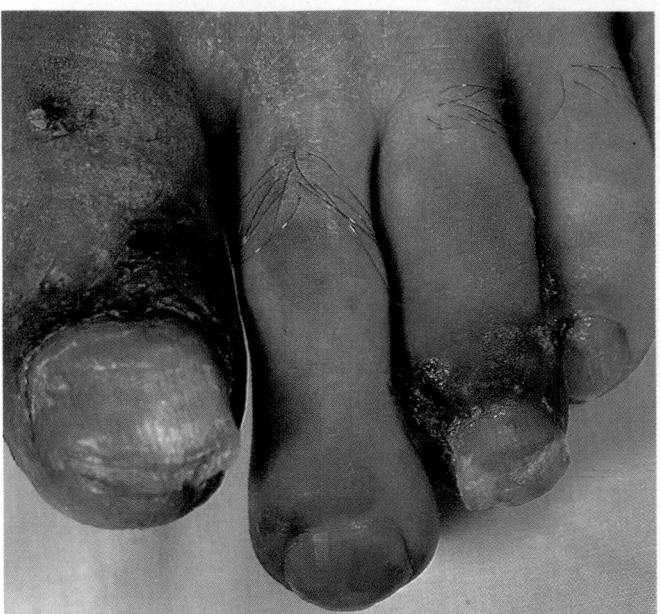

Figure 2–5. Classical Kaposi's sarcoma. Plaque stage.

Hyperpigmented purple, indurated periungual lesions of Kaposi's sarcoma on the toes with some ulceration. These lesions could be mistaken for early gangrene which can be seen in patients with peripheral vascular insufficiency.

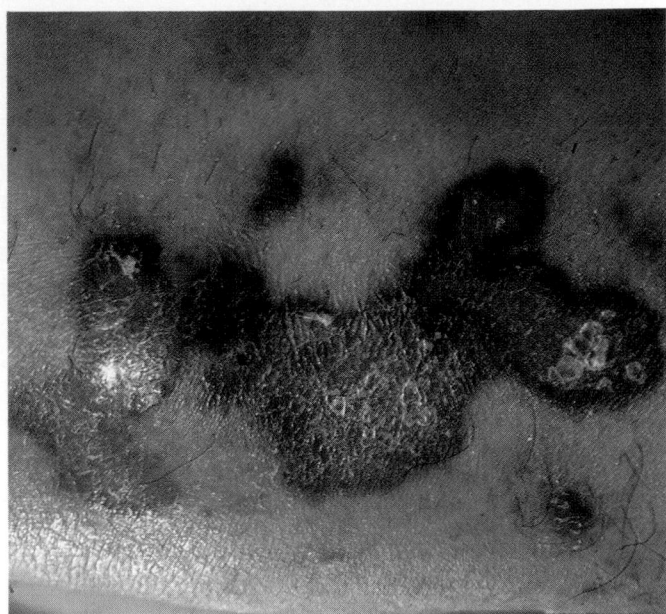

Figure 2–6. Classical Kaposi's sarcoma. Plaque stage.

Multiple, brown to purple, serpiginous plaque-stage lesions of Kaposi's sarcoma with hyperpigmented borders, located on the lower extremity. Such lesions may occur in patients with long-standing disease.

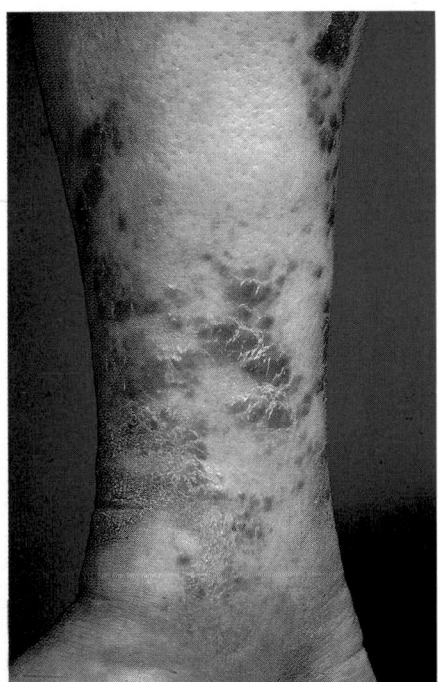

Figure 2–7. Classical Kaposi's sarcoma. Plaque stage.

Clusters of pink to violet plaque and papular tumors of long-standing duration on the lower leg.

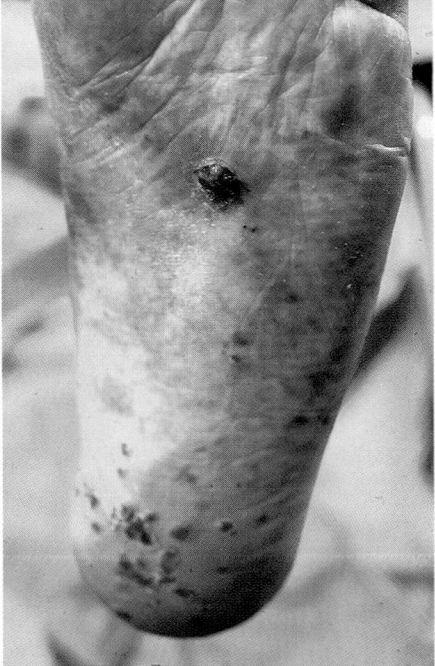

Figure 2–8. Classical Kaposi's sarcoma. Nodular stage.

There are multiple red and purple individual and clustered papular lesions of Kaposi's sarcoma on the heel of the foot. The isolated nodular tumor on the metatarsal region of the sole of the foot had been denuded following superficial trauma. Although these lesions look highly vascular, they do not bleed excessively when cut or bruised.

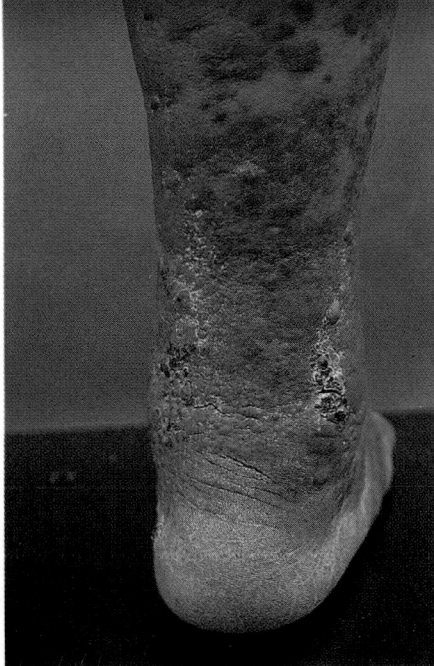

Figure 2–9. Classical Kaposi's sarcoma. Plaque and nodular stage.

Multiple pink to lavender plaques, papules, and nodules associated with chronic nonpitting edema. Some ulceration on the surface of tumor nodules is present on the ankle region.

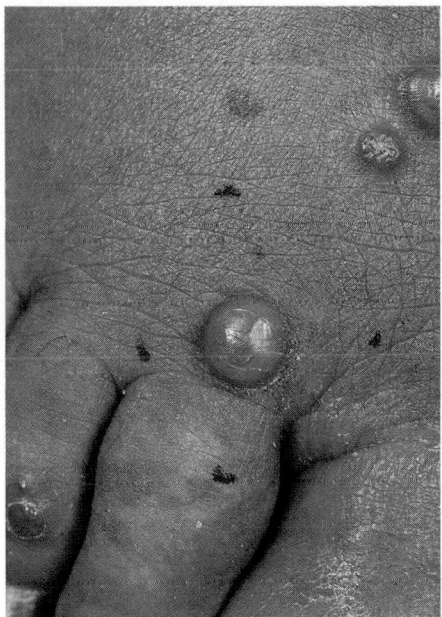

Figure 2–10. Classical Kaposi's sarcoma. Nodular stage.

Discrete dome-shaped pearly opalescent nodules of Kaposi's sarcoma on the dorsum of the foot and the toes.

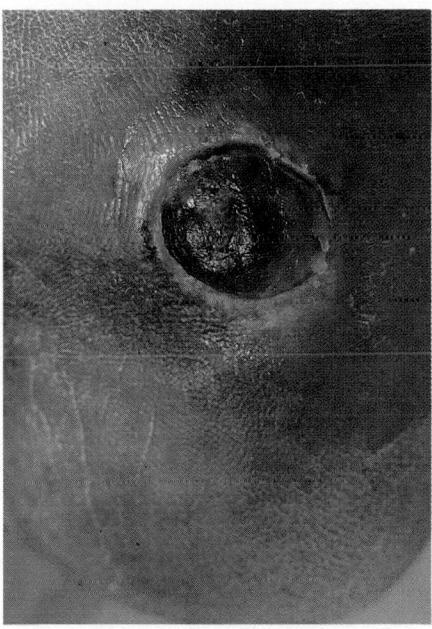

Figure 2–11. Classical Kaposi's sarcoma. Nodular stage.

A well-demarcated round nodular tumor on the sole of the foot near the lateral margin of the heel extruding through a collar of callous tissue. The surface of this tumor was denuded owing to friction while wearing shoes, a common complication seen with lesions in this location.

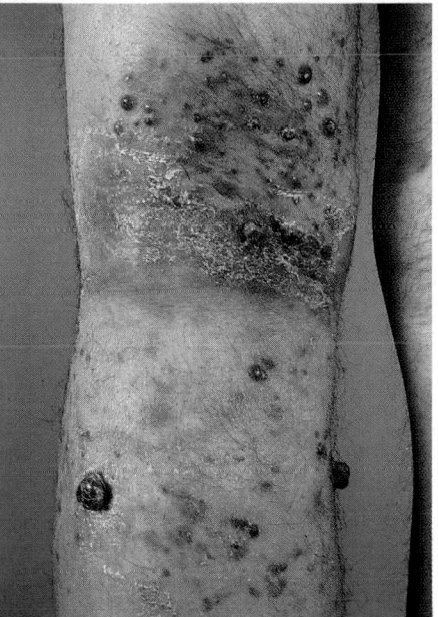

Figure 2–12. Classical Kaposi's sarcoma. Nodular stage.

Multiple deep purple to brown-black nodular tumors on the calf and popliteal fossa, associated with lymphedema.

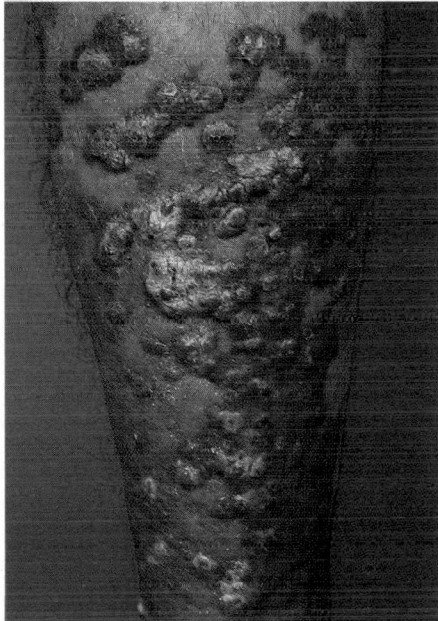

Figure 2–13. Classical Kaposi's sarcoma. Nodular stage.

Long-standing advanced disease on the lower extremity. Coalescing brown to violet plaque-to-nodular lesions of Kaposi's sarcoma with overlying adherent hyperkeratotic scales.

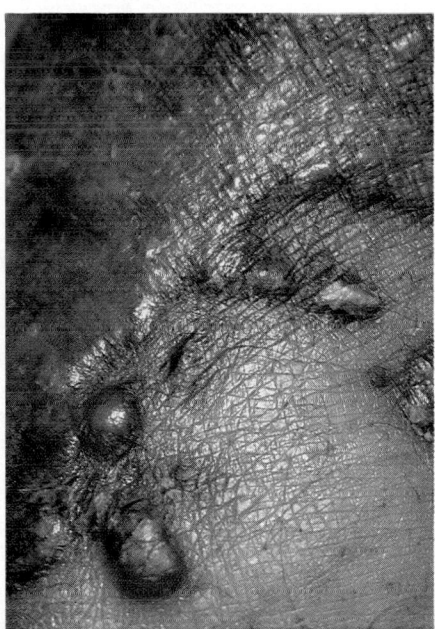

Figure 2–14. Classical Kaposi's sarcoma. Nodular stage.

A close-up view of a markedly indurated blue to purple plaque stage lesion of Kaposi's sarcoma with well-demarcated border and evolving nodular elements.

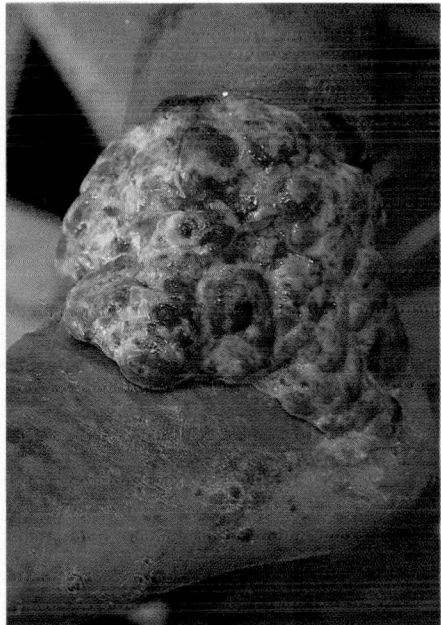

Figure 2–15. Classical Kaposi's sarcoma. Nodular stage.

A grumous, exophytic fungating tumor of Kaposi's sarcoma on the ankle region of a patient who had his disease for 17 years. The local tumor invasion of the underlying subcutaneous muscle and bone observed in this case is unusual for the classical type of disease. The tumor regressed following local radiation treatment.

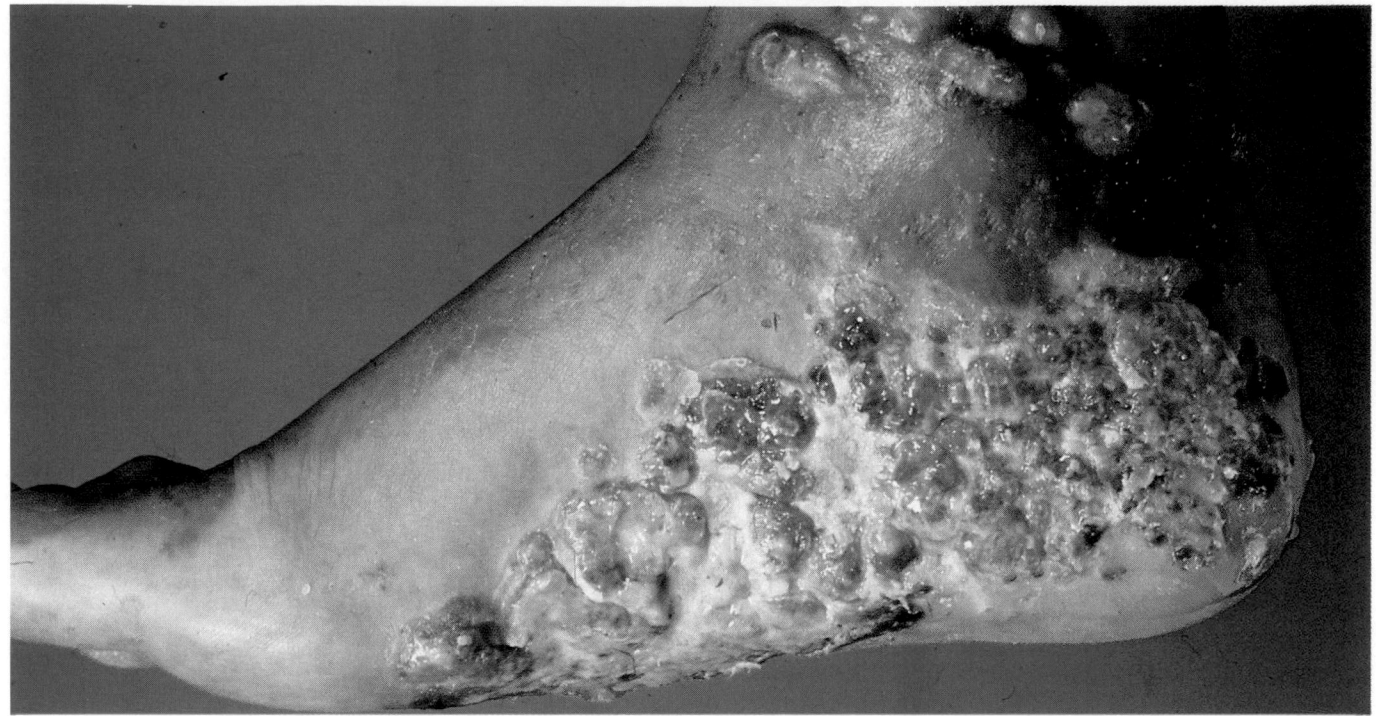

Figure 2–16. Classical Kaposi's sarcoma. Nodular stage.

A long-standing case of Kaposi's sarcoma involving the lower extremity with ulceration of the tumor on the arch of the foot. There are rounded nodules extending over the ankle. These tumors responded very well to local radiation therapy.

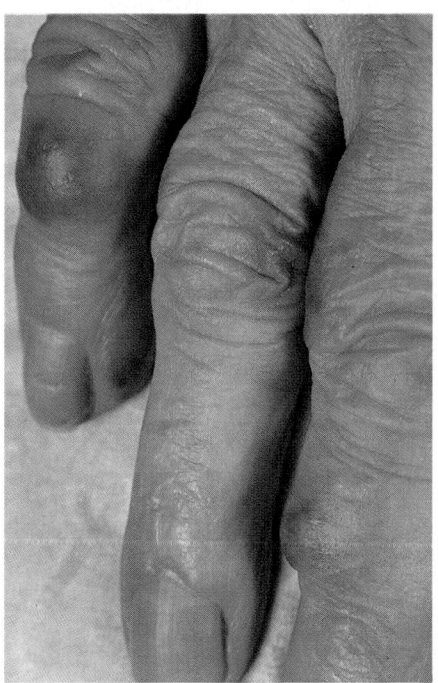

Figure 2–17. Classical Kaposi's sarcoma. Nodular stage.

Advanced, disseminated disease. Late-appearing, violet-colored nodular lesions of Kaposi's sarcoma on the fingers in a patient with disease on the lower extremities of several years' duration.

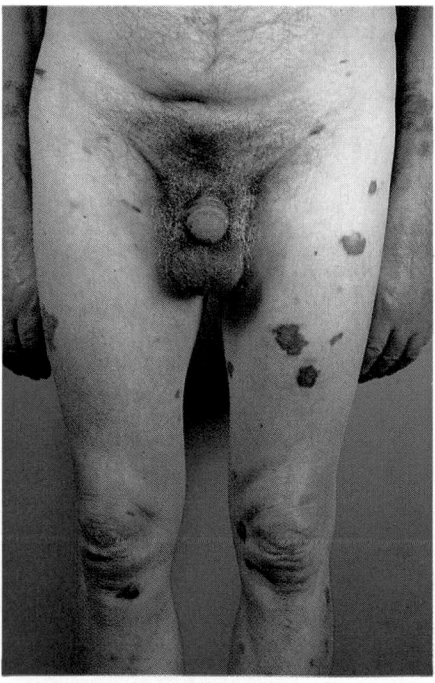

Figure 2–18. Classical Kaposi's sarcoma. Plaque stage.

An elderly Ashkenazic Jewish male who had Kaposi's sarcoma for 12 years with gradual development of multiple irregularly shaped, elevated plaque lesions ranging in color from red to deep purple, widely distributed over his body.

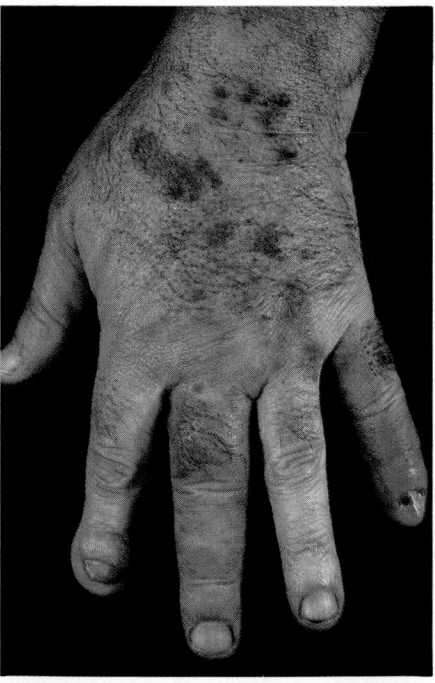

Figure 2–19. Classical Kaposi's sarcoma. Patch, plaque, and nodular stage.

Advanced, disseminated Kaposi's sarcoma, with purple macular, plaque, and papular lesions, which appeared simultaneously and late in the course of this patient's disease on the dorsum of the hand.

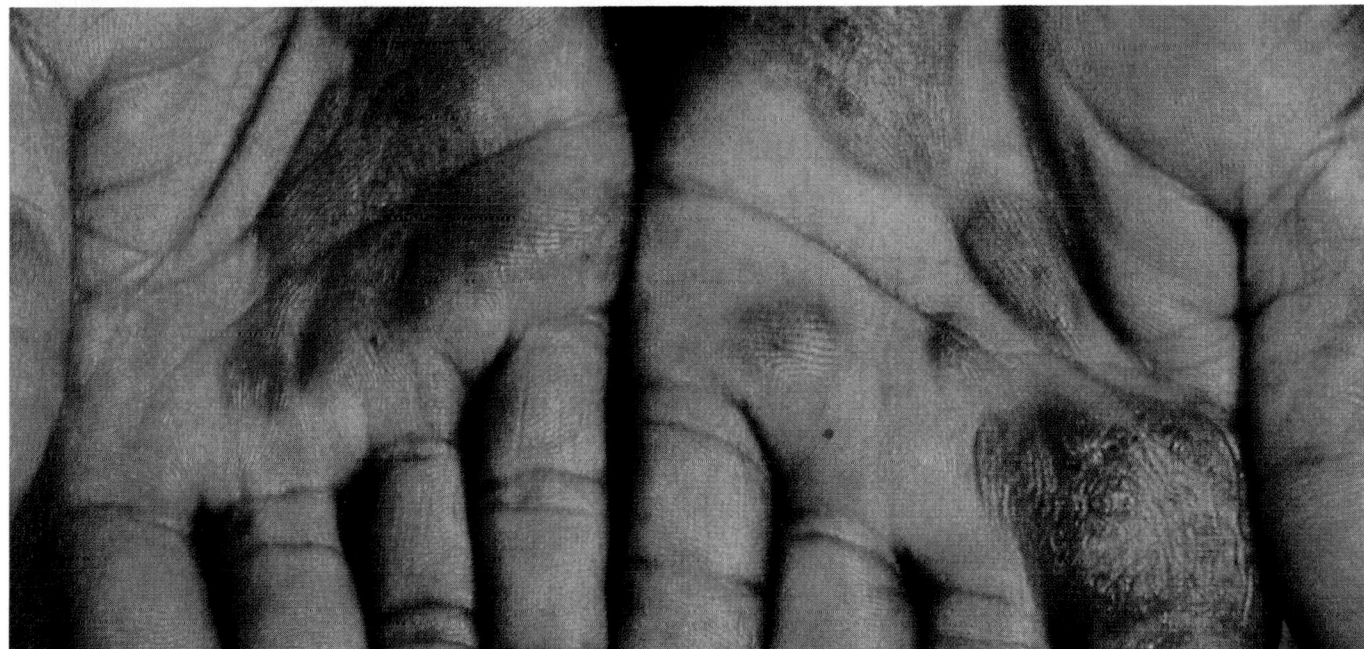

Figure 2–20. Classical Kaposi's sarcoma. Plaque stage.
Advanced disease with thickened violet to brown confluent plaques of Kaposi's sarcoma on the palms of both hands.

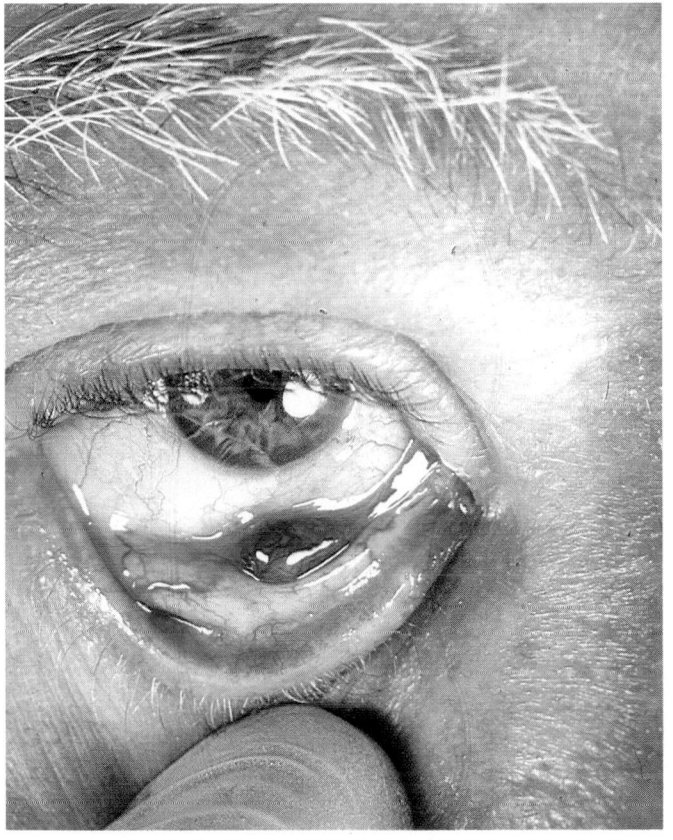

Figure 2–21. Classical Kaposi's sarcoma. Nodular stage.
An unusual red nodular tumor of Kaposi's sarcoma on the conjunctivum in an elderly patient with long-standing and widespread disease.

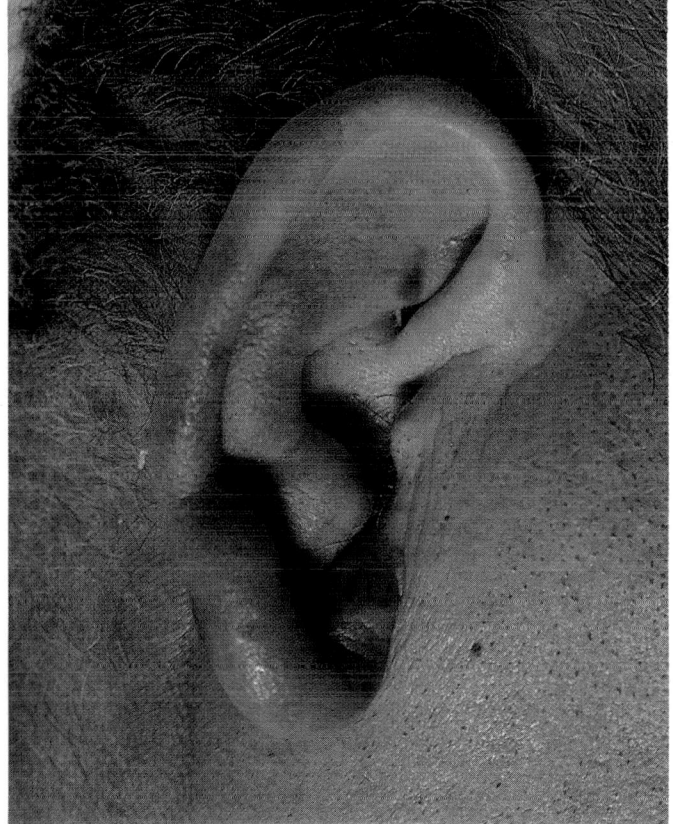

Figure 2–22. Classical Kaposi's sarcoma. Nodular stage.
A 53 year old male with a Kaposi's sarcoma tumor involving the ear lobe and a few papular lesions on the other portions of the ear. The ear is an uncommon site of involvement in patients with the classical form of the disease.

Endemic Kaposi's Sarcoma in Africa
(Figures 2–23 to 2–38)

In the early 1950s, there was a resurgence of interest in this rare neoplasm resulting from a report of 43 cases of Kaposi's sarcoma among the Bantu tribesmen of South Africa.[3] Shortly thereafter, a remarkably high prevalence of Kaposi's sarcoma was recognized among the black populations in a geographic belt across equatorial Africa, including Zaire, Kenya, Uganda, Zimbabwe, Chad, and Gabon.[28, 29] In these countries, Kaposi's sarcoma is now considered a common neoplastic disease. At the First International Cancer Conference on Kaposi's sarcoma held in Kampala, Uganda in 1962, it was reported that this disease accounted for approximately 9 per cent of all cancers seen in Uganda.[3] Geographically, Kaposi's sarcoma is found to be endemic in the same regions of equatorial Africa, as is another neoplasm, Burkitt's lymphoma, a malignant tumor closely associated with the Epstein-Barr virus. However, Kaposi's sarcoma is seen more frequently in regions of higher altitudes in this geographic area.[29–31] The incidence of Kaposi's sarcoma in the white and Asian populations living in these same regions was found to be extremely low and was comparable to the incidence of classical Kaposi's sarcoma seen in North America and Europe in these same groups.[32]

Four distinct variants of endemic Kaposi's sarcoma are observed in Africa. Three variants are as follows: (1) a *benign nodular* type, which resembles the classical localized indolent disease pattern; (2) an *aggressive* form, characterized by large, fungating and infiltrative skin lesions in which the tumors commonly invade and destroy underlying subcutaneous soft tissues and bone; (3) a rapidly and widely disseminated *florid* type of disease. These three variants of endemic Kaposi's sarcoma seen in African adults occur with a male-to-female ratio of about 17 to 1, which is almost comparable to that observed in the classical form of the disease in North America and Europe. However, the black African patients are significantly younger than their European counterparts, ranging in age between 25 and 40 years.[3]

The fourth variant of endemic Kaposi's sarcoma is an extremely uncommon and unusually virulent, generalized *lymphadenopathic* form seen predominantly in prepubescent black children between 1 and 15 years of age (mean: 3 years), with a male-to-female ratio of 3 to 1.[4, 19, 28, 29, 32, 33] This pediatric form of the disease is characterized by rapid disseminated lymph node and visceral involvement, usually in the absence of cutaneous lesions. Clinically, the lymphadenopathic variety of endemic African Kaposi's sarcoma closely resembles the behavior of an untreated generalized lymphoma and runs an unrelenting malignant course. Lymphadenopathic Kaposi's sarcoma seen in these children is usually fatal within one to three years, despite the use of aggressive therapeutic regimens, including radiation and combination systemic chemotherapy, to which the classical and the other endemic forms of Kaposi's sarcoma seen in adults usually respond.[28, 29]

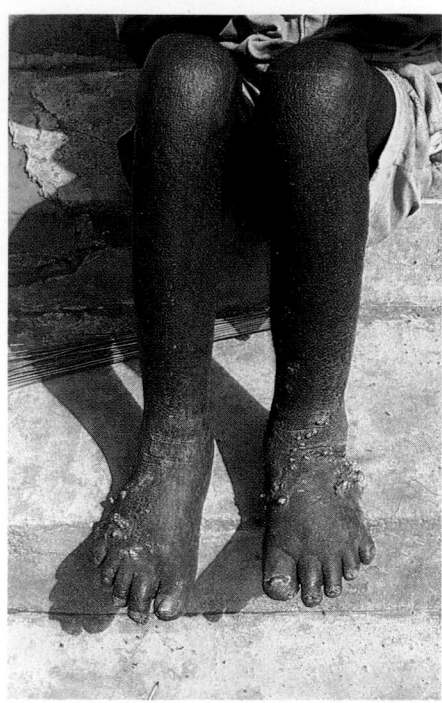

Figure 2–23. Endemic Kaposi's sarcoma (Africa). Benign nodular type.

A 45 year old man from Cameroun who has numerous indolent nodular lesions of Kaposi's sarcoma on both lower extremities of several years' duration associated with chronic lymphedema. This patient's disease resembled the classical variety of Kaposi's sarcoma seen in individuals of eastern European and Mediterranean origins. (Courtesy of P. L. Gigase, MD, Antwerp, Belgium.)

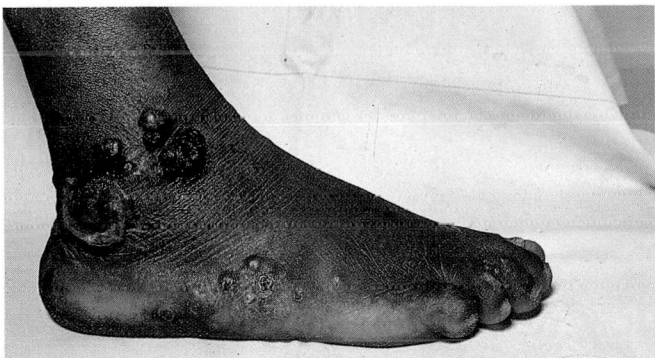

Figure 2–24. Endemic Kaposi's sarcoma (Africa). Benign nodular type.

There are multiple brown to black pearly tumor nodules seen on the lower extremity of this 36 year old black African male, with a large ulceration of the skin overlying the ankle region. The lesions were present for several years. (Courtesy of A. Templeton, MD, Chicago, and C. Olweny, MD, Makerere University Medical School, Kampala, Uganda.)

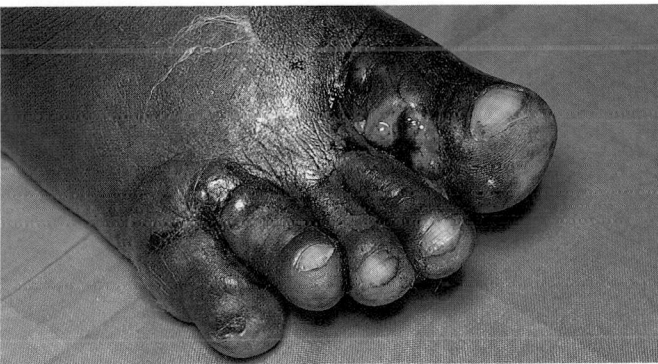

Figure 2–25. Endemic Kaposi's sarcoma (Africa). Local aggressive type.

A 27 year old male who had his disease for three years. There is a denuded, ulcerated, nodular tumor located on the great toe of his foot, which has locally invaded the subcutaneous tissues and bone. A similar tumor was present between the fourth and fifth toes on the same foot. (Courtesy of J. Ziegler, MD, San Francisco, and C. Olweny, MD, Makerere University Medical School, Kampala, Uganda.)

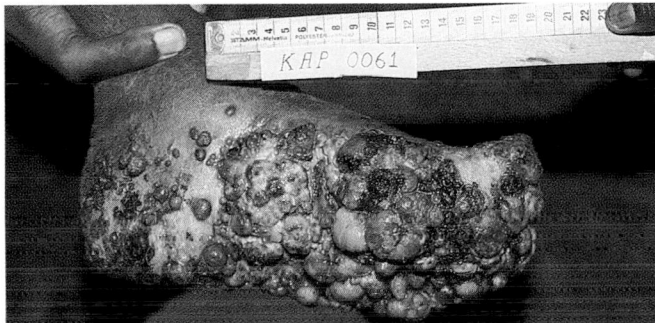

Figure 2–26. Endemic Kaposi's sarcoma (Africa). Aggressive type.

A 34 year old male from Zaire with multiple and coalescent nodular tumors on the sole of the foot of three years' duration. The extensive involvement of the foot and toes included local invasion of the subcutaneous tissue and bone. The tumors vary from deep purple to black in color. The surfaces of several of the nodules are ulcerated. The patient's serum was found to be seronegative for HIV. (Courtesy of P. L. Gigase, MD, Antwerp, Belgium.)

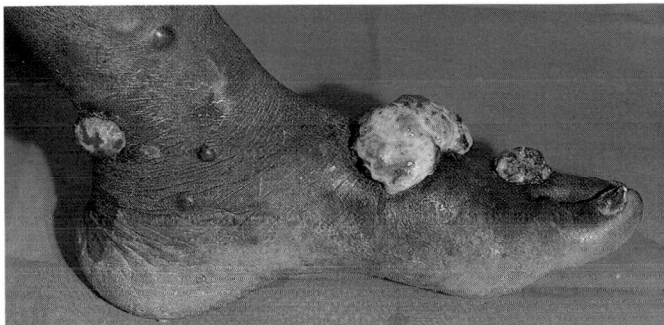

Figure 2–27. Endemic Kaposi's sarcoma (Africa). Nodular aggressive type.

Numerous large exophytic ulcerated tumors, as well as smaller nonulcerated smooth nodules of Kaposi's sarcoma located on the lower leg and foot. (Courtesy of C. Olweny, MD, Makerere University Medical School, Kampala, Uganda.)

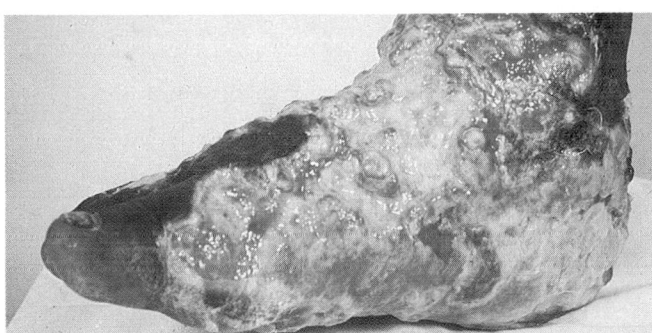

Figure 2–28. Endemic Kaposi's sarcoma (Africa). Nodular aggressive type.

A 43 year old black African male with the locally aggressive and invasive form of Kaposi's sarcoma. There is extensive ulceration of the skin of the foot and invasion of the underlying bone and soft tissues. (Courtesy of C. Vogel, MD, Miami.)

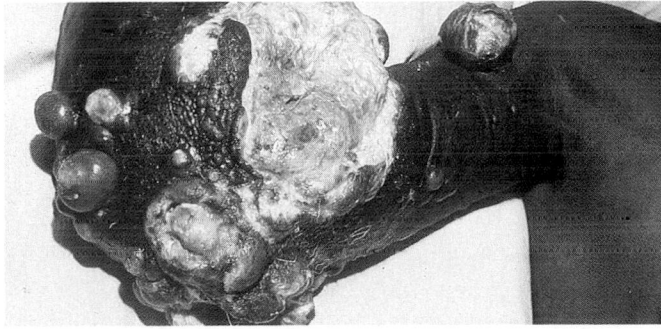

Figure 2–29. Endemic Kaposi's sarcoma (Africa). Local aggressive type.

Massive destructive locally invasive nodular lesions of Kaposi's sarcoma involving the entire arm with a huge ulcerated mass occupying the antecubital fossa. Multiple large exophytic ulcerated and nonulcerated tumor nodules are present on the shoulder and arm. (Courtesy of C. Vogel, MD, Miami, and C. Olweny, MD, Makerere University Medical School, Kampala, Uganda.)

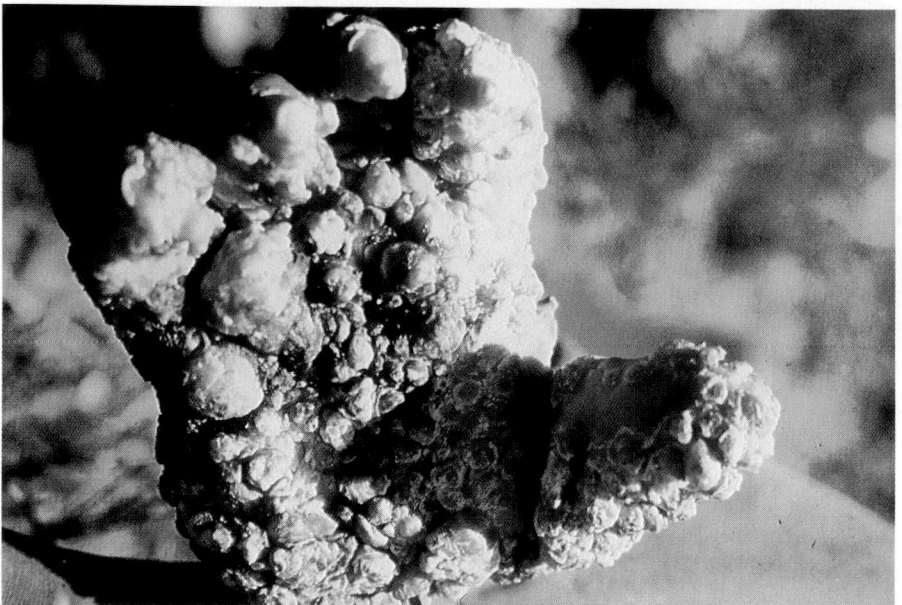

Figure 2–30. Endemic Kaposi's sarcoma (Africa). Local aggressive type.

The entire hand of this adult black man from Zaire is totally covered with multiple confluent nodular skin tumors, which had invaded and destroyed the subcutaneous tissue and bone, especially in the fingers. Such aggressive lesions are reported to respond to palliative radiation therapy; however, damage to the underlying tissue and bone is not reversible. (Courtesy of C. Vogel, MD, Miami.)

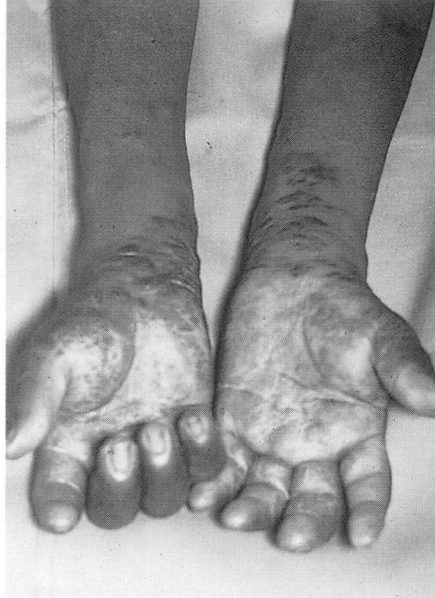

Figure 2–31. Endemic Kaposi's sarcoma (Africa). Florid type.

Multiple widely and rapidly disseminating nodules of Kaposi's sarcoma, seen on both forearms and palmar surfaces, on a 35 year old black Ugandan. The tumor was found to infiltrate bone and soft tissues. The patient also had visceral involvement. (Courtesy of C. Olweny, MD, Makerere University Medical School, Kampala, Uganda.)

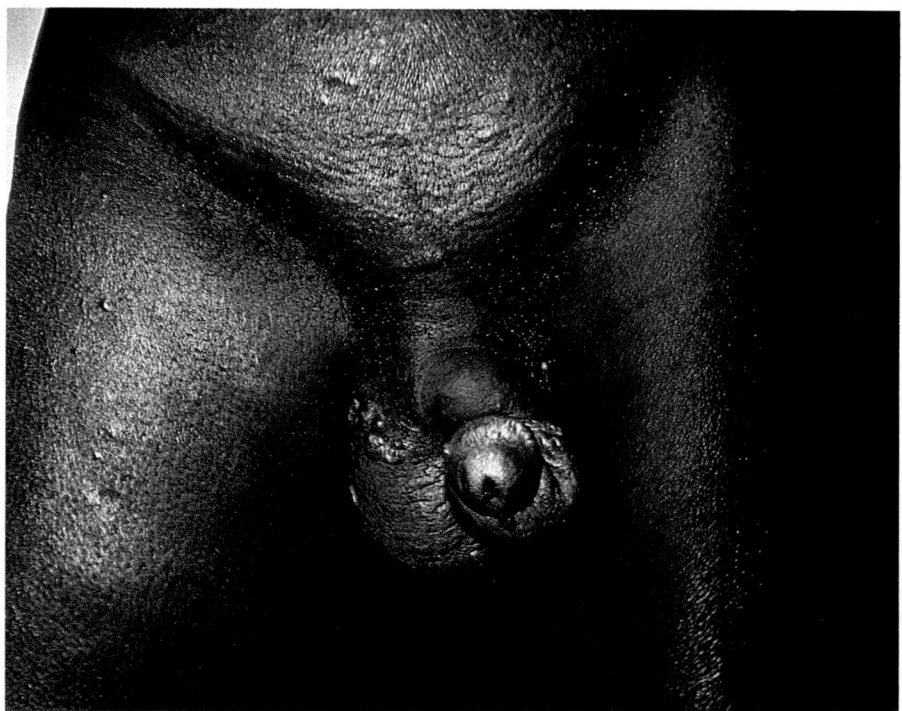

Figure 2–32. Endemic Kaposi's sarcoma (Africa). Florid type.

A 45 year old black African male from Zaire with widespread Kaposi's sarcoma, including involvement of the inguinal nodes, first diagnosed in 1974. The disease ran a slowly progressive course. His serum HIV antibody status is unknown. (Courtesy of J. Ziegler, MD, San Francisco, and C. Olweny, MD, Makerere University Medical School, Kampala, Uganda.)

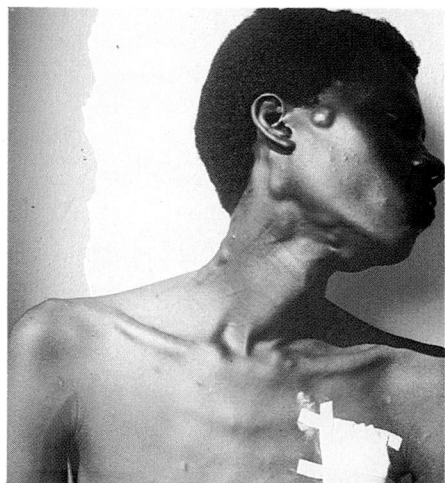

Figure 2–33. Endemic Kaposi's sarcoma (Africa). Florid type.

A 35 year old black African male from Burundi with numerous cutaneous nodular lesions of Kaposi's sarcoma. The enlarged lymph nodes on his neck below the mandibular angle near his ear were infiltrated with Kaposi's sarcoma. Lymphadenopathic involvement is rarely seen in adults with this neoplasm. Although his clinical disease behaved like that seen in a patient with AIDS, this individual was seronegative to HIV. (Courtesy of P. L. Gigase, MD, Antwerp, Belgium.)

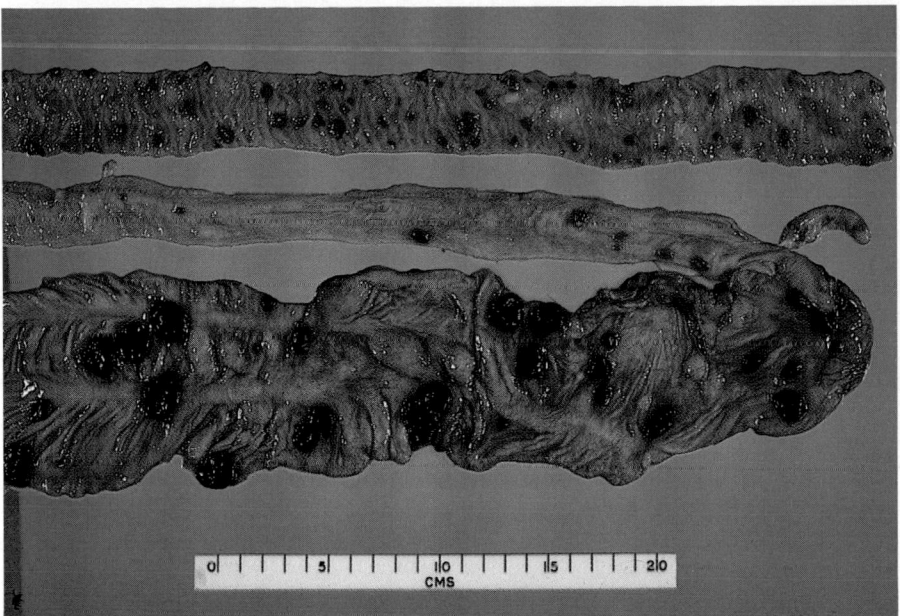

Figure 2–34. Endemic Kaposi's sarcoma (Africa). Florid type.

Gross pathologic specimen of the small and large intestines studded with red to black tumor nodules of Kaposi's sarcoma. (Courtesy of A. Templeton, MD, Chicago, and Makerere University Medical School, Kampala, Uganda.)

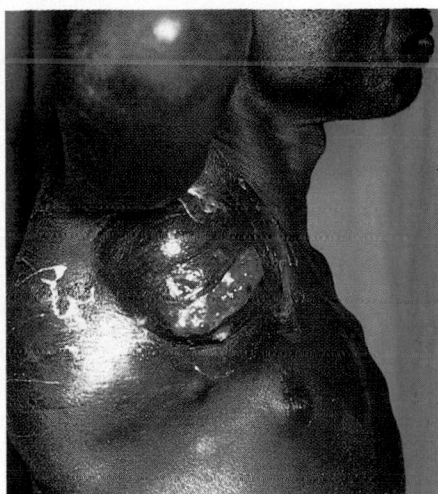

Figure 2–35. Endemic Kaposi's sarcoma (Africa). Florid type.

A black adult male with grossly enlarged axillary lymphadenopathy due to Kaposi's sarcoma. Lymph node involvement sometimes occurs in adults with the florid type of endemic disease but is more commonly seen in the pediatric population with the lymphadenopathic variety of Kaposi's sarcoma. (Courtesy of C. Olweny, MD, and A. Templeton, MD, Chicago, and Makerere University Medical School, Kampala, Uganda.)

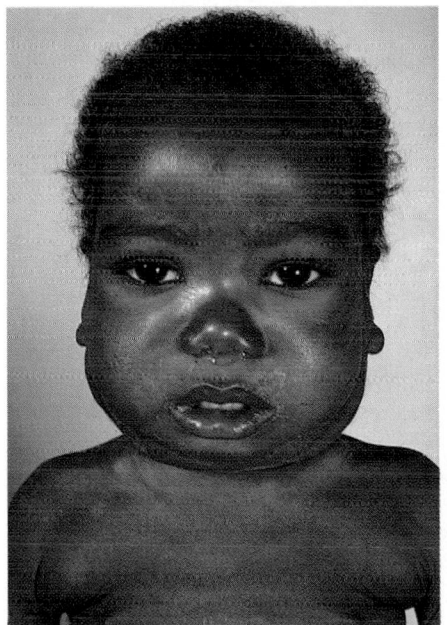

Figure 2–36. Endemic Kaposi's sarcoma (Africa). Lymphadenopathic type.

A 2 year old boy with disseminated lymph node involvement with facial edema due to obstruction of lymphatic drainage. Also present is bilateral axillary adenopathy. The lymphadenopathic variety of the disease is primarily seen in children. Skin lesions are extremely uncommon in children with this form of the disease. (Courtesy of A. Templeton, MD, Chicago, and Makerere University Medical School, Kampala, Uganda.)

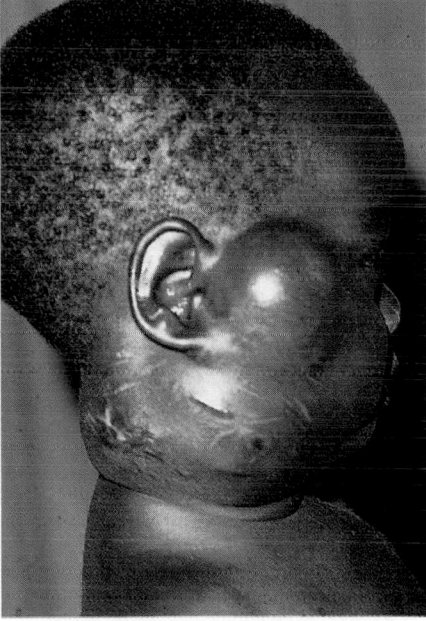

Figure 2–37. Endemic Kaposi's sarcoma (Africa). Lymphadenopathic type.

An 18 month old boy with massive preauricular and cervical lymphadenopathy due to Kaposi's sarcoma. The lymphadenopathic form of the disease responds poorly to either chemotherapy or radiation therapy. (Courtesy of C. Olweny, MD, Makerere University Medical School, Kampala, Uganda.)

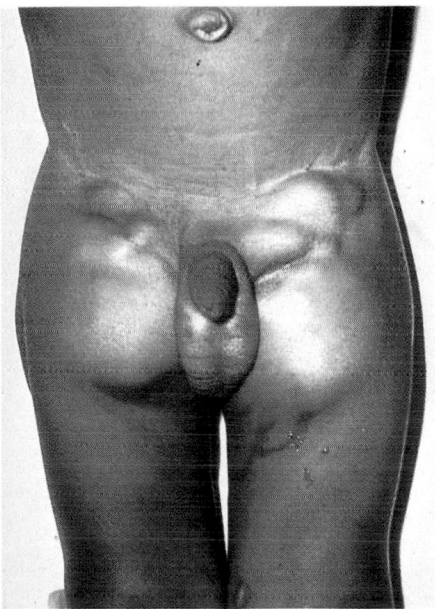

Figure 2–38. Endemic Kaposi's sarcoma (Africa). Lymphadenopathic type.

A 3 year old black African male with bilateral inguinal and femoral lymph node enlargement due to Kaposi's sarcoma. (Courtesy of C. Vogel, MD, Miami, and Makerere University Medical School, Kampala, Uganda.)

Kaposi's Sarcoma in Iatrogenically Immunosuppressed Patients

In the 1960s, a number of immunosuppressed renal allograft recipients receiving prednisone and azathioprine were found to develop Kaposi's sarcoma. There are also reports of this neoplasm occurring in patients with diseases such as temporal arteritis and systemic lupus erythematosus, who had been treated with immunosuppressive medications, such as systemic steroids and cyclophosphamide.[6, 7, 34–37]

The Kaposi's sarcoma that develops in these iatrogenically immunosuppressed individuals usually remains limited to a few localized skin lesions, although widespread dissemination with visceral involvement may occur. These patients have ranged in age from 23 to 59 years (mean: 42 years) with a male-to-female ratio of 2.3 to 1.[37] The lesions have been reported to develop between 2.5 and 101 months (mean: 16.5 months) after the onset of immunosuppressive therapy. It is important to emphasize that some of these drug-induced immunosuppressed patients who developed Kaposi's sarcoma experienced a partial or complete regression of the tumors when their immunosuppressive treatment regimen was re-duced, changed, or discontinued.[37, 38] In one study of 58 renal transplant patients who developed Kaposi's sarcoma, 40 had lesions limited to the skin and mucous membranes, and 18 also had visceral involvement. Of the 40 patients with only mucocutaneous lesions, 23 experienced remission of their Kaposi's sarcoma after discontinuation of, or changes in, their immunosuppressive therapy. The prognosis for those patients with visceral involvement, however, was poor. Immunosuppressed renal transplant recipients were also found to have an increased incidence of lymphoid malignancies, similar to the increased occurrence of lymphomas observed in patients with classical Kaposi's sarcoma.[37, 39, 40]

Epidemic, AIDS-Associated Kaposi's Sarcoma
(Figures 2–39 to 2–66)

Between the late fall of 1979 and the spring of 1981, 26 cases of a previously undescribed, unusually aggressive, and disseminated form of Kaposi's sarcoma were observed in apparently healthy, sexually active homosexual and bisexual young men in New York City and California.[8] Simultaneously and independently, five cases of a rare opportunistic infection, *Pneumocystis carinii* pneumonia, were also reported to have occurred in young homosexual men in Los Angeles.[41] These observations heralded the recognition of an epidemic of several devastating diseases which were to characterize AIDS. Kaposi's sarcoma and *Pneumocystis carinii* pneumonia remain the most common neoplastic and infectious manifestations of AIDS in the United States and Europe.[8, 9, 11, 24, 41, 42] In contrast to the older patients with classical Kaposi's sarcoma who are most often in the fifth to seventh decades of life, those with the AIDS-associated variant of this neoplasm range in age from 19 to 64 years, with a mean age of 37.7 years.[51]

Kaposi's sarcoma, *Pneumocystis carinii* pneumonia, and other life-threatening opportunistic infections were previously known to occur in the setting of defective cell-mediated immunity such as in patients with congenital immunodeficiencies, lymphoreticular malignancies, renal transplant recipients, or other patients receiving immunosuppressive chemotherapy. The sudden epidemic occurrence of Kaposi's sarcoma and unusual opportunistic infections among previously healthy individuals who had no recognizable cause of immunosuppression suggested a common underlying newly acquired immunologic disorder.

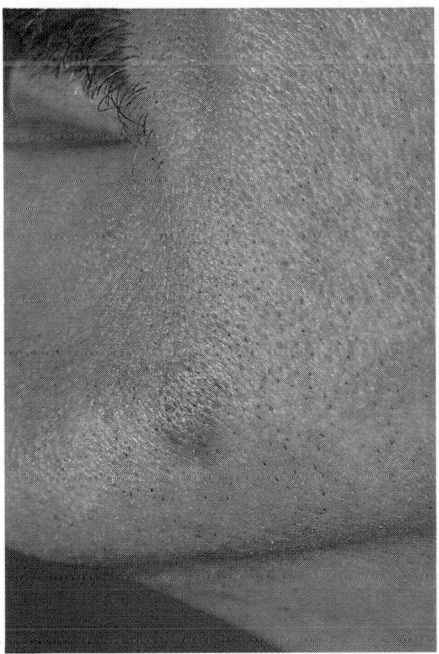

Figure 2–39. Epidemic Kaposi's sarcoma. Patch stage.

This totally asymptomatic faint pink macular lesion of Kaposi's sarcoma spontaneously appeared on the side of this patient's chin. Similar patch-stage lesions developed at distant sites on the patient's body at about the same time.

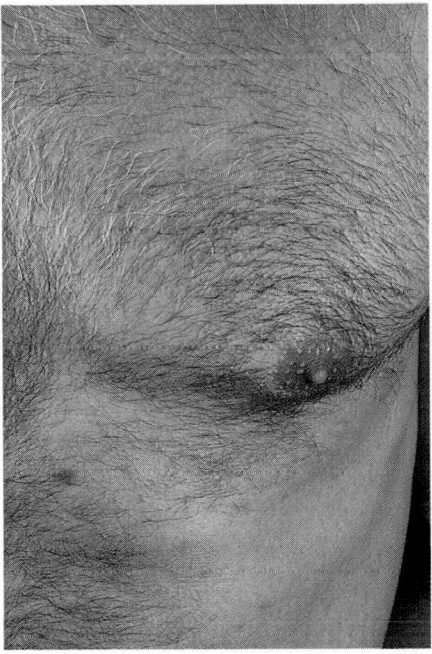

Figure 2–40. Epidemic Kaposi's sarcoma. Patch stage.

A 44 year old otherwise healthy, homosexual male with a single flat red macule of Kaposi's sarcoma on his lower chest.

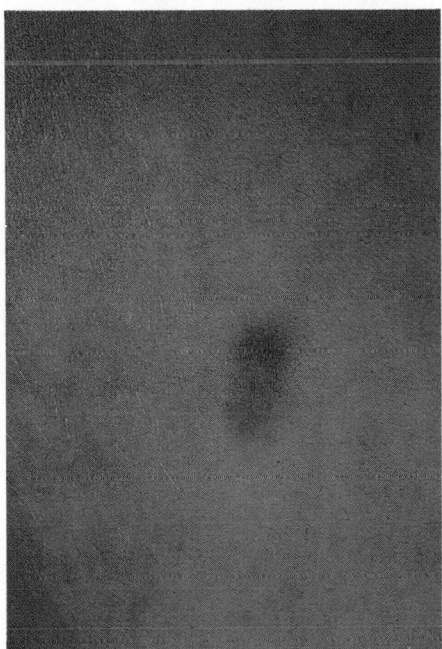

Figure 2–41. Epidemic Kaposi's sarcoma. Patch stage.

An elongated flat lesion on the trunk, which varied in color from pink to red, was initially ignored because the patient thought that this "spot" represented a minor bruise. As this skin lesion became darker in color, other macules developed at distant sites. The patient sought medical attention at that time.

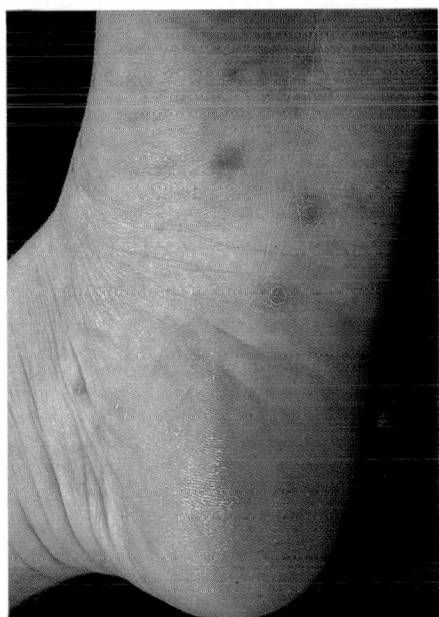

Figure 2–42. Epidemic Kaposi's sarcoma. Patch stage.

A 23 year old homosexual male with multiple flat, tawny pink lesions on the sole and ankle of the foot. Initially, the lesions were thought to represent secondary syphilis. There were several other cutaneous lesions of a similar nature widely disseminated over the rest of his body.

Figure 2–43. Epidemic Kaposi's sarcoma. Patch stage.

A single light brown flat macular lesion on the palm of the hand. The biopsy confirmed the diagnosis of Kaposi's sarcoma.

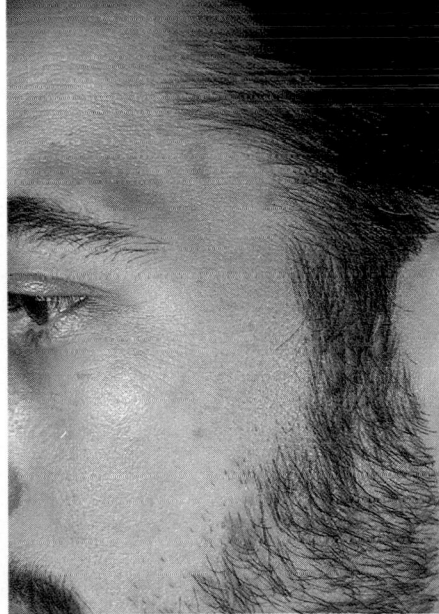

Figure 2–44. Epidemic Kaposi's sarcoma. Patch stage.

Multiple patch-stage lesions on the temple and bearded areas of the face. The lesions were slightly irregular in shape and widely dispersed over the rest of the body.

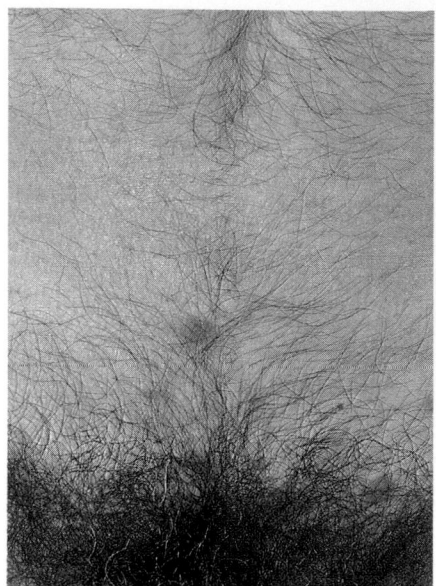

Figure 2–45. Epidemic Kaposi's sarcoma. Patch stage.

A 39 year old homosexual male with multiple reddish macules on the lower abdomen and pubic region.

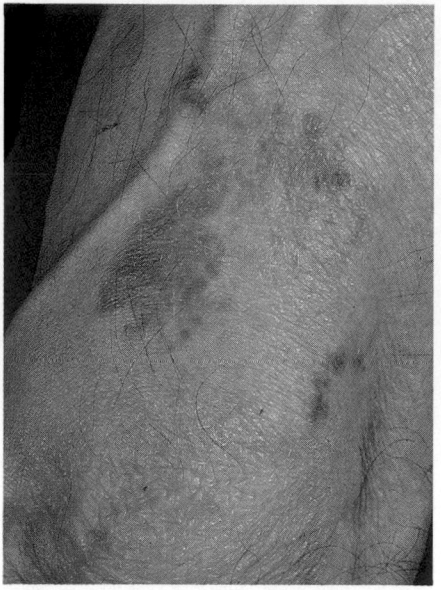

Figure 2–46. Epidemic Kaposi's sarcoma. Patch stage.

These red, flat, irregularly shaped lesions were initially mistaken for bruises. When additional lesions developed, a diagnosis of Kaposi's sarcoma was confirmed by biopsy.

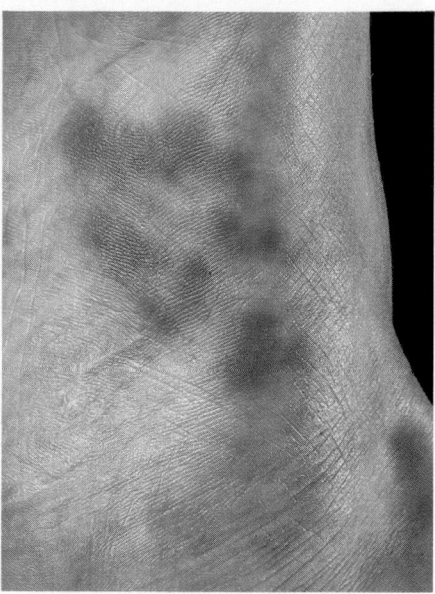

Figure 2–47. Epidemic Kaposi's sarcoma. Patch stage.

These tawny to pink coalescing macules on the ankle region were thought to be secondary to trauma. They were asymptomatic and were only diagnosed as Kaposi's sarcoma when the patient developed multiple other lesions on distant sites of his body.

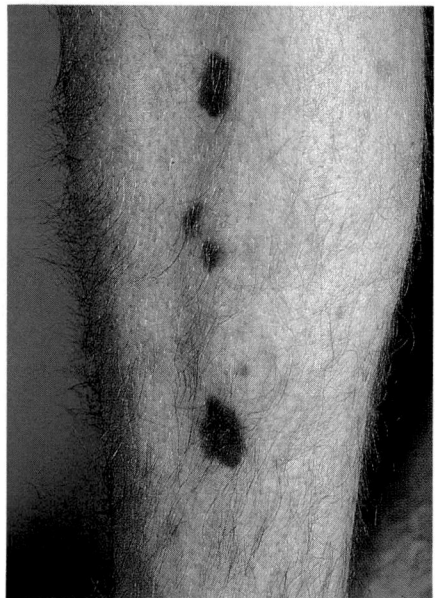

Figure 2–48. Epidemic Kaposi's sarcoma. Patch stage.

Several flat, blue-black macular lesions of Kaposi's sarcoma on the lower leg had been present for two years.

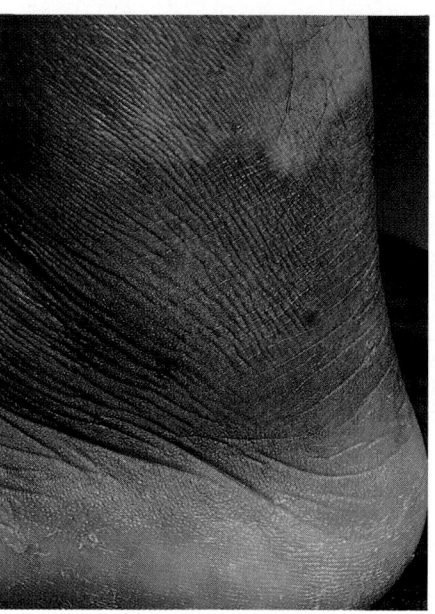

Figure 2–49. Epidemic Kaposi's sarcoma. Patch stage.

This large, asymptomatic, hyperpigmented patch of Kaposi's sarcoma on the ankle region of a mulatto homosexual male was ignored by the patient and remained undiagnosed for several months until the patient suddenly developed a life-threatening opportunistic infection with toxoplasmosis.

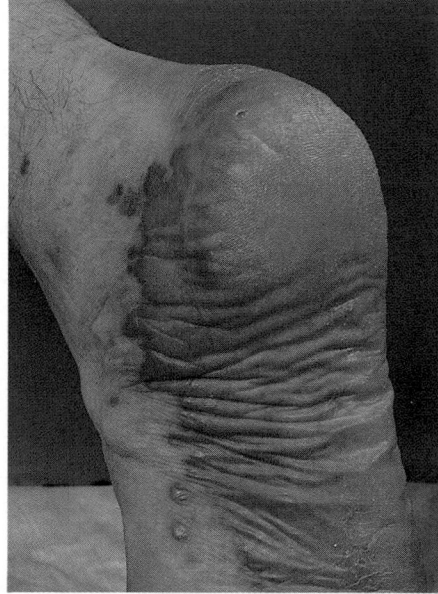

Figure 2–50. Epidemic Kaposi's sarcoma. Patch stage.

A large, pink confluent flat lesion of Kaposi's sarcoma, located on the sole of the foot extending from the heel. Numerous satellite lesions are also present on the ankle and at the border of this patch-stage lesion. This lesion, which had been present for several months, was initially thought to represent a tinea pedis infection that did not respond to topical antifungal medication. The diagnosis of Kaposi's sarcoma was confirmed by biopsy. This resembles the classical variety of the tumor (see Figure 2–1).

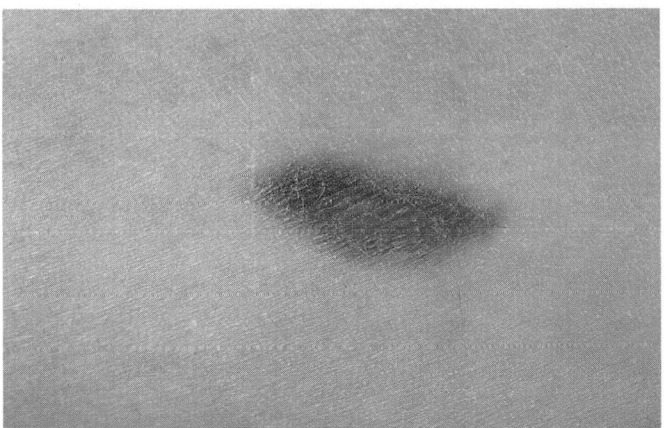

Figure 2–51. Epidemic Kaposi's sarcoma. Patch-to-plaque stage.

A close-up view of a violet to brown, hyperpigmented elliptic, slightly indurated lesion on the trunk.

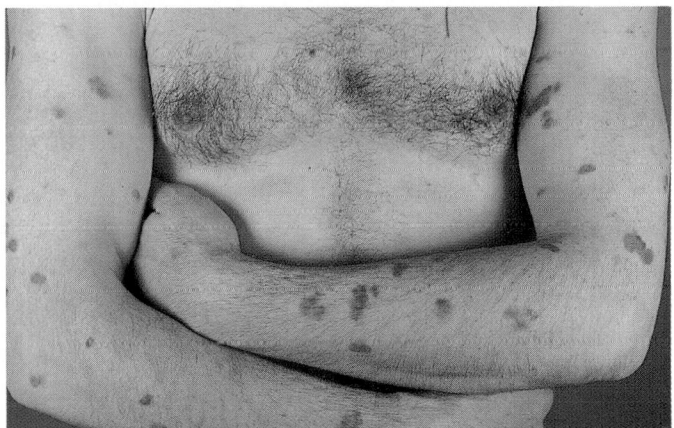

Figure 2–52. Epidemic Kaposi's sarcoma. Plaque stage.

Multiple elongated and irregularly shaped violet to brown plaque lesions of Kaposi's sarcoma on the upper extremities.

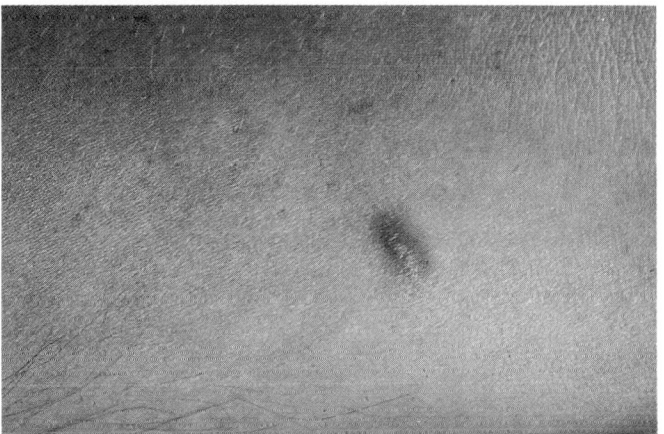

Figure 2–53. Epidemic Kaposi's sarcoma. Plaque stage.

A raised fusiform violaceous lesion on the upper arm of a patient who developed this lesion several months after experiencing his first bout of *Pneumocystis carinii* pneumonia.

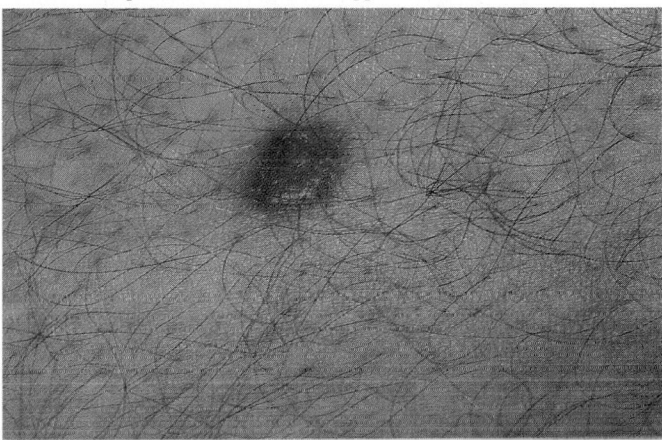

Figure 2–54. Epidemic Kaposi's sarcoma. Plaque stage.

An elevated red to brown polygonal lesion that became increasingly pigmented over several months, especially at the peripheral margin.

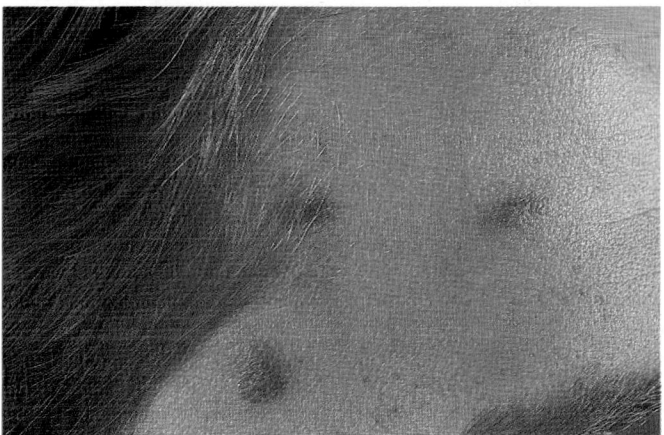

Figure 2–55. Epidemic Kaposi's sarcoma. Plaque stage.

Three ovoid, indurated, red to purple plaques found on the temple. The diagnosis of Kaposi's sarcoma was initially made in this patient several months earlier, when a lymph node biopsy was performed, and proved to have foci of tumor.

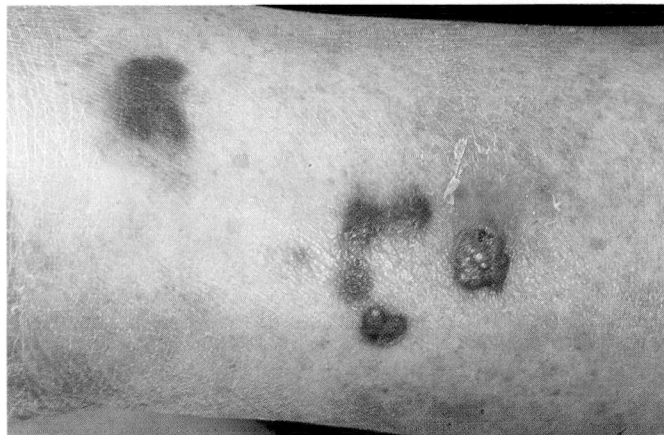

Figure 2–56. Epidemic Kaposi's sarcoma. Plaque stage.

Multiple dark brown to black lesions had been present on the skin of this patient's arm for approximately eight months. These lesions resemble malignant melanoma.

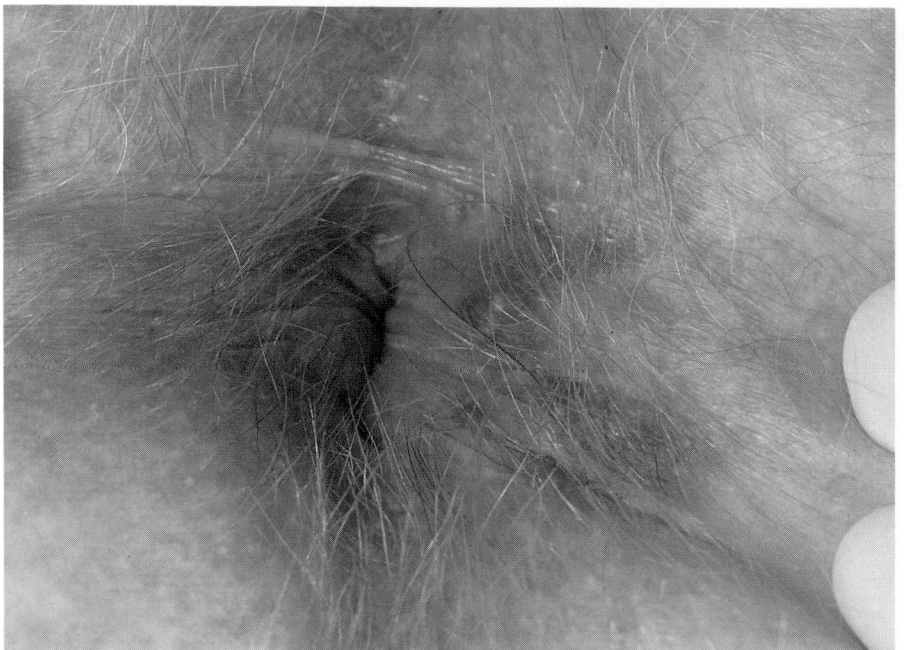

Figure 2–57. Epidemic Kaposi's sarcoma. Plaque stage.

A 40 year old homosexual male with two lavender, irregularly shaped, asymptomatic plaque lesions of Kaposi's sarcoma on the right side of the perianal skin. The patient also had several other mucocutaneous lesions of Kaposi's sarcoma. On colonoscopy, nodules of Kaposi's sarcoma were also found.

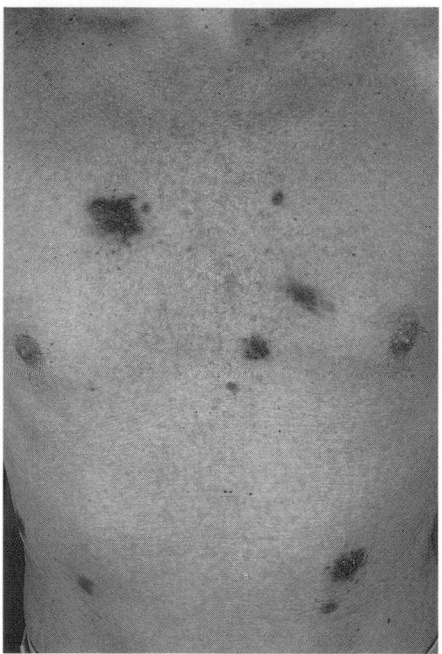

Figure 2–58. Epidemic Kaposi's sarcoma. Plaque stage.

Multiple large plaque lesions of Kaposi's sarcoma. Several of the lesions are surrounded by a yellowish halo similar to that observed in resolving bruises or ecchymoses of the skin. This halo is frequently observed associated with lesions of epidemic Kaposi's sarcoma.

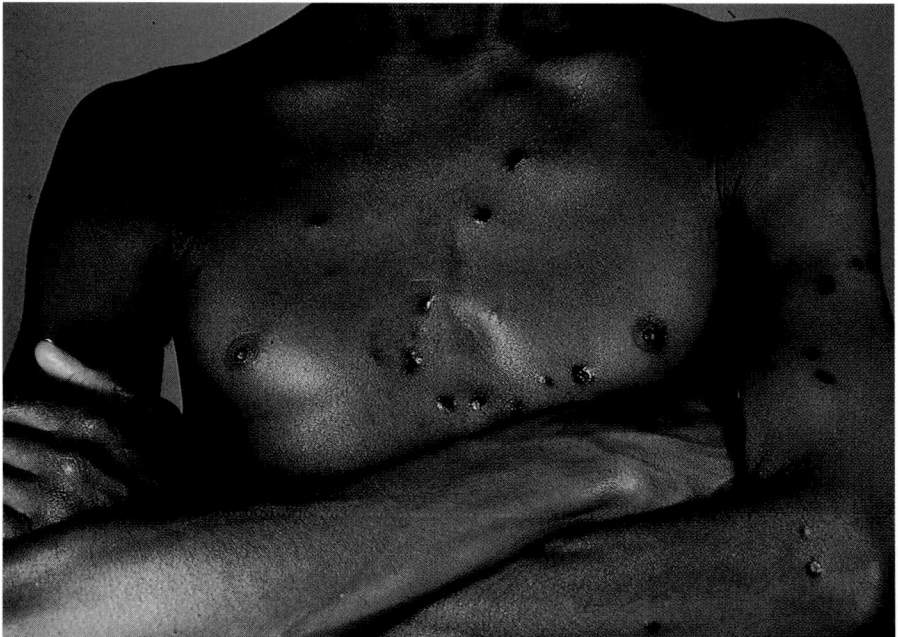

Figure 2–59. Epidemic Kaposi's sarcoma. Plaque stage.

This AIDS patient was an intravenous drug user who developed widely disseminated black, papular skin lesions. Kaposi's sarcoma is uncommon in intravenous drug users with AIDS, and is much more prevalent among the homosexual population at risk. In dark-skinned individuals, the lesions of Kaposi's sarcoma rapidly become hyperpigmented.

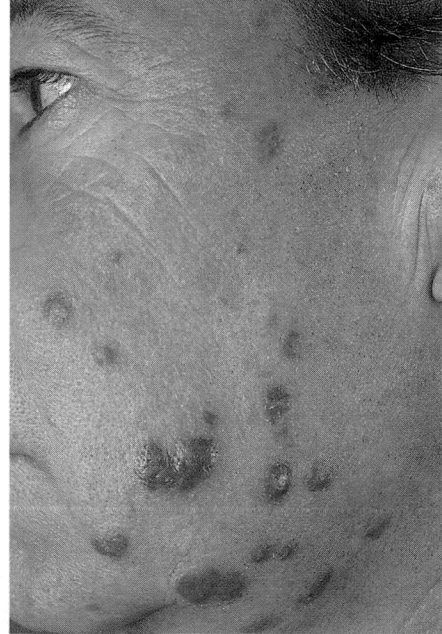

Figure 2–60. Epidemic Kaposi's sarcoma. Plaque-to-nodular stage.

A 60 year old homosexual Hispanic male presented with patch and plaque lesions on his face, some of which were developing into nodules. With time, several of the lesions coalesced.

1

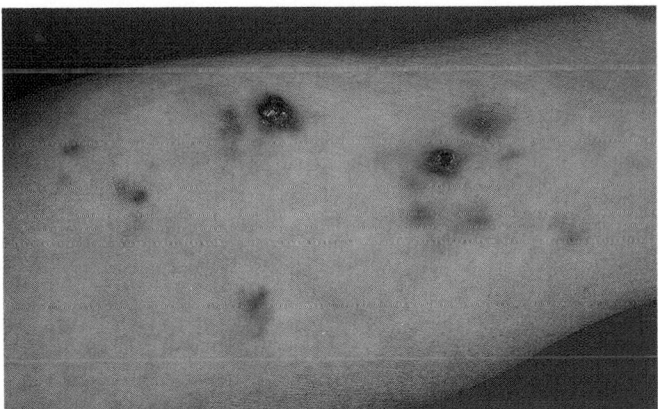

Figure 2–61. Epidemic Kaposi's sarcoma. Patch, plaque, and nodular stages.

Multiple cherry red lesions of Kaposi's sarcoma in various stages (patch, plaque, and nodule) may appear concurrently in the same region. New lesions usually continue to develop during the course of the illness.

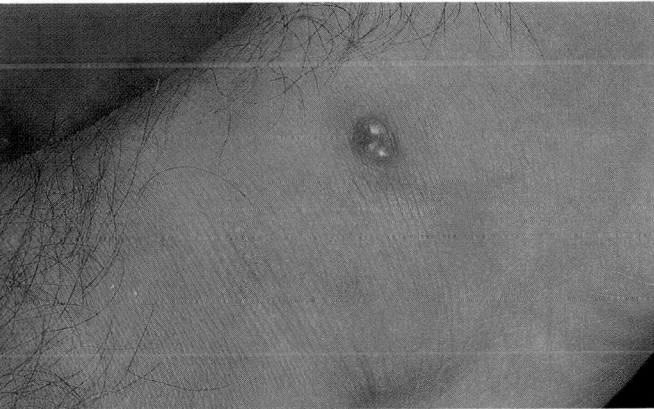

Figure 2–62. Epidemic Kaposi's sarcoma. Nodular stage.

A singular opalescent, pearl-like tumor nodule appeared in the skin of the antecubetal fossa of an otherwise asymptomatic 22 year old HIV-seropositive homosexual male.

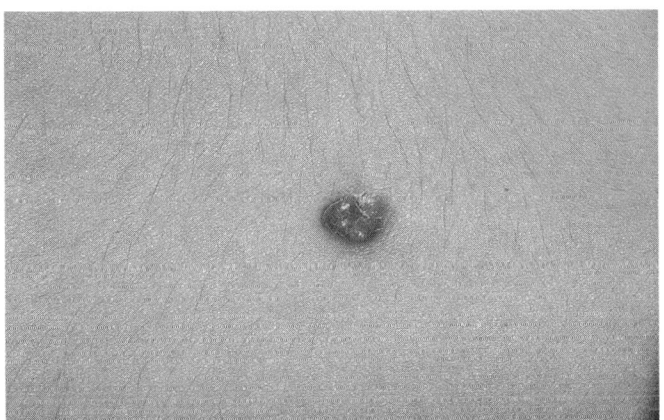

Figure 2–63. Epidemic Kaposi's sarcoma. Nodular stage.

An isolated dark red translucent loculated nodular skin tumor, which was the presenting lesion of Kaposi's sarcoma in this patient. This lesion could be mistaken for a basal cell carcinoma.

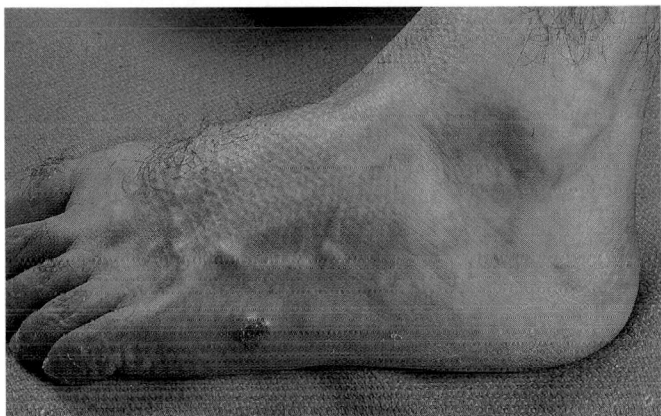

Figure 2–64. Epidemic Kaposi's sarcoma. Nodular stage.

A solitary extruding nodular tumor present on the lateral margin of the foot, which is reminiscent of the typical tumor often seen in patients with classical Kaposi's sarcoma.

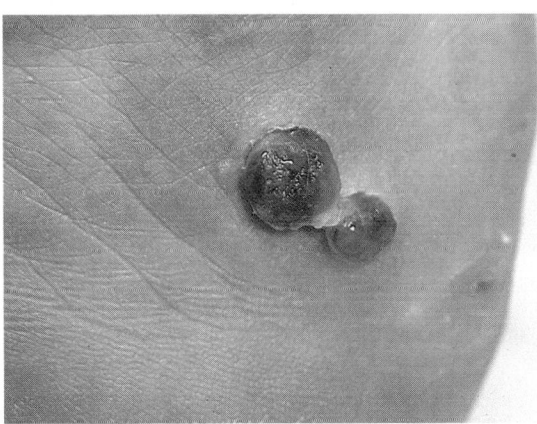

Figure 2–65. Epidemic Kaposi's sarcoma. Nodular stage.

Two adjacent nodular lesions which appeared on the lateral margin of the heel below the ankle and progressed from flat red macules to protruding nodules within a month. The surfaces of these nodules are denuded.

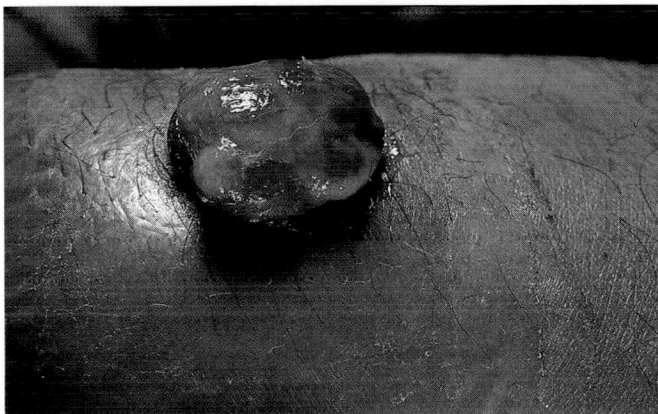

Figure 2–66. Epidemic Kaposi's sarcoma. Nodular stage.

A solitary tumor nodule located on the finger of a light-skinned black man with AIDS was one of many widespread lesions which developed over a five month period. The surfaces of such elevated lesions are prone to superficial trauma.

The diagnosis of AIDS frequently has been made by the chance discovery of one or multiple skin lesions of Kaposi's sarcoma in an otherwise totally asymptomatic individual. New multifocal lesions often develop anywhere on the skin and mucosal surfaces and may continue to appear throughout the course of the disease. Similar to classical Kaposi's sarcoma, the morphologic appearance of the lesions of AIDS-associated Kaposi's sarcoma vary from flat macular *patches* to indurated papules and *plaques* or elevated *nodules* (Figures 2–67 to 2–76). When compared to the usually slow-growing round tumors of the classical disease, most often found on the lower extremities, the lesions of epidemic Kaposi's sarcoma have a more varied configuration; they are commonly oval, elongated, and fusiform, and are often irregular in shape. As the lesions become more numerous, they tend to develop rapidly in a widely disseminated, bilateral, strikingly symmetric pattern of distribution along the lines of skin cleavage (Langer's lines). This phenomenon had not been previously observed in the other forms of Kaposi's sarcoma.

The early faint, asymptomatic lesions of AIDS-associated Kaposi's sarcoma can be easily ignored or misdiagnosed by both the patient and the examining physician. Frequently overlooked but commonly involved anatomic sites include the oropharyngeal mucosa, the posterior auricular regions of the scalp, and the ear lobes. The nose is a frequent site of lesion involvement as well (Figures 2–77 to 2–110).

The early, often discrete *patch*-stage lesions of epidemic Kaposi's sarcoma may be mistaken for bruises, purpura, diffuse cutaneous hemorrhages such as those seen in patients with leukemia, flat heman-

giomas, pigmented nevi, or melanomas. The evolving Kaposi's sarcoma lesions often become elevated, developing into papules or thickened *plaques*. These raised, often widely disseminated tumor lesions can resemble the dermatologic eruptions of other diseases such as secondary syphilis, pityriasis rosea, lichen planus, sarcoidosis, eruptive xanthomas, insect bites, papular urticaria, urticaria pigmentosa, intradermal nevi, or cutaneous metastases of systemic malignancies, melanomas, carcinomas, or cutaneous lymphomas. Eventually, the neighboring patch and plaque-stage lesions may coalesce and continue to enlarge into *nodular* tumors. The differential diagnosis of these nodular tumors includes benign pedunculated nevi, neurofibromas, dermatofibromas, pyogenic granulomas, glomus tumors, hemangiomas or malignant angiosarcomas, basal cell carcinomas, melanomas and cutaneous metastases of internal malignancies, or lymphomas of the skin.[24] The mucocutaneous lesions of other diseases, which may be easily mistaken for Kaposi's sarcoma, are illustrated and discussed in Chapter 5.

Epidemic Kaposi's sarcoma involving lymph nodes or visceral organs including the gastrointestinal tract, lung, liver, kidney, and spleen has been reported, even in the absence of visible skin or oral lesions.[23, 43, 44] The development of persistent, generalized lymphadenopathy has frequently been associated with HIV infection. Histologic examination of enlarged lymph nodes in such patients usually shows an atypical hyperplasia of the nodal structure; however, microscopic foci of Kaposi's sarcoma may also be detected.[43, 44] Gastrointestinal lesions of Kaposi's sarcoma, from the oropharynx to the anus, may be detected radiographically or by endoscopic examination.[23]

The lesions of epidemic Kaposi's sarcoma may occur before or after the development of constitutional symptoms such as fever, night sweats, unexplained weight loss, chronic diarrhea, malaise, and fatigue; the occurrence of opportunistic infections; or neurologic manifestations due to HIV infection.[26, 45, 46]

A study involving the first 212 patients with AIDS-associated Kaposi's sarcoma diagnosed and followed at New York University Medical Center was conducted between 1981 and 1986. The patients who presented with only AIDS-associated Kaposi's sarcoma in the absence of constitutional symptoms or opportunistic infections, and who had greater than 300 T-helper lymphocytes per cu mm in their peripheral blood, had the best prognosis, with a mean survival of 32 months. The individuals who had neither constitutional symptoms nor an opportunistic infection, but had an absolute T-helper cell count of less than 300 cells per cu mm, were found to have a mean survival of 24 months. Those patients who presented with constitutional symptoms at the time of diagnosis of Kaposi's sarcoma had a mean survival of 14 months, regardless of their absolute T-helper cell counts. Patients who developed an opportunistic infection within three months of their diagnosis of Kaposi's sarcoma had the poorest prognosis, with a mean survival of seven months. These data show that in patients with AIDS-associated Kaposi's sarcoma, the absolute number of T-helper cells and the presence or development of constitutional symptoms or opportunistic infections are predictive of the patient's prognosis for survival. It appears that Kaposi's sarcoma alone is rarely the direct cause of death in these patients. Rather, it is the development of infectious complications to which patient death is most often attributed.[47]

In addition to Kaposi's sarcoma, patients with symptomatic HIV infection frequently develop other chronic, often severe, skin conditions including generalized unrelenting pruritus, folliculitis, hives, psoriasiform or seborrheic dermatitis, impetigo, oral and intertriginous candidiasis, and other fungal infections of the skin and nails. Persistent condylomata acuminata, ulcerative anogenital herpes simplex, generalized molluscum contagiosum, and severe herpes zoster are common viral skin infections that can appear at any time during the course of the illness and may represent the earliest clinical signs of an underlying HIV-induced immunodeficiency in a previously "healthy" individual.[48] A newly described entity known as oral "hairy" leukoplakia has been reported only in patients with HIV infection. This unique lesion may be viral in origin and has been found to be closely associated with the Epstein-Barr virus.[49, 50] These HIV-related skin conditions are discussed and illustrated in Chapter 6.

As of July 13, 1987, there were 37,785 adult patients with diagnosed AIDS in the United States, of whom 7736 (20.5 per cent) had Kaposi's sarcoma. One of the most intriguing epidemiologic observations is that 95 per cent of all cases of AIDS-associated Kaposi's sarcoma in the United States have been diagnosed among homosexual and bisexual men. Of these homosexual men with Kaposi's sarcoma, 9.4 per cent were also known to be intravenous drug users. The remaining 5 per cent of AIDS-associated Kaposi's sarcoma cases have been reported among heterosexual men and women with AIDS. Three per cent of heterosexual intravenous drug abusers with AIDS developed Kaposi's sarcoma. Kaposi's sarcoma was also reported to occur within the other risk groups with the following frequencies: transfusion recipients, 3.5 per cent; hemophiliacs, 1.5 per cent; heterosexual contacts of individuals at known risk, 1.9 per cent; individuals born in countries where most AIDS cases have no identified risk (i.e., Haiti, Central Africa), 8.5 per cent; and patients with no identified risk fac-

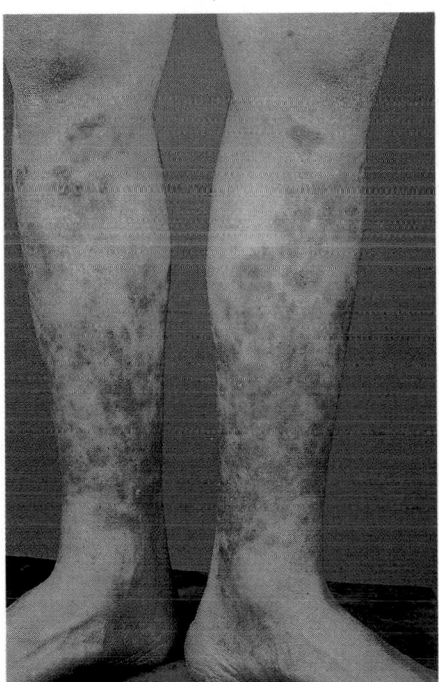

Figure 2–67. Epidemic Kaposi's sarcoma. Plaque stage.

A 35 year old homosexual male with Kaposi's sarcoma primarily located on the lower extremities. As his disease progressed, new lesions developed in the same region and the early discrete pink macules became confluent, indurated, and hyperpigmented. This distribution of lesions resembles the most frequent clinical presentation of classical Kaposi's sarcoma.

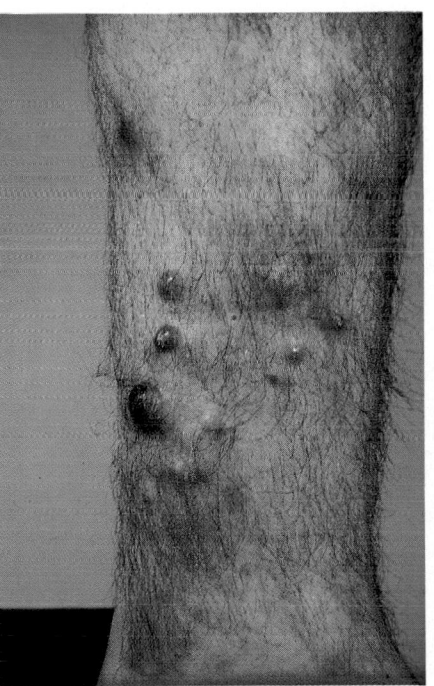

Figure 2–68. Epidemic Kaposi's sarcoma. Nodular stage.

A 47 year old homosexual male of Italian extraction with multiple nodular lesions of Kaposi's sarcoma ranging in color from pink to brown on both lower extremities present since 1980. The original diagnosis of classical Kaposi's sarcoma was changed to epidemic (AIDS-associated) Kaposi's sarcoma in 1982 when he developed *Pneumocystis carinii* pneumonia. A stored serum sample from 1979 was found to contain antibodies to HIV.

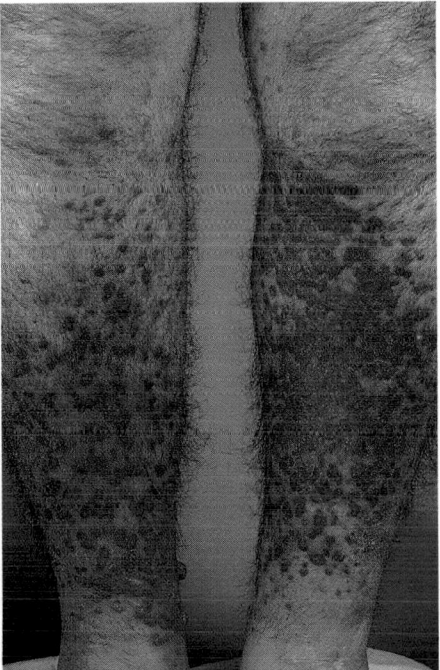

Figure 2–69. Epidemic Kaposi's sarcoma. Plaque stage.

This 39 year old homosexual male of Mediterranean extraction developed multiple dark brown to purple plaque and nodular lesions predominantly located on the lower extremities, associated with chronic lymphedema. There is a subset of patients with epidemic Kaposi's sarcoma in whom the lesions tend to be localized to the lower extremities, a pattern that is similar to the typical classical variant of the disease (see classical pattern observed in Figure 2–13).

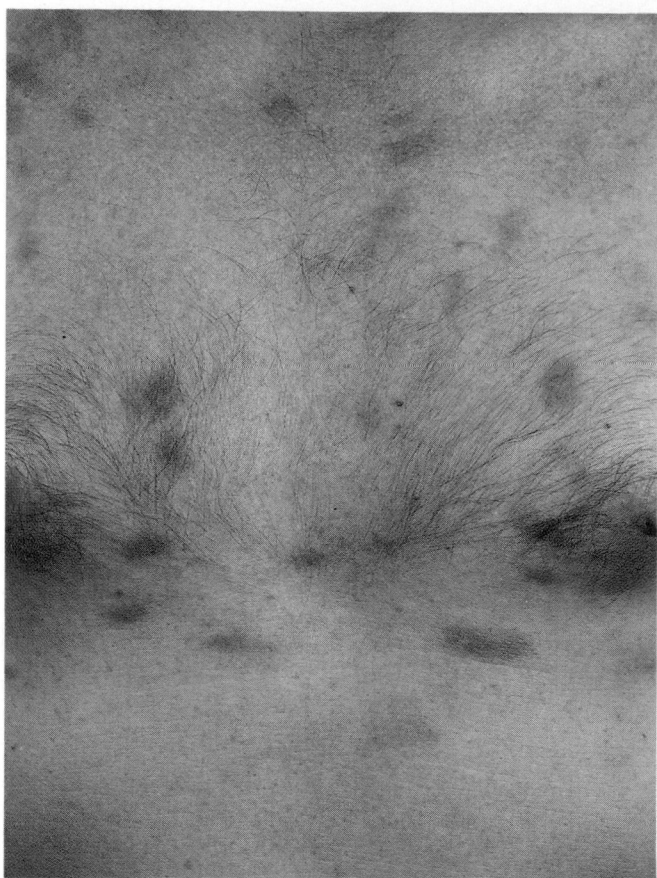

Figure 2–70. Epidemic Kaposi's sarcoma. Patch-to-plaque stage.

A 33 year old homosexual male with bilateral dark pink to violet elongated lesions of Kaposi's sarcoma symmetrically and widely distributed over his entire body. The lesions resemble dabs of paint spattered on the skin surface. It is interesting to note that the lesions conform to the creases of the skin (lines of Langer).

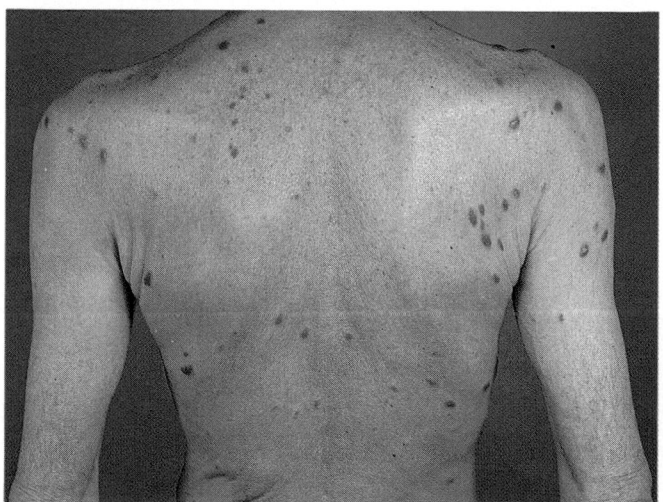

Figure 2–72. Epidemic Kaposi's sarcoma. Plaque stage.

A 58 year old Hispanic homosexual male intravenous drug user with multiple symmetric purple plaques, which developed rapidly over his trunk and extremities. Many of the lesions appear to follow the creases of the skin (lines of Langer).

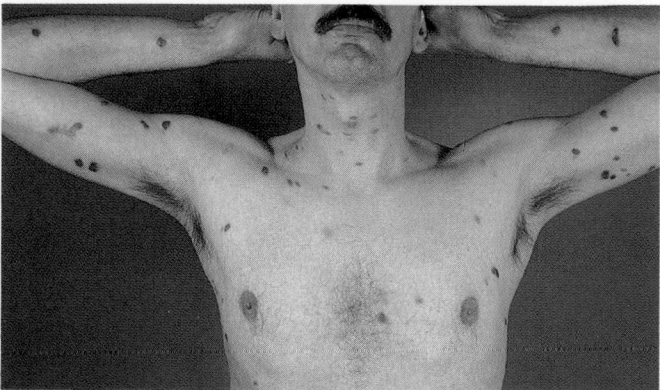

Figure 2–71. Epidemic Kaposi's sarcoma. Plaque stage.

A 41 year old homosexual male with widespread, symmetric cutaneous patches, plaques, and nodules of Kaposi's sarcoma, present for approximately one year. Some of the lesions have an elongated ovoid shape, and they vary in color from red to brown.

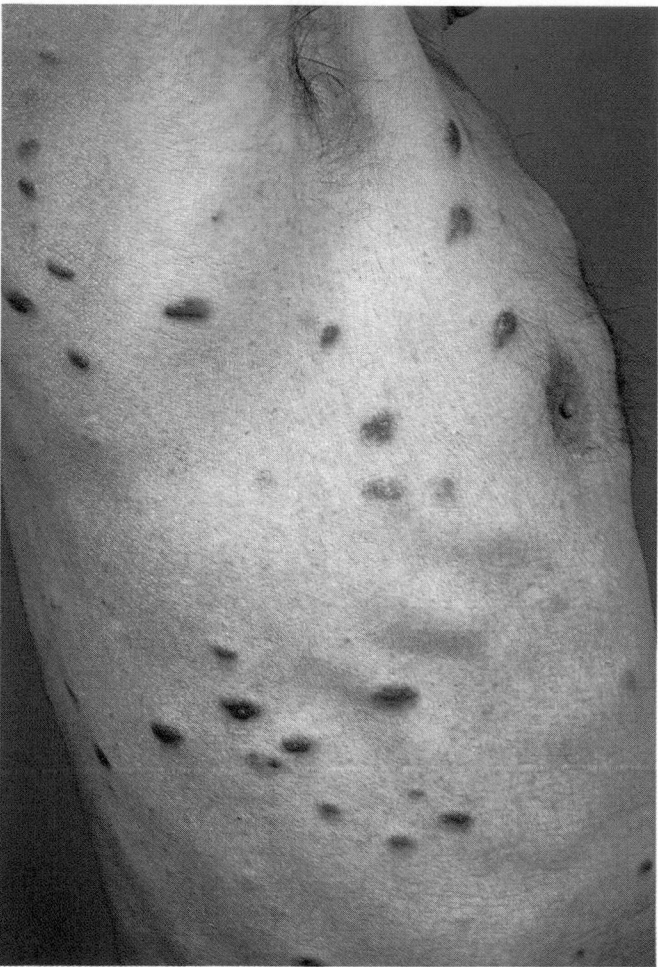

Figure 2–73. Epidemic Kaposi's sarcoma. Plaque-to-nodular stage.

Widely disseminated fusiform plaque lesions distributed symmetrically in a swirled pattern. They vary in color from dark red to violet. Some hyperpigmentation of the lesions is also evident.

tors, 9.1 per cent. In addition, 11 cases of Kaposi's sarcoma have been reported among the 527 children with AIDS (2.1 per cent). All these children had parents with AIDS or at known risk for the development of AIDS. Whereas the overall male:female ratio of the prevalence of epidemic Kaposi's sarcoma is 106:1, a large degree of the male predominance may be explained by the greater prevalence of the disease among homosexual men. When comparing heterosexual men and women with known primary risk factors (i.e., intravenous drug use, transfusion recipients), the relative risks of development of epidemic Kaposi's sarcoma are almost equal.[51, 52]

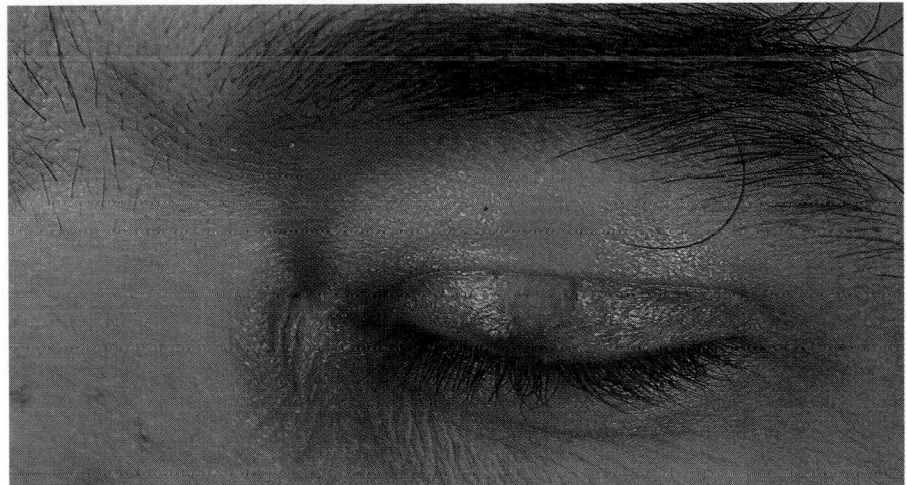

Figure 2–74. Epidemic Kaposi's sarcoma. Plaque stage.

A slightly indurated papular lesion on the upper eyelid of a patient with epidemic Kaposi's sarcoma. Initially, the lesion was thought to represent a stye and was examined by an ophthalmologist who eventually biopsied the lesion when it did not respond to conventional therapy.

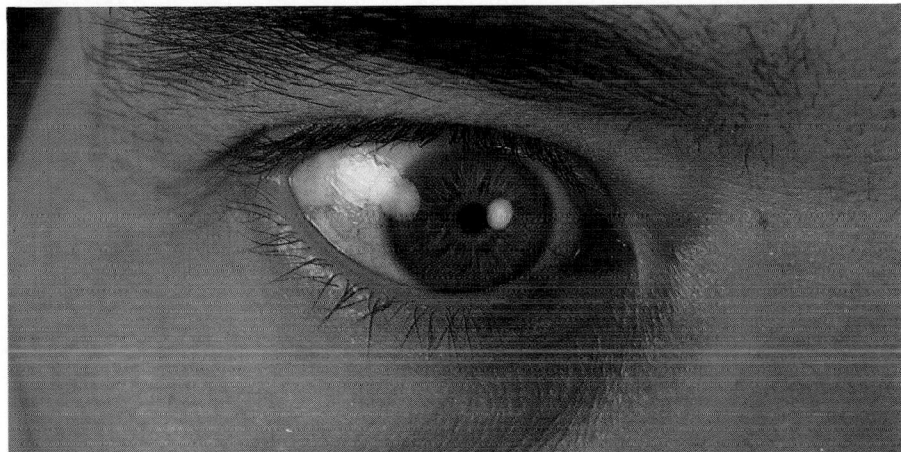

Figure 2–75. Epidemic Kaposi's sarcoma. Patch stage.

A linear red lesion on the lower eyelid margin of this bisexual male was one of many lesions present on the patient's skin. The lesion rapidly developed into a tumor nodule, which responded favorably to local radiation therapy.

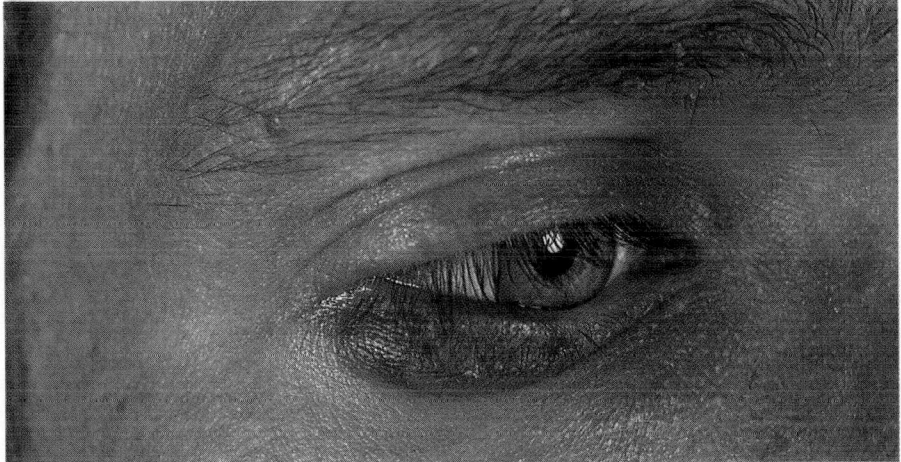

Figure 2–76. Epidemic Kaposi's sarcoma. Plaque stage.

Indurated violaceous lesion involving the lateral lower eyelid.

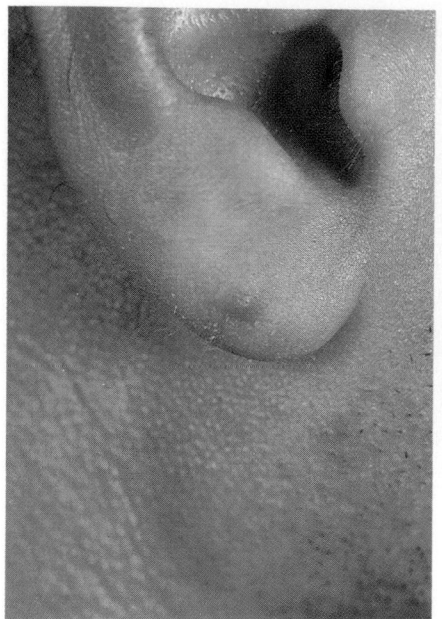

Figure 2–77. Epidemic Kaposi's sarcoma. Nodular stage.

A 29 year old homosexual male with epidemic Kaposi's sarcoma. The patient presented with multiple faint macular lesions on his trunk and hard palate and this asymptomatic pink solitary nodule on the ear lobe. Lesions on the ear have been reported rarely in the classical or endemic African forms of the disease.

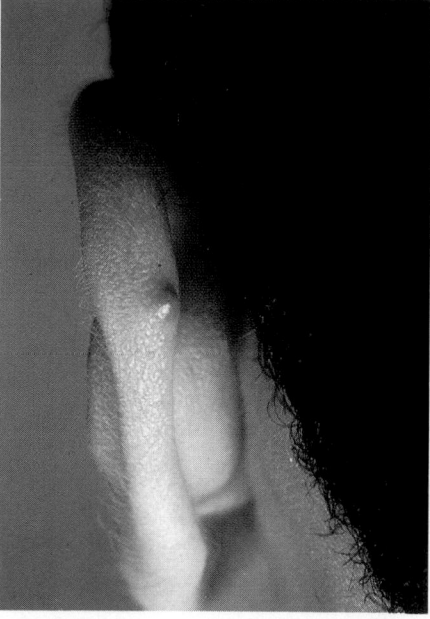

Figure 2–78. Epidemic Kaposi's sarcoma. Nodular stage.

A 30 year old bisexual Hispanic male intravenous drug user with a red tumor nodule present on the pinna of the ear.

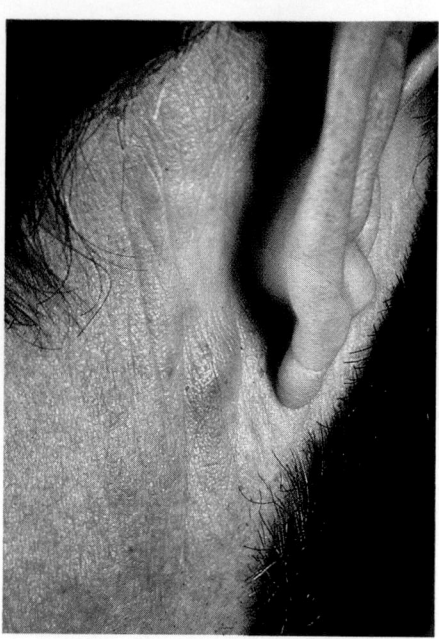

Figure 2–79. Epidemic Kaposi's sarcoma. Nodular stage.

A faint bluish posterior auricular skin nodule. This is a common, frequently overlooked site for Kaposi's sarcoma lesions to appear in patients with AIDS.

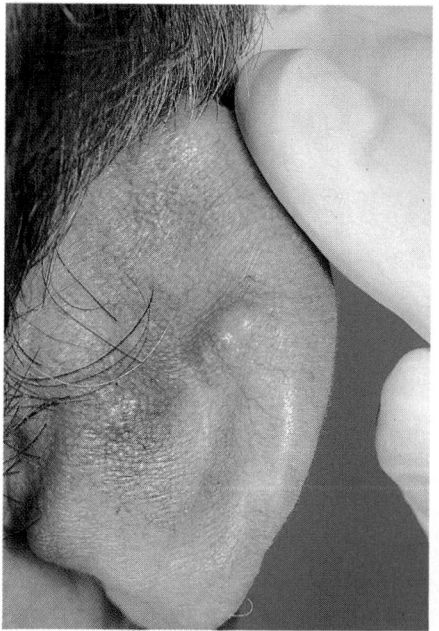

Figure 2–80. Epidemic Kaposi's sarcoma. Nodular stage.

Two opalescent bluish-colored asymptomatic nodules on the back of the ear.

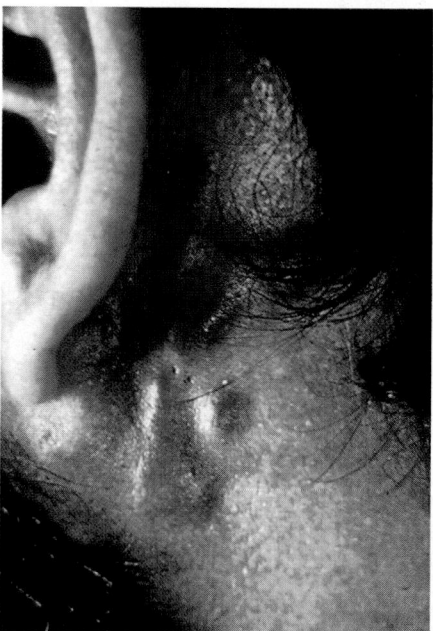

Figure 2–81. Epidemic Kaposi's sarcoma. Plaque stage.

A cluster of irregularly shaped red indurated plaques of Kaposi's sarcoma located behind the ear.

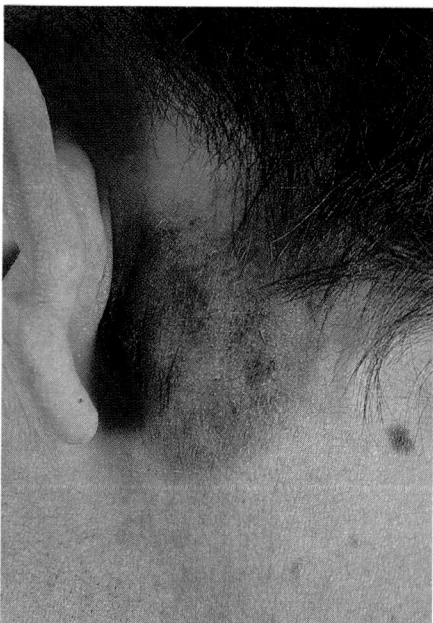

Figure 2–82. Epidemic Kaposi's sarcoma. Patch stage.

A large pink macular lesion with variegated pigmentation located behind the ear. This lesion resembles a superficial spreading melanoma. There is a small brown flat nevus just posterior to the tumor which had been present since childhood.

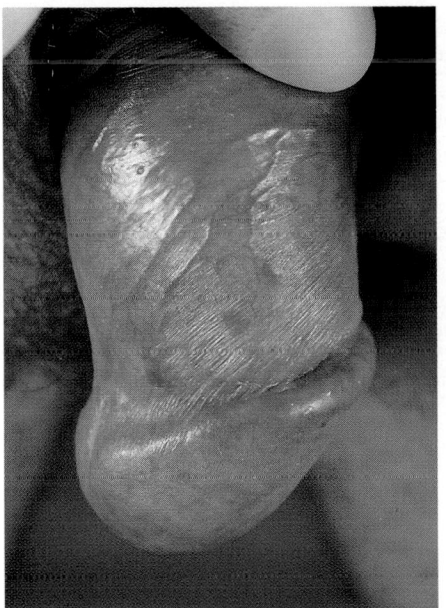

Figure 2–83. Epidemic Kaposi's sarcoma. Patch stage.

A 42 year old Hispanic with three asymptomatic faint red macules of Kaposi's sarcoma present on the inner surface of the retracted foreskin.

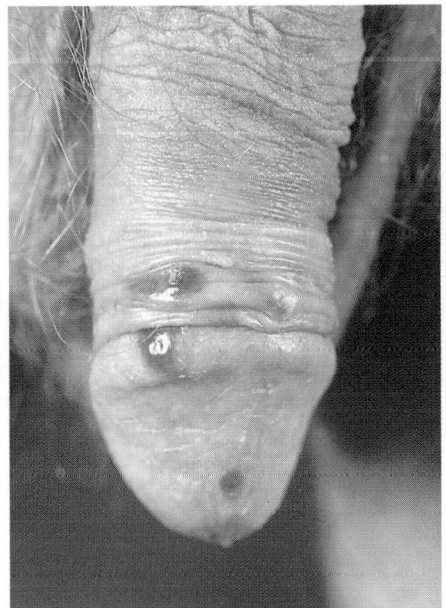

Figure 2–84. Epidemic Kaposi's sarcoma. Plaque stage.

Slightly indurated red papules seen on the inner aspect of the retracted foreskin and glans. These lesions resemble those of lichen planus or secondary syphilis.

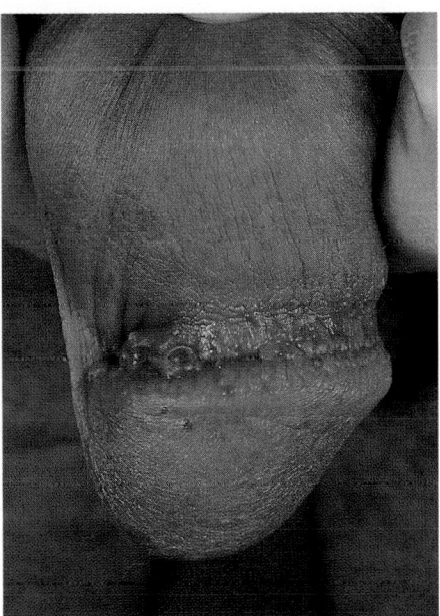

Figure 2–85. Epidemic Kaposi's sarcoma. Nodular stage.

Multiple red pinpoint and nodular lesions present along the coronal sulcus of the penis. The patient was initially thought to have condylomata acuminata. It was only after unsuccessful treatment with topical podophyllum that a biopsy was performed, which surprisingly revealed a diagnosis of Kaposi's sarcoma.

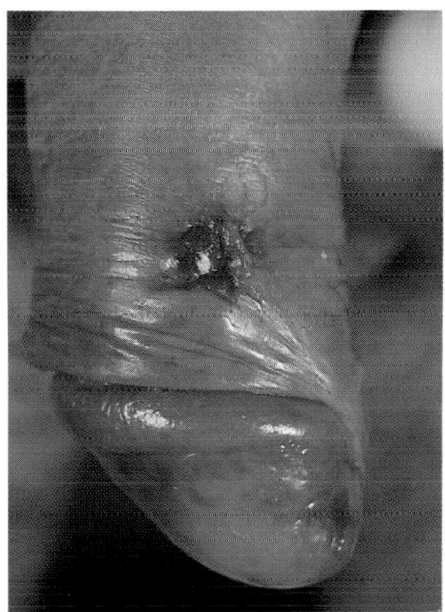

Figure 2–86. Epidemic Kaposi's sarcoma. Nodular stage.

A deep brown nodule of Kaposi's sarcoma on the lateral shaft of the penis. In addition, there is a purple macular lesion on the glans penis.

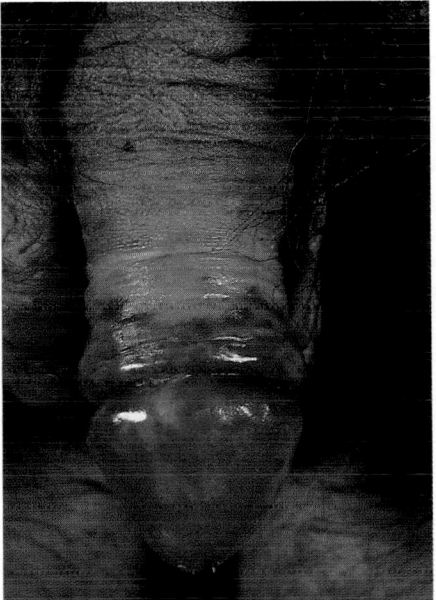

Figure 2–87. Epidemic Kaposi's sarcoma.

A 37 year old Caucasian male with an advanced infiltrative lesion of Kaposi's sarcoma involving the entire glans and distal shaft of the penis. The lesion caused severe pain when the patient developed an erection and eventually caused urethral obstruction. On autopsy, the tumor was found to invade the corpus cavernosus.

The incidence of Kaposi's sarcoma among homosexual men with AIDS in the United States has steadily decreased each year since 1981. In 1981, 44 per cent of homosexual men with AIDS presented with Kaposi's sarcoma, with or without concurrent opportunistic infections. In 1985, 36 per cent of homosexual men with AIDS presented with the tumor, and in 1987 approximately 20 per cent.[53] It has been suggested that the remarkable decreasing reported incidence of Kaposi's sarcoma in this population may be due to changes in sexual practices, a reduction in the number of sexual partners, and possibly a decline in the use of recreational drugs, especially inhalant amyl or butyl nitrites, which were particularly popular among homosexual men at the onset of the AIDS epidemic.[52] However, one cannot be certain that this decline in the incidence of Kaposi's sarcoma among patients with AIDS is not a reporting artifact. Although collected in the same manner for six years, these epidemiologic data are derived from surveillance reports of the clinical manifestations of AIDS at the time of diagnosis and may not include those cases in whom Kaposi's sarcoma develops later in the course of the illness. It is also possible that physicians are making a clinical diagnosis of Kaposi's sarcoma without the biopsy confirmation, which is required by the CDC for surveillance reporting purposes.

Although Kaposi's sarcoma *per se* is rarely the direct cause of death in AIDS patients, there are clinical circumstances that warrant local or systemic treatment of Kaposi's sarcoma in this patient population. Tumors requiring local therapy include cosmetically disturbing lesions such as those on the face and other visible parts of the body, and large ulcerating or painful lesions. These may be successfully treated with local radiation therapy, as this tumor is extremely radiosensitive. Other local treatment modalities that have been used in anecdotal and uncontrolled trials include electrocauterization, surgical excision, and intralesional injections of vinblastine or bleomycin. The application of liquid nitrogen cryotherapy to the early smaller skin lesions of Kaposi's sarcoma may be effective in eliminating such tumors. Occasionally individual lesions of epidemic Kaposi's sarcoma have been observed to disappear spontaneously, even when new lesions may continue to appear at distant sites.

In patients with symptomatic Kaposi's sarcoma involving visceral organs such as the lungs or gastrointestinal tract, rapidly progressive and disseminated mucocutaneous disease, or problematic mucocutaneous lesions unresponsive to local treatment, the disease may respond to systemic therapy with chemotherapeutic agents such as Adriamycin, etoposide, bleomycin, or vinblastine as single agents or in combination, resulting in temporary reduction in the size of existing tumors and possibly retarding the development of new lesions. In addition, the systemic administration of the biologic response modifier alpha interferon has been shown to cause tumor regression in some AIDS patients with Kaposi's sarcoma.[54-56] Although treatments may provide transient palliation, systemic chemotherapy has not been shown to influence the overall survival of these patients. With the exception of these situations, therapeutic efforts in patients with AIDS-related Kaposi's sarcoma should concentrate on treatment of the various life-threatening opportunistic infections to which they are prone, the control of the underlying infection with HIV, and reconstitution of their depleted immune functions.

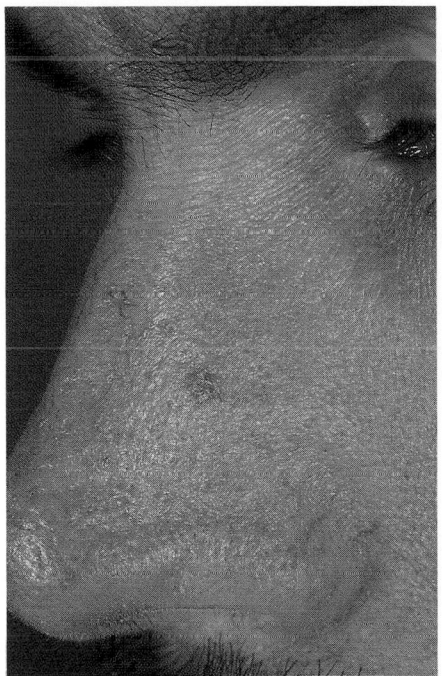

Figure 2–88. Epidemic Kaposi's sarcoma. Patch stage.

An isolated lavender macule of Kaposi's sarcoma on the side of the nose. Such early lesions could easily be overlooked or ignored by the patient and examining physician.

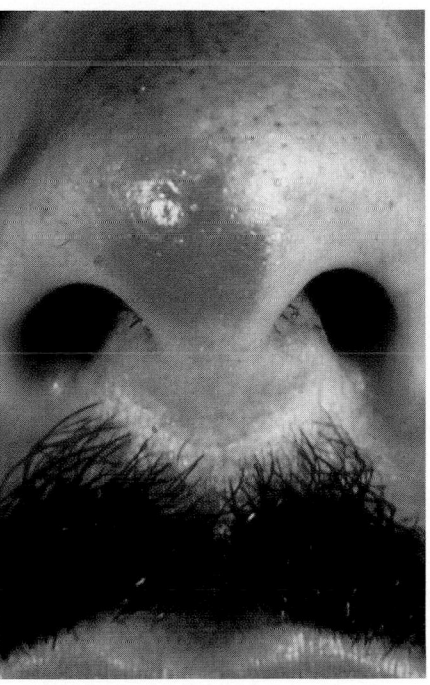

Figure 2–89. Epidemic Kaposi's sarcoma. Patch stage.

This erythematous patch-stage lesion on the nose of a 32 year old homosexual male was originally thought to be the result of an insect bite.

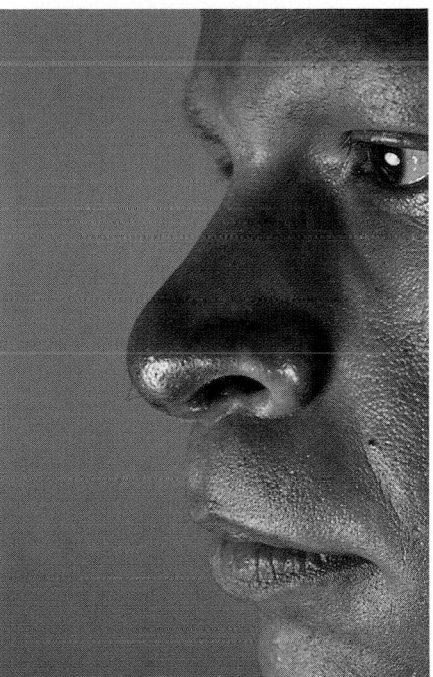

Figure 2–90. Epidemic Kaposi's sarcoma. Patch stage.

Large confluent hyperpigmented lesion of Kaposi's sarcoma in a mulatto homosexual male. Such lesions in dark-skinned individuals rapidly become hyperpigmented.

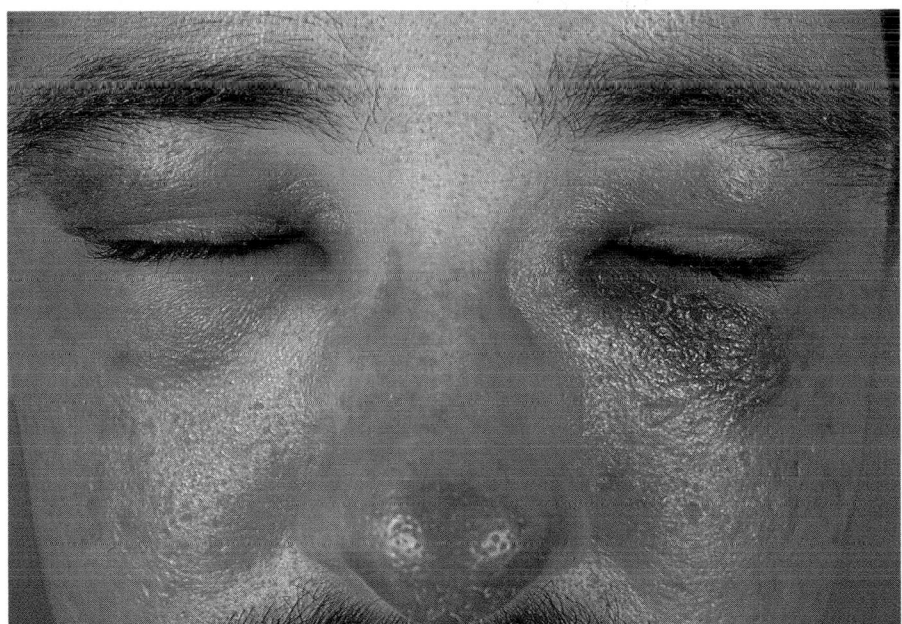

Figure 2–91. Epidemic Kaposi's sarcoma. Advanced disease.

Pink plaque stage lesion on the skin of the tip of the nose that infiltrated into the nasal mucosa. The patient also has a large bluish purple macular lesion below his left eye and bilateral periorbital edema due to lymphatic obstruction, with yellowish discoloration.

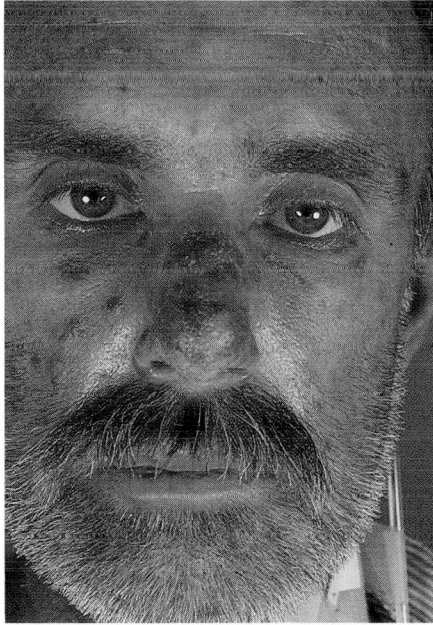

Figure 2–92. Epidemic Kaposi's sarcoma. Advanced disease.

A patient with widely disseminated mucocutaneous lesions of Kaposi's sarcoma. This picture illustrates infiltrative violaceous tumor involvement of the nose. Also note the tiny cherry red tumor nodule on the inner canthus of the right eye.

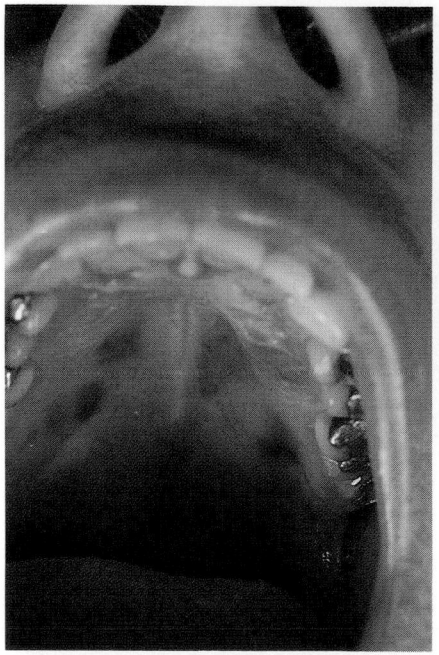

Figure 2–93. Epidemic Kaposi's sarcoma. Patch stage.

Several discrete asymptomatic violet macular lesions on the hard palate. Oral lesions, common in patients with epidemic Kaposi's sarcoma, are rarely reported in patients with classical or endemic African forms of this neoplasm.

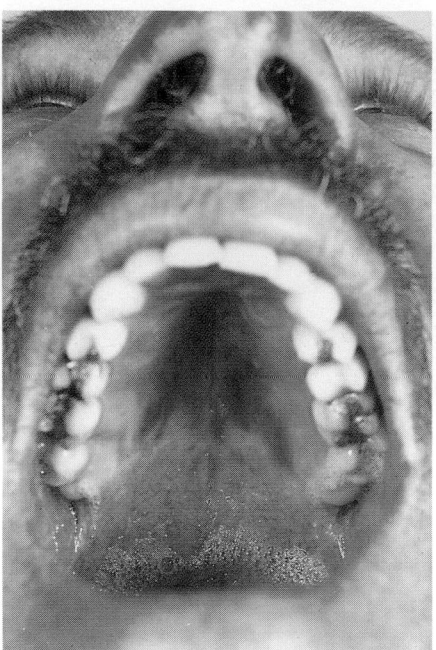

Figure 2–94. Epidemic Kaposi's sarcoma. Patch stage.

Large confluent macule of Kaposi's sarcoma on the hard palate. The macular lesions are almost always asymptomatic.

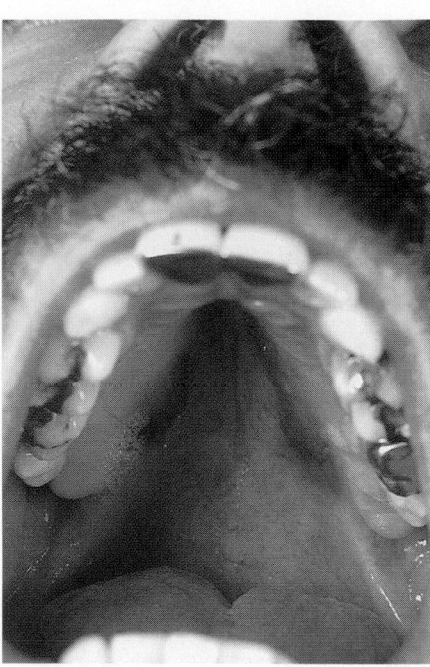

Figure 2–95. Epidemic Kaposi's sarcoma. Plaque stage.

Violet symmetric indurated plaques of Kaposi's sarcoma on the hard palate of a homosexual male. These were among the earliest lesions to develop in this patient.

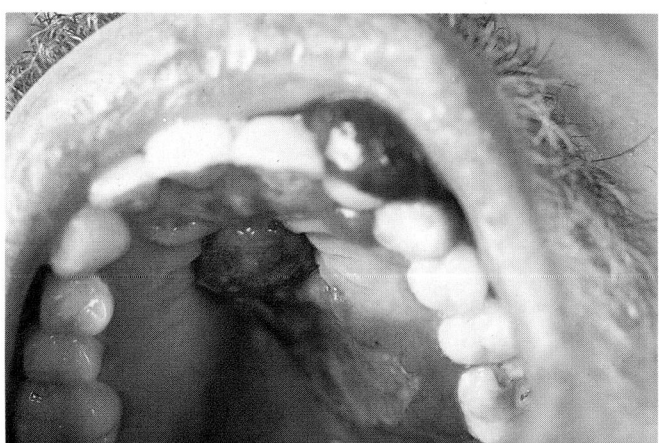

Figure 2–96. Epidemic Kaposi's sarcoma. Nodular stage.

Extensive Kaposi's sarcoma of the oral cavity with a large purple nodular tumor on the hard palate and a red gingival nodular lesion extending over the left incisor. Also present is a chronic oral ulcer on the mucosa of the hard palate due to herpes simplex virus.

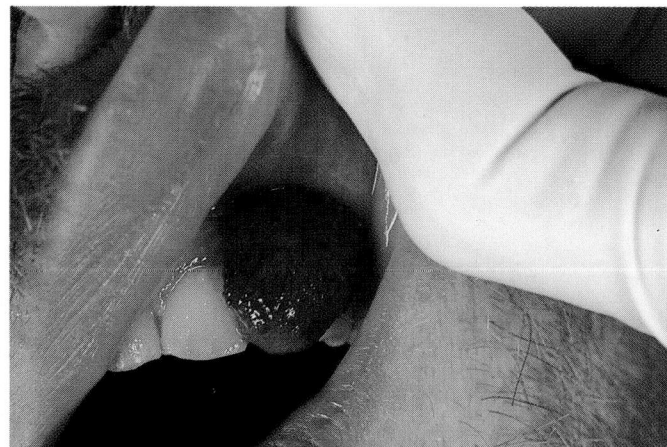

Figure 2–97. Epidemic Kaposi's sarcoma. Nodular stage.

A close-up view of the large deep red stalactite-like tumor extending from the gingiva over the incisor tooth (also seen in Figure 2–60).

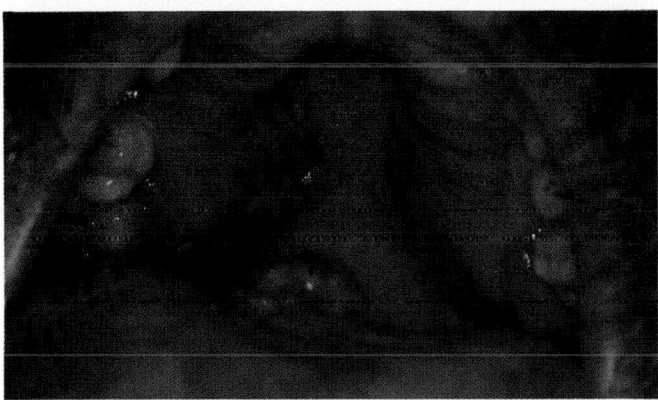

Figure 2–98. Epidemic Kaposi's sarcoma. Nodular stage.

Bilateral symmetric pink to purple nodular tumors on the hard palate. Also present is a nodular lesion on the tongue. Kaposi's sarcoma involving the tongue has been reported rarely.

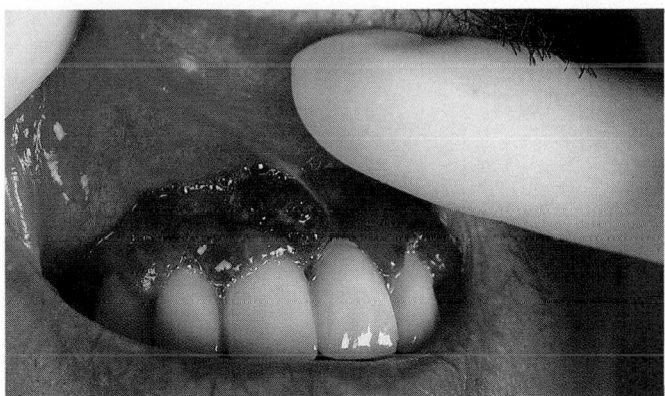

Figure 2–99. Epidemic Kaposi's sarcoma. Nodular stage.

Multiple nodular red and purple lesions of Kaposi's sarcoma extensively involving the gingiva.

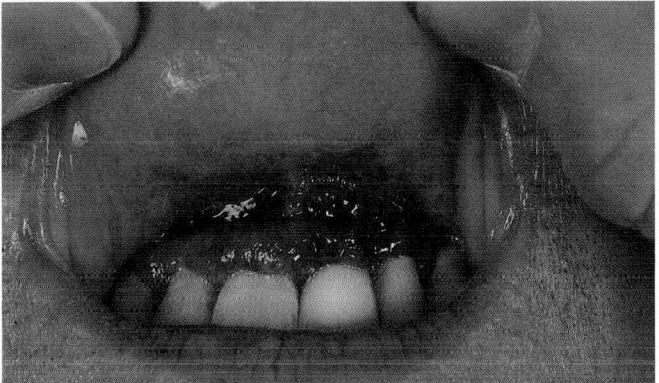

Figure 2–100. Epidemic Kaposi's sarcoma. Nodular stage.

Numerous hemorrhagic-appearing deep red lesions located on the lower gingiva extending onto the labial mucosa.

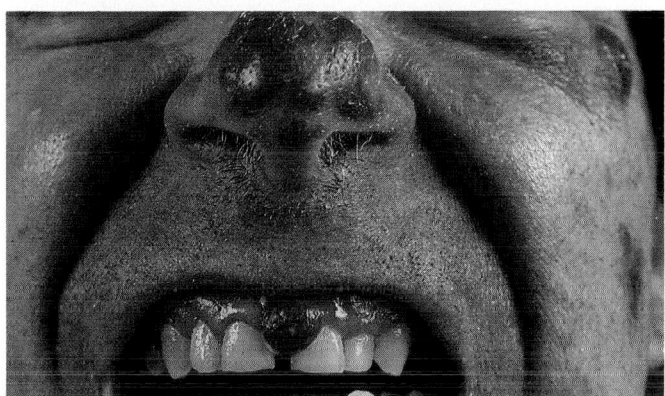

Figure 2–101. Epidemic Kaposi's sarcoma. Plaque and nodular stages.

A homosexual male with advanced stage disease with widely disseminated deep purple plaque and nodular tumor lesions of the skin and oral mucosa.

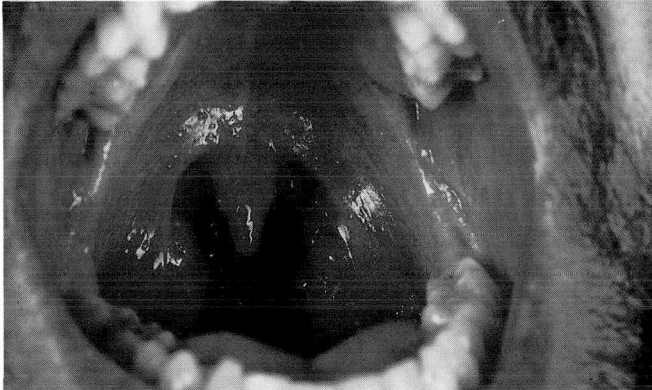

Figure 2–102. Epidemic Kaposi's sarcoma. Nodular stage.

Bilateral enlarged erythematous tonsils, found at tonsillectomy to be due to Kaposi's sarcoma. (Courtesy of N. Cohen, MD, New York University Medical Center.)

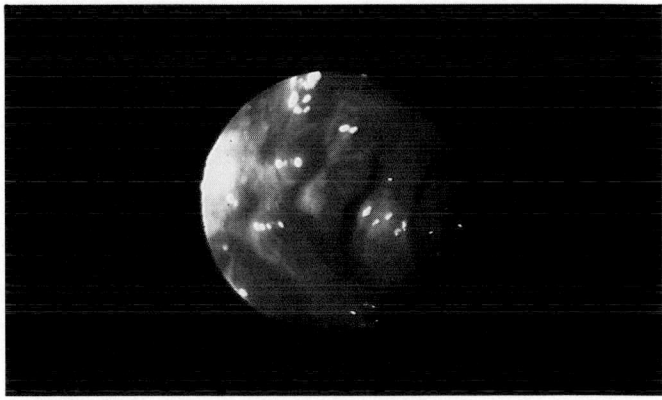

Figure 2–103. Epidemic Kaposi's sarcoma. Nodular stage.

Nodular lesions detected in the esophagus by endoscopy examination. At autopsy the patient was found to have numerous nodular lesions extending throughout the entire gastrointestinal tract. (Courtesy of L. Horowitz, MD, Department of Medicine, New York University Medical Center.)

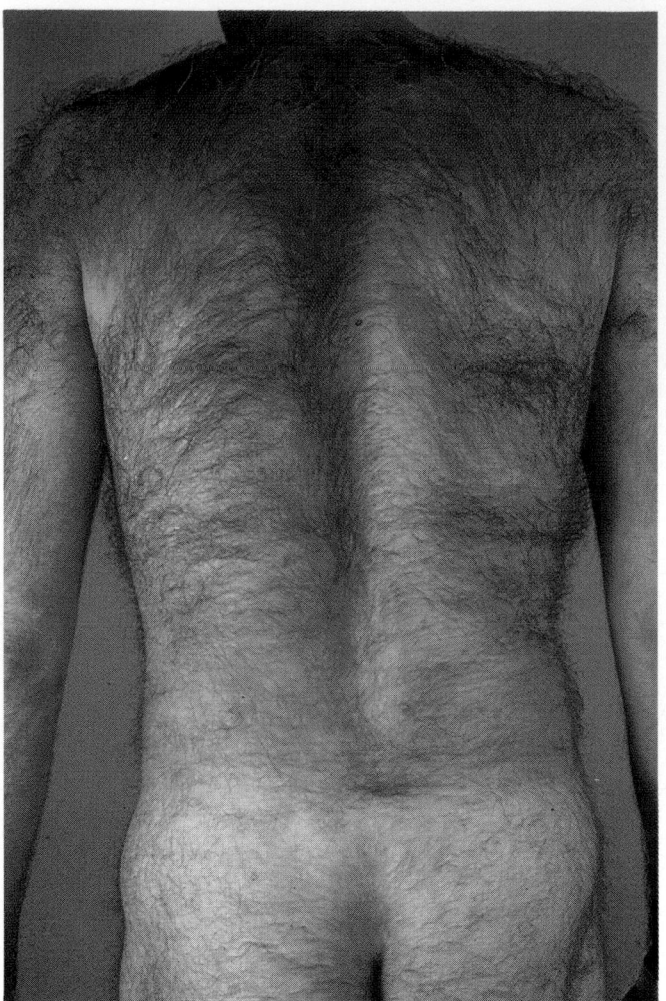

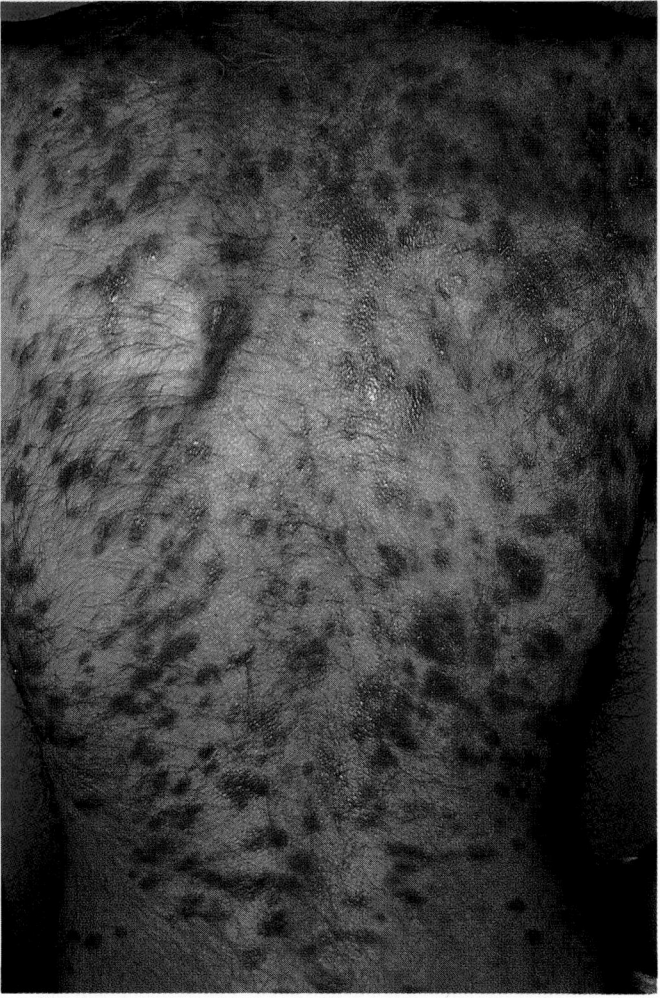

Figure 2–104. Epidemic Kaposi's sarcoma.

This photograph of the back of a 36 year old homosexual male who was one of the earliest AIDS patients seen at New York University Medical Center in early 1981 who presented with only a few macular lesions of Kaposi's sarcoma on his face and oral mucosa. There were no lesions on his back at that time.

Figure 2–105. Epidemic Kaposi's sarcoma. Plaque-stage lesion.

A follow-up photograph of the back of the same patient seen in Figure 2–104, taken six months later, illustrates the rapid development of widely disseminated purple plaques of Kaposi's sarcoma over his skin.

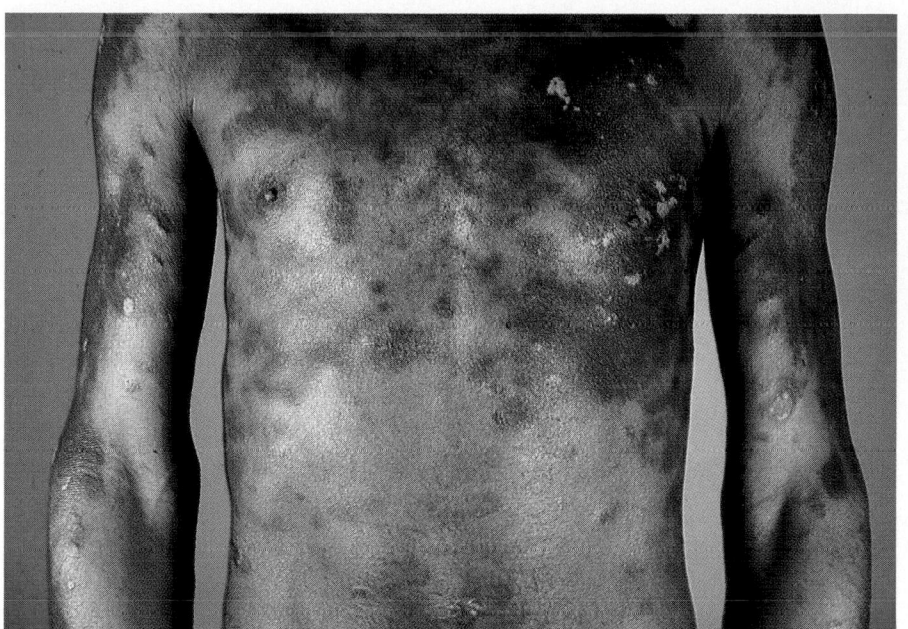

Figure 2–106. Epidemic Kaposi's sarcoma.

A 31 year old black male with extensive hyperpigmented confluent patch and plaque lesions of Kaposi's sarcoma on his trunk and upper extremities. Coincidentally, there are some hypopigmented areas representing long-standing vitiligo.

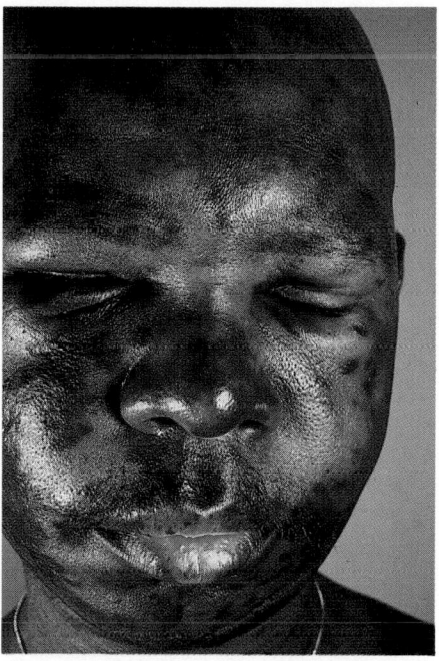

Figure 2–107. Epidemic Kaposi's sarcoma.

This photograph shows the face of the same patient seen in Figure 2–106. The large confluent lesions extended over his face and scalp were associated with marked facial edema, due to invasive lymphatic obstruction.

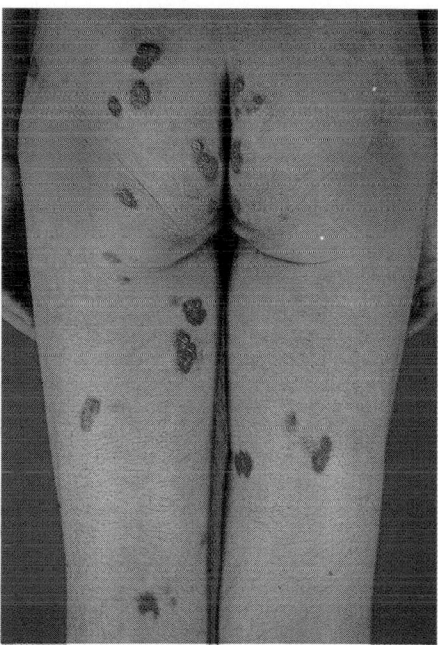

Figure 2–108. Epidemic Kaposi's sarcoma. Plaque stage.

A 24 year old homosexual male with Kaposi's sarcoma of two years' duration. The patient is markedly cachectic following multiple opportunistic infections. There are widespread hyperpigmented purple to brown-black plaques on the lower extremities and buttocks, some with superficial surface erosions.

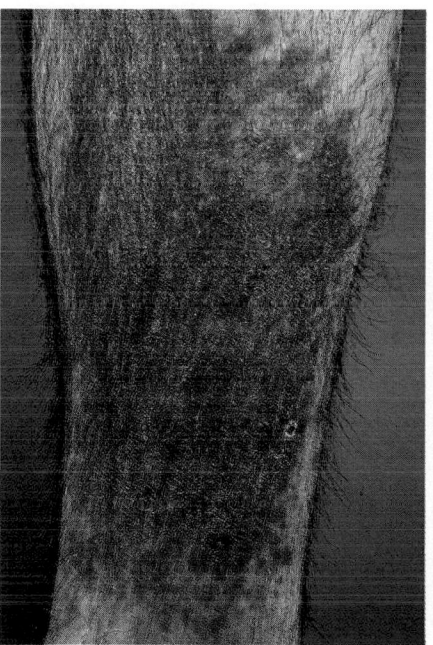

Figure 2–109. Epidemic Kaposi's sarcoma. Plaque stage.

A 37 year old homosexual male with Kaposi's sarcoma for two years. As his disease progressed, macular and plaque-stage lesions increased in both size and number, coalescing to form this large confluent deep purple tumor involving a large area of the pretibial region.

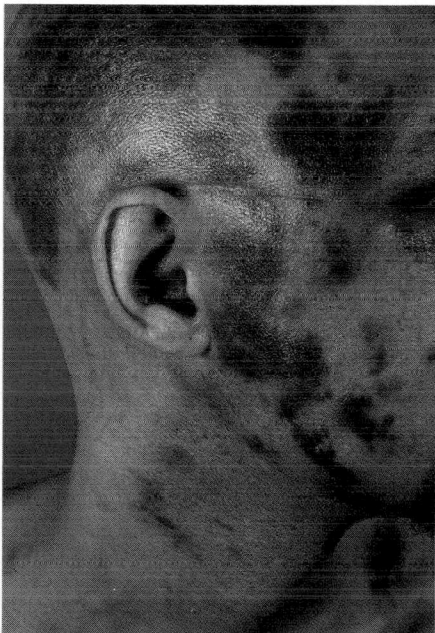

Figure 2–110. Epidemic Kaposi's sarcoma. Plaque stage.

Advanced disease with widespread, large deep purple to brown confluent plaque lesions of Kaposi's sarcoma on the head and neck in a 37 year old homosexual male.

AIDS-Associated Kaposi's Sarcoma in Africa

(Figures 2–111 to 2–117)

In 1983 the diagnoses of the first cases of AIDS in black Africans were confirmed.[57] These patients were young, sexually active, heterosexual men and women with severe chronic wasting illness, opportunistic infections, or Kaposi's sarcoma who were either recent immigrants to Belgium, or came from Africa to Belgium specifically for medical attention.[57] They were natives of equatorial African nations such as Zaire, Rwanda, Zambia, and Uganda. As of May 1988, 38 countries in Africa have reported 13% of the world's total AIDS cases.[58] Retrospective HIV seroepidemiologic studies of stored serum samples suggest that HIV infection already existed in Africa in the early 1970s, as compared to the United States, where the antibodies to HIV were not detected in stored sera specimens taken prior to 1978.[59]

The epidemiologic features and clinical manifestations of HIV infection and AIDS observed in Africa appear to differ from those seen in Europe and the United States.[60] HIV infection in Africa is believed to be primarily a heterosexually transmitted disease occurring with equal frequency among men and women. As the incidence of HIV infection among African women increases, so does the rate of perinatal transmission and the number of HIV-infected children. A manifestation of HIV infection seen more commonly in Africa is a wasting illness referred to as "slim disease," characterized by chronic diarrhea, fever, and weight loss. The frequencies of several of the opportunistic infections associated with AIDS in Africa appear to differ from those observed in the United States and Europe. Specifically, there is an increased incidence of severe, often disseminated, *Mycobacterium tuberculosis* infections in African AIDS victims and a lower incidence of reported cases of *Pneumocystis carinii* pneumonia, the most prevalent opportunistic infection seen among AIDS patients in the United States and Europe.

In addition to the endemic variety of Kaposi's sarcoma, AIDS-related Kaposi's sarcoma also occurs in Africa. Clinically, the AIDS-related Kaposi's sarcoma in Africa behaves differently from the previously recognized endemic varieties of African Kaposi's sarcoma seen in young adults. The AIDS-related Kaposi's sarcoma seen in Africa follows a fulminant disseminated course similar to epidemic Kaposi's sarcoma observed in Europe and the United States. It appears to be more virulent than the indolent nodular but less invasive than the locally aggressive endemic African forms of Kaposi's sarcoma. Although features of AIDS-related African Kaposi's sarcoma and the endemic lymphadenopathic variety are similar, the lymphadenopathic variety seen in infants has not, to date, been associated with HIV infection.[61] Epidemic, HIV-related African Kaposi's sarcoma frequently involves lymph nodes and visceral organs and is less responsive to palliative therapy than the endemic Kaposi's sarcoma. The epidemic form of AIDS-related Kaposi's sarcoma in Africa has been reported to occur with a male-to-female ratio of 17 to 5 in Zambia, and 3 to 1 in Uganda.[62] As in other parts of the world, most AIDS patients in Africa succumb to the multiple opportunis-

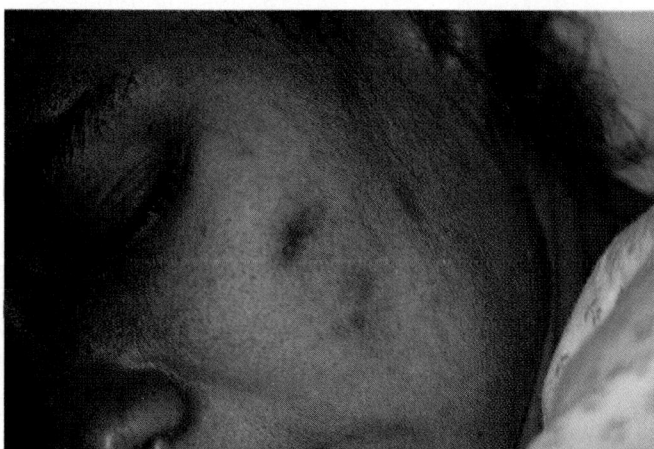

Figure 2–111. Epidemic Kaposi's sarcoma (Africa). Patch stage.

An HIV seropositive black woman from Zaire, who developed widely disseminated red to purple macular lesions of Kaposi's sarcoma on her skin. (Courtesy of N. Clumeck, MD, Brussels, Belgium.)

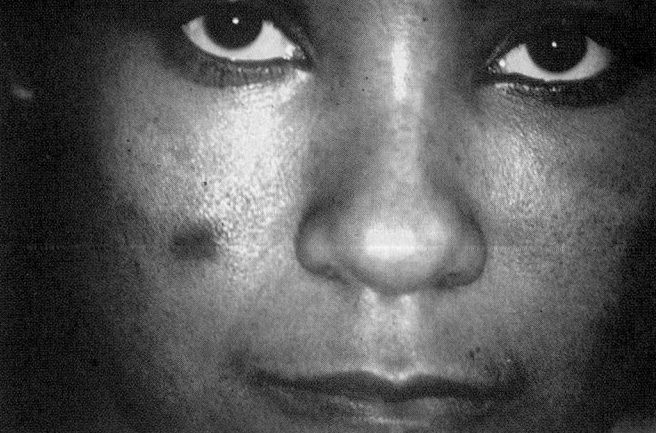

Figure 2–112. Epidemic Kaposi's sarcoma (Africa). Plaque stage.

The patient has a purple ovoid plaque of Kaposi's sarcoma on her left cheek. Other skin lesions were present, widely distributed over the rest of her body. (Courtesy of N. Clumeck, MD, Brussels, Belgium.)

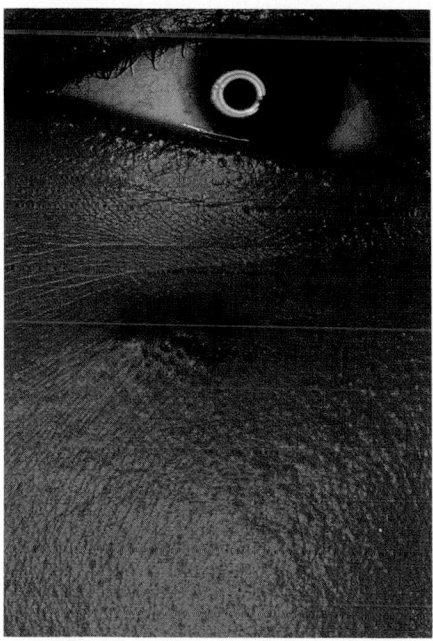

Figure 2–113. Epidemic Kaposi's sarcoma (Africa). Plaque stage.

A 27 year old black female from Zaire who sought medical attention in Brussels, Belgium, when she noted the development of asymptomatic purple to black nodules of Kaposi's sarcoma on her skin. The patient was found to have serum antibodies to HIV. Illustrated here is a lesion of Kaposi's sarcoma on her cheek, just below the eye. (Courtesy of N. Clumeck, MD, Brussels, Belgium.)

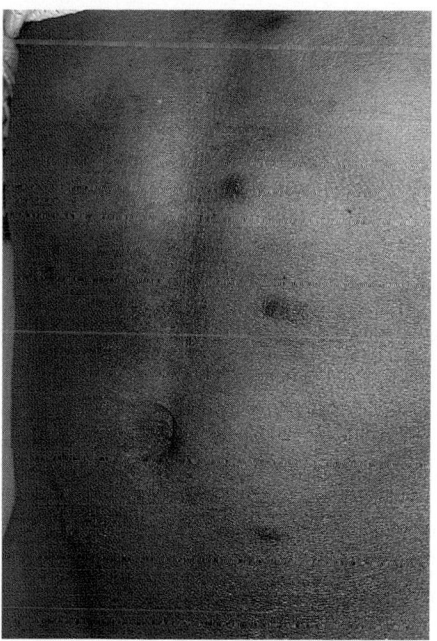

Figure 2–114. Epidemic Kaposi's sarcoma (Africa). Plaque and nodular stage.

Plaque and nodular lesions over the abdomen in this young black male from Zaire who was seropositive for HIV antibodies. There is considerable confusion between the incidence of the endemic form and of the epidemic AIDS-associated varieties of Kaposi's sarcoma seen in Africa. (Courtesy of N. Clumeck, MD, Brussels, Belgium.)

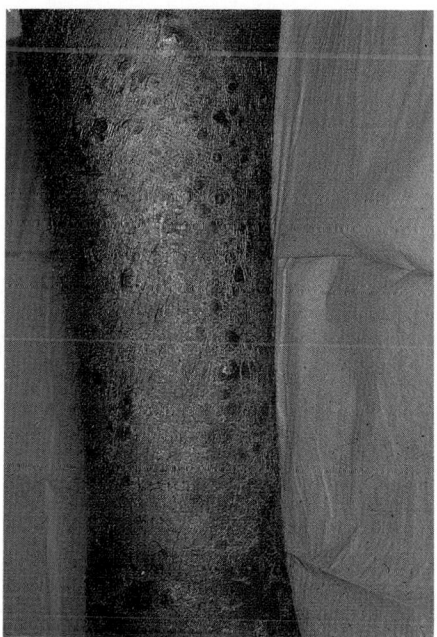

Figure 2–115. Epidemic Kaposi's sarcoma (Africa). Plaque stage.

A 37 year old black male from central Africa with AIDS-associated Kaposi's sarcoma rapidly developed multiple dark brown to black plaque-stage lesions which were widely disseminated over his body. During the fulminant course of his brief illness, he developed multiple opportunistic infections. (Courtesy of N. Clumeck, MD, Brussels, Belgium.)

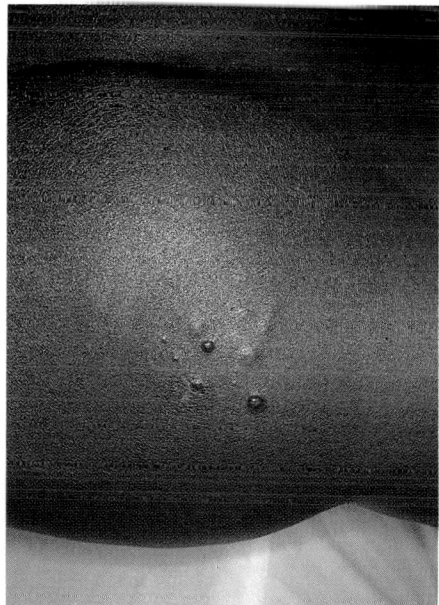

Figure 2–116. Epidemic Kaposi's sarcoma (Africa). Nodular stage.

A cluster of purplish-brown nodules on the side of the hip and buttock of this young black male from Zaire who was HIV antibody seropositive. (Courtesy of N. Clumeck, MD, Brussels, Belgium.)

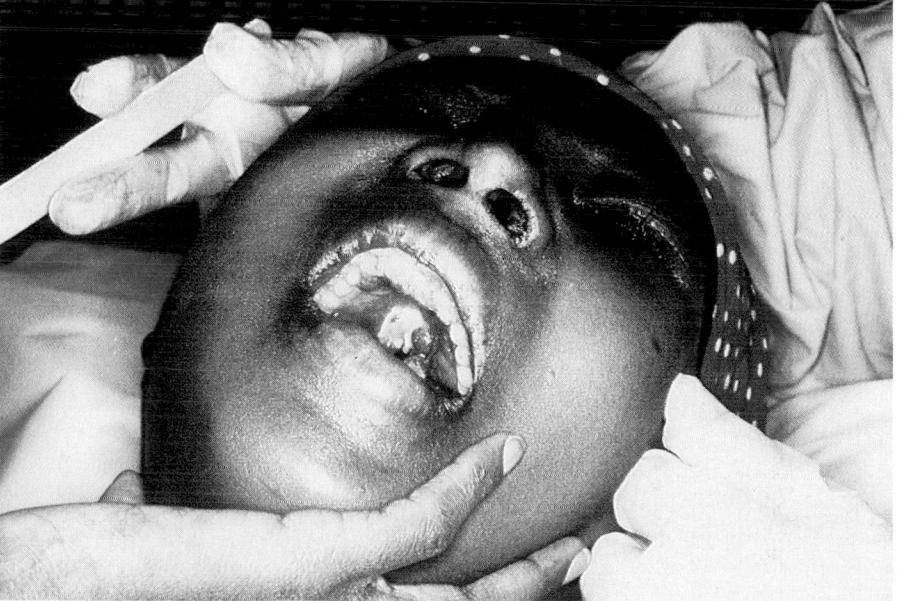

Figure 2–117. Epidemic Kaposi's sarcoma (Africa). Nodular stage.

A 36 year old black female with nodular tumors of Kaposi's sarcoma on the hard palate who had come from Zaire to Belgium for treatment. Other lesions were present on her skin as well. (Courtesy of N. Clumeck, MD, Brussels, Belgium.)

Table 2–1. Epidemiology of Kaposi's Sarcoma Variants

Type	Population at Risk	Age at Onset (Years)	Male:Female Ratio
Classical	Eastern European Jewish and Mediterranean backgrounds	50–80	10–15:1
Endemic African			
1. Benign nodular	Black African adults	25–40	17:1
2. Aggressive	"	"	"
3. Florid	"	"	"
4. Lymphadenopathic	Black African children	2–15 (Mean:3)	3:1
Iatrogenic immunosuppression	Patients on azathioprine, cyclosporine, and corticosteroids; renal transplant recipients; systemic lupus erythematosus; temporal arteritis	20–60 (Mean:42)	2.3:1
Epidemic AIDS-related	Homosexual men (95%), other risk groups (5%)	18–65 (Mean:37)	106:1

Table 2–2. Clinical Characteristics of Kaposi's Sarcoma Variants

Type	Predominant Mucocutaneous Lesions	Mucocutaneous Distribution	Lymph Node Involvement	Visceral Involvement	Behavior
Classical	Some patches, mostly plaques and nodules usually rounded	Usually confined to lower extremities; disseminated lesions; late in course of disease	Rare	Sometimes	Indolent—gradual increase in number of lesions often associated with lymphedema; visceral lesions occur late, often discovered at autopsy; survival—10 to 15 years
Endemic African					
1. Benign nodular	Papules and nodules	Multiple localized tumors, most commonly seen on lower extremities	Rare	Rare	Indolent, resembles classical type disease; survival—8 to 10 years
2. Aggressive	Large exophytic nodules and fungating tumor	Most often located on the extremities	Rare	Sometimes	Progressive development of multiple lesions with invasion and destruction of underlying subcutaneous tissues and bone; survival—5 to 8 years
3. Florid	Nodules	Widely disseminated	Sometimes	Sometimes	Rapidly progressive; locally aggressive and invasive, early visceral involvement; survival—3 to 5 years
4. Lymphadeno-pathic	Rarely manifests lesions	Minimal	Always	Frequent	Rapidly progressive; survival—2 to 3 years
Iatrogenic immunosuppression	Patches, plaques, and nodules	Usually localized to the extremities; rarely disseminated	Rare	Sometimes	Indolent; occasional tumor regression after immunosuppressive therapy is discontinued
Epidemic (HIV-associated)	Patches, plaques, nodules; often fusiform and irregular	Multifocal, widely disseminated, often symmetric; frequent oral lesions	Frequent	Frequent	Rapidly progressive; survival—2 months to 5 years (median: 18 months)

tic infections to which they are susceptible.

Understandably, there has been considerable confusion related to the overlap of the concurrent presence of AIDS-related Kaposi's sarcoma and the widespread endemic non-AIDS-related form of this tumor occurring simultaneously among black Africans. Seroepidemiologic studies performed in 1984 and 1985 in Zaire did not show any HIV serum antibody in patients with endemic Kaposi's sarcoma in that region.[63, 64] Furthermore, patients with the endemic African Kaposi's sarcoma were not found to be immunodeficient by standard laboratory parameters.[65] In another 1985 study of patients with Kaposi's sarcoma in Uganda and Zambia who were initially considered to have the endemic form of the neoplasm and were free of the other clinical manifestations of AIDS, 17 per cent were found to have serum antibodies to HIV.[62] Of those patients with Kaposi's sarcoma who eventually developed systemic symptoms commonly associated with AIDS, 90 per cent were found to be seropositive for antibodies to HIV.[62]

Because the identical histopathologic picture is observed in both the AIDS-associated and the endemic form of Kaposi's sarcoma, some of these African cases originally thought to represent the endemic disease have been reclassified as having the AIDS-associated form of the disease for the purposes of epidemiologic surveillance when the patients were found to have serum antibodies to HIV.[59] The increasing prevalence of HIV infection in Africa will further complicate efforts to distinguish the previously described endemic African forms of Kaposi's sarcoma from the HIV-infected black patients who may also develop this neoplasm.

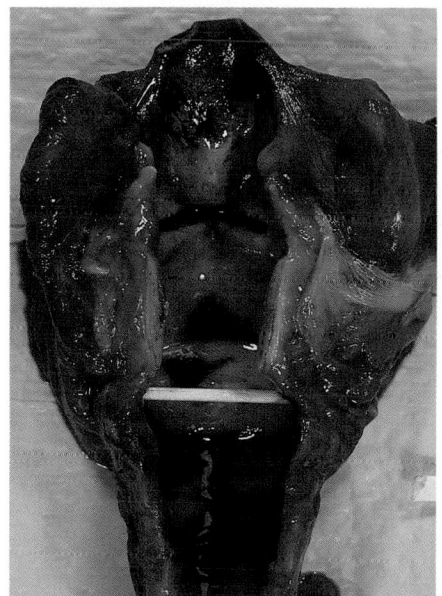

Figure 2–118. Autopsy, disseminated Kaposi's sarcoma.

A 47 year old homosexual male with disseminated Kaposi's sarcoma and a history of multiple, recurrent opportunistic infections. Autopsy revealed extensive cutaneous Kaposi's sarcoma and visceral organ involvement including tracheobronchial tree, liver, spleen, gastrointestinal tract, and lymph nodes. Multiple flat to slightly raised black hemorrhagic lesions of Kaposi's sarcoma were present in the supraglottic and infraglottic regions of the larynx and in the trachea. (Courtesy of Dr. John Li. Northcentral Bronx Hospital, New York.)

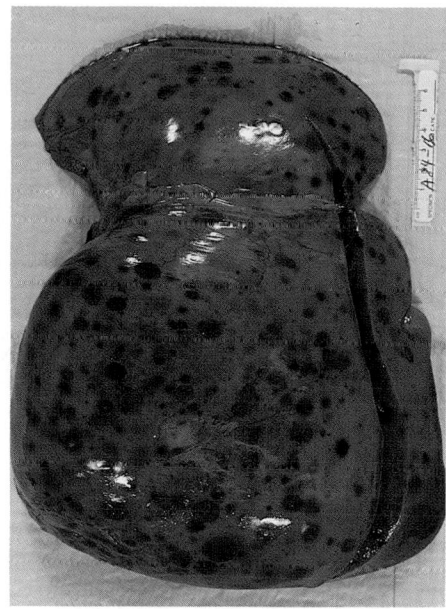

Figure 2–119. Autopsy, disseminated Kaposi's sarcoma.

Autopsy of patient in Figure 2–117 shows an external view of the liver revealing numerous flat red-purple areas of Kaposi's sarcoma in both lobes. (Courtesy of Dr. John Li. Northcentral Bronx Hospital, New York.)

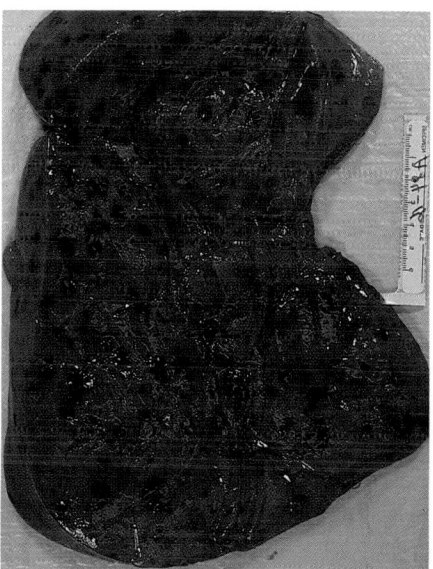

Figure 2–120. Autopsy, disseminated Kaposi's sarcoma.

Cut surface view of the liver of patient shown in Figure 2–117 shows the organ to be studded with hemorrhagic foci of Kaposi's sarcoma. (Courtesy of Dr. John Li. Northcentral Bronx Hospital, New York.)

Figure 2–121. Autopsy, disseminated Kaposi's sarcoma.

Cut surface of the spleen of patient in Figure 2–117 revealing multiple nodules of Kaposi's sarcoma. (Courtesy of Dr. John Li. Northcentral Bronx Hospital, New York.)

Etiology of Kaposi's Sarcoma

In considering the possible etiologies of Kaposi's sarcoma in patients with AIDS, a clear distinction must be made between (1) certain behavioral activities and particular cofactors which may be closely associated with infection with HIV and (2) those factors which may predispose to the development of Kaposi's sarcoma in an HIV-infected individual.[66] Practices such as engaging in sex with multiple partners and other specific sexual activities, such as anal receptive intercourse, have been associated with increased risk of HIV infection. Previous and perhaps repeated exposure to one or more infectious agents including syphilis and viruses such as cytomegalovirus, Epstein-Barr virus, herpes simplex virus, and hepatitis B may "prime" or activate the T-helper cells. Activation of T-helper lymphocytes, the primary target cell of HIV, may render them more susceptible to this infection.

Macrophages have recently been recognized to also be infected with HIV and may serve as a reservoir for HIV in the infected host.

The aforementioned observation that 95 per cent of AIDS-associated Kaposi's sarcoma occurs among homosexual or bisexual men led to the search for possible yet unidentified cofactors peculiar to the homosexual life-style which may predispose to the development of Kaposi's sarcoma in certain HIV-infected individuals. Hypothetically, such potential contributory factors related to epidemic Kaposi's sarcoma may play a role in the development of this neoplasm in other settings such as classical, endemic, or iatrogenic immunosuppression-related disease. Potential cofactors for the development of Kaposi's sarcoma in a sub-set of HIV-infected homosexual men which are under investigation include genetic predisposition; environmental factors; history of past or current infection with various bacteria, or viruses; and the use of recreational drugs. Of these, the associations with the genetic marker human leukocyte antigen (HLA)-DR5, past or current infection with cytomegalovirus, and the recreational use of inhaled volatile nitrites have received the most attention.[66]

The possible role of genetic factors in the development of Kaposi's sarcoma has been suggested by the increased prevalence of the classic form of Kaposi's sarcoma among men of Eastern European and Mediterranean backgrounds. The frequency of HLA-DR5 has been found to be greater in patients from these ethnic groups than in other Caucasians (64 per cent as compared to 23 per cent general background frequency).[9] An early immunogenetic study of AIDS patients with Kaposi's sarcoma seen at New York University Medical Center showed a relationship between the frequency of HLA-DR5 among AIDS patients and the development of Kaposi's sarcoma. Between 1980 and 1981, the frequency of HLA-DR5 was found to be 41.2 per cent, which was significantly higher in the patients with AIDS-associated Kaposi's sarcoma, as compared to the incidence of this allele in age- and sex-matched control subjects, which was 23 per cent.[9] This association was independent of ethnic background of the AIDS patients.[9, 67] However, as the size of the population increased, the association was no longer statistically significant. In 1982 and 1983 the frequency of the DR5 allele among AIDS patients with Kaposi's sarcoma was found to be decreased to 36 and 27 per cent, respectively, approaching the 23 per cent frequency that was seen in the control population.

Cytomegalovirus infection is well known to cause immunosuppression in humans and animals, and it has been postulated for many years to play an etiologic role in all forms of Kaposi's sarcoma.[68] Higher titers of serum antibodies to cytomegalovirus were found in patients with endemic African and classical Kaposi's sarcoma than in controls.[69] A high prevalence of serum antibodies to cytomegalovirus has been observed in two other groups of patients at risk for development of Kaposi's sarcoma—HIV-infected homosexual men and renal transplant recipients.[70] However, integrated cytomegalovirus DNA sequences were not identified in 11 of 13 biopsies of AIDS-related Kaposi's sarcoma tumors examined.[71] Furthermore, cytomegalovirus DNA was also not identified by DNA hybridization studies, electron microscopy, or immunohistologic studies in biopsy specimens from African individuals with endemic Kaposi's sarcoma, even though most of the individuals had serologic evidence of previous or concurrent cytomegalovirus infection.[66, 72]

Volatile nitrites (e.g., amyl nitrite, butyl nitrite) were reported to have been commonly used in the 1970s and early 1980s particularly by homosexual men as a recreational drug during sexual activity. Several epidemiologic studies indicated a possible association between the use of amyl nitrite and the development of Kaposi's sarcoma among homosexual men. The frequency and quantity of nitrite use has been directly correlated with the number of different sexual partners.[52, 73]

The etiology of Kaposi's sarcoma remains a mystery. It has been suggested that the uncontrolled abnormal endothelial hyperplasia that results in multifocal Kaposi's sarcoma tumors may possibly be due to an endogenous endothelial growth factor which may be produced in certain predisposed individuals who are immunosuppressed.[74] It has also been proposed that yet another undiscovered virus or perhaps the expression of an oncogene and the induction of an endogenous growth factor may be responsible for the multifocal uncontrolled abnormal endothelial cell proliferation that results in this disseminated opportunistic neoplasm in certain immunosuppressed hosts.[75]

In the 100 years following the initial description of Kaposi's sarcoma, the information that we have gathered about the tumor has brought with it many as yet unanswered questions. The initial observation that the tumors occurred more commonly in elderly men of Mediterranean and Eastern European Jewish origin suggested the importance of genetic factors. The recognition of an endemic variant of the tumor in Africa raised the issue of possible environmental or infectious cofactors. When in the 1960s the tumor was found to occur in immunocompromised patients, and later in 1981 when cases of AIDS-associated Kaposi's sarcoma were first reported, investigators sought to define the interrelationships between all these possible cofactors. The prevalence of this tumor in the immunocompromised host (especially the male homosexual in whom 95 per cent of all AIDS-associated Kaposi's sarcoma has been observed) suggests possible life-style–related, environmental, or infectious cofactors in its etiology. The fact that this endothelial tumor has a multifocal distribution with a predilection for the skin and especially lower extremities sets it apart from other neoplasms, and broaches the possible role of a unique pathogenic mechanism, perhaps one mediated by oncogene expression or by a specific growth factor.

Kaposi's sarcoma remains a medical curiosity over 100 years after its discovery. The epidemic occurrence of this tumor as the major neoplastic manifestation of AIDS provides us with a unique opportunity to study the roles of these possible cofactors in its development. It is our hope that the focused efforts of the medical and scientific community on this tumor and AIDS will lead us to a better understanding of the neoplastic process in general and possibly the development of new treatment modalities for this and other malignant tumors.

References

1. Kaposi M: Idiopathiches multiples pigment sarcom der Haut. Arch Dermatol Syphil 4:265–272, 1872.
2. Flotte TJ, Hatcher VA, Friedman-Kien AE: Factor VIII–related antigen in Kaposi's sarcoma of young homosexual men. Arch Dermatol 120:180–182, 1984.
3. Oettle AG: Geographical and racial differences in the frequency of Kaposi's sarcoma as evidence of environmental or genetic causes. Acta Unio Int Contra Carcum 18:330–363, 1962.
4. Davies JNP, Loethe F: Kaposi's sarcoma in African children. Acta Unio Int Contra Carcum 18:394–399, 1962.
5. Olweny CLM, Kaddumukasa AA, Atine I, et al: Childhood Kaposi's sarcoma: Clinical features and therapy. Br J Cancer 33:555–560, 1976.
6. Harwood AR, Osoba D, Hofstader SL, et al: Kaposi's sarcoma in recipients of renal transplants. Am J Med 67:759–765, 1979.
7. Penn I: Kaposi's sarcoma in organ transplant recipients. Transplantation 27:8–11, 1979.
8. Friedman-Kien AE, Laubenstein L, Marmor M, et al: Kaposi's sarcoma and Pneumocystis pneumonia among homosexual men–New York and California. MMWR 30:250–252, 1981.
9. Friedman-Kien AE: Disseminated Kaposi-like sarcoma syndrome in young homosexual men. J Am Acad Dermatol 5:468–470, 1981.
10. Gottlieb MS, Schroff R, Schanker HM, et al: Pneumocystic carinii pneumonia and mucosal candidiasis in previously healthy homosexual men: Evidence of a new acquired cellular immunodeficiency. N Engl J Med 305:1425, 1981.
11. Hymes K, Cheung T, Greene JB, et al: Kaposi's sarcoma in homosexual men. Lancet 2:598, 1981.
12. Centers for Disease Control Task Force on Kaposi's Sarcoma and Opportunistic Infections: Epidemiological aspects of the current outbreak of Kaposi's sarcoma and opportunistic infections. N Engl J Med 306:248–252, 1982.
13. Gottlieb GJ, Ackerman AB: Kaposi's sarcoma: An extensively disseminated form in young homosexual men. Hum Pathol 13:10, 1982.
14. Cox H, Helwig EB: Kaposi's sarcoma. Cancer 12:289–298, 1959.
15. Safai B, Good RA: Kaposi's sarcoma: A review and recent developments. CA 31:2–12, 1981.
16. Reynolds WA, Winkelmann RK, Soule EII: Kaposi's sarcoma: A clinicopathological study with particular reference to its relationship to the reticuloendothelial system. Medicine 44:419–433, 1965.
17. Safai B, Good RA: Kaposi's sarcoma: A review and recent developments. Cancer 31:2–12, 1981.
18. Rothman S: Remarks on sex, age, and racial distribution of Kaposi's sarcoma and on possible pathogenic factors. Acta Unio Int Contra Carcum 18:326–329, 1962.
19. Templeton AC: Kaposi's sarcoma. In Andrade R, Cumport SL, Popkin GL, et al (eds): Cancer of the Skin: Biology, Diagnosis, and Management. Philadelphia, W. B. Saunders Co., 1976.
20. Epstein E: Kaposi's sarcoma and parapsoriasis en plaque in brothers. JAMA 219:1477–1478, 1972.
21. Krigel RL, Friedman-Kien AE: Kaposi's sarcoma in AIDS. In DeVita VT Jr, Hellman S, Rosenberg SA (eds): AIDS: Etiology, Diagnosis, Treatment and Prevention. Philadelphia, J. B. Lippincott Company, 1985, pp 185–211.
22. Rothman S: Some clinical aspects of Kaposi's sarcoma in the European and North American population. Acta Unio Int Contra Carcum 18:364–371, 1962.
23. Horowitz L, Stern JO, Segarra S: Gastrointestinal manifestations of Kaposi's sarcoma and AIDS. In Friedman-Kien AE, Laubenstein LJ (eds): AIDS: The Epidemic of Kaposi's Sarcoma and Opportunistic Infections. New York, Masson Publishing USA, 1984.
24. Friedman-Kien AE, Ostreicher R: Overview of classical and epidemic Kaposi's sarcoma. In Friedman-Kien AE, Laubenstein LJ (eds): AIDS. The Epidemic of Kaposi's Sarcoma and Opportunistic Infections. New York, Masson Publishing USA, 1984, pp 23–34.
25. Safai B, Mike V, Giraldo G, et al: Association of Kaposi's sarcoma with secondary primary malignancies. Possible etiopathogenic implications. Cancer 45:1472–1479, 1980.
26. Friedman-Kien AE, Laubenstein L, Rubinstein P, et al: Disseminated Kaposi's sarcoma in homosexual men. Ann Intern Med 96(I):693–700, 1982.
27. Muggia FM: Treatment of classical Kaposi's sarcoma: A new look. In Friedman-Kien AE, Laubenstein LJ (eds): AIDS: The Epidemic of Kaposi's Sarcoma and Opportunistic Infections. New York, Masson Publishing USA, 1984, p 57.
28. Loethe F, Murray JF: Kaposi's sarcoma: Autopsy findings in the African. Acta Unio Int Contra Carcum 18:429–451, 1962.

29. Olweny CLM: Epidemiology and clinical features of Kaposi's sarcoma in tropical Africa. *In* Friedman-Kien AE, Laubenstein LJ (eds): AIDS: The Epidemic of Kaposi's Sarcoma and Opportunistic Infections. New York, Masson Publishing USA, 1984, pp 35–40.

30. Taylor JF, Templeton AC, Vogel CL, et al: Kaposi's sarcoma in Uganda: A clinicopathological study. Int J Cancer 8:122, 1971.

31. Simpson DM, Snider WD, Nielsen S, et al: Neurologic complications of acquired immune deficiency syndrome: Analysis of 50 patients. *In* Friedman-Kien AE, Laubenstein LJ (eds): AIDS: The Epidemic of Kaposi's Sarcoma and Opportunistic Infections. New York, Masson Publishing USA, 1984, pp 213–234.

32. Hood AF, Farmer ER, Weiss RA: Kaposi's sarcoma. Johns Hopkins Med J 151:222–230, 1980.

33. Slavin G, Cameron HM, Forbes C, et al: Kaposi's sarcoma in east African children: A report of 51 cases. J Pathol 100:187, 1970.

34. Klepp O, Dahl O, Stenwig JT: Association of Kaposi's sarcoma and prior immunosuppressive therapy. Cancer 42:2626–2630, 1978.

35. Gange RW, Wilson-Jones E: Kaposi's sarcoma and immunosuppresive therapy: An appraisal. Clin Exp Dermatol 3:135, 1978.

36. Kapadia SB, Krause JR: Kaposi's sarcoma after long-term alkylating agent therapy for multiple myeloma. South Med J 70:1011–1013, 1977

37. Klein MB, Pereira FA, Kantor I: Kaposi's sarcoma complicating systemic lupus erythematosus treated with immunosuppression. Arch Dermatol 110:602, 1974.

38. Leung F, Fam AG, Osoba D: Kaposi's sarcoma complicating corticosteroid therapy for temporal arthritis. Am J Med 71:320–322, 1981.

39. Myers BD, Kessler E, Levi D, et al: Kaposi's sarcoma in kidney transplant recipients. Arch Intern Med 133:307–311, 1974.

40. Gatti RA, Good RA: Occurrence of malignancy in immunodeficiency diseases: A literature review. Cancer 28:89, 1971.

41. Centers for Disease Control: *Pneumocystis* pneumonia. Los Angeles. MMWR 30:250–252, 1981.

42. Centers for Disease Control: Follow-up on Kaposi's sarcoma and *Pneumocystis* pneumonia. MMWR 30:409, 1981.

43. Mildvan D, Mathur U, Enlow R, et al: Persistent generalized lymphadenopathy among homosexual males. MMWR 31:249–251, 1982.

44. Metroka CE: Generalized lymphadenopathy in homosexual men. *In* Friedman-Kien AE, Laubenstein LJ (eds): AIDS: The Epidemic of Kaposi's Sarcoma and Opportunistic Infections. New York, Masson Publishing USA, 1984, pp 73–79.

45. Friedman-Kien AE, Greene J: Acquired immune deficiency syndrome. *In* Petersdorf RG, Adams RD, Brouswald E, Isselbacher KJ, Marttin JB, Wilson JD (eds): Harrison's Principles of Internal Medicine Update, IV. New York, McGraw-Hill Book Co., 1984.

46. Navia BA, Jordan BD, Price RW: The AIDS dementia complex: I. Clinical features. Ann Neurol 19:517–524, 1986.

47. Chachoua A, Krigel RL, Friedman-Kien AE, Lafleur F, Ostreicher R, Speer M, Laubenstein LJ, Wernz J, Rubinstein P, Zang E: Prognostic factors and staging classification of patients with epidemic Kaposi's sarcoma (in preparation).

48. Hatcher V: Mucocutaneous infections in acquired immune deficiency syndrome. *In* Friedman-Kien AE, Laubenstein LJ (eds): AIDS: The Epidemic of Kaposi's Sarcoma and Opportunistic Infections. New York, Masson Publishing USA, 1984, pp 245–252.

49. Greenspan D, Greenspan JS, Conant MA, et al: Oral "hairy" leukoplakia in male homosexuals: Evidence of association with papillomavirus and herpes group virus. Lancet 2:831–836, 1984.

50. Greenspan JS, Greenspan D, Lennette ET, et al: Replication of Epstein-Barr virus within the epithelial cells of oral "hairy" leukoplakia, an AIDS-associated lesion. N Engl J Med 313:1564–1571, 1985.

51. Morgan M, CDC, AIDS Branch, Division of Biostatistics, 1987. Personal communication.

52. Haverkos HW: Kaposi's sarcoma and nitrite inhalants. Adv Biochem Ther 1988 (in press).

53. Haverkos HW, Drotman DP, Morgan M: Prevalence of Kaposi's sarcoma among patients with AIDs. N Engl J Med 312:1518, 1985.

54. Krown SE, Real FX, Cunningham-Rundles S, et al: Interferon in the treatment of Kaposi's sarcoma. Letter to the Editor. N Engl J Med 309:923, 1983.

55. Groopman JE, Gottlieb MS, Goodman J, et al: Recombinant alpha-2 interferon therapy for Kaposi's sarcoma associated with the acquired immune deficiency syndrome. Ann Intern Med 100:671, 1984.

56. Rios A, Mansell P, Dewell G, et al: The use of lymphoblastoid interferon in the treatment of acquired immunodeficiency syndrome related Kaposi's sarcoma (abstract). Proc Am Soc Clin Oncol 3:63, 1984.

57. Clumeck N, Sonnet J, Taelman H, et al: Acquired immunodeficiency syndrome in African patients. N Engl J Med 310:492, 1984.

58. Update: Acquired Immunodeficiency Syndrome (AIDS)-Worldwide. MMWR 37:286–295, 1988.

59. Piot P, Plummer FA, Rey M, et al: Retrospective seroepidemiology of AIDS virus infection in Nairobi populations. Conference on AIDS/SIDA, Paris, France, June 1986.

60. Clumeck N: Epidemiological correlation between African AIDS and AIDS in Europe. Infection 14(3):97–99, 1986.

61. Bayley AC: Aggressive Kaposi's sarcoma in Zambia, 1983. Lancet i:1318, 1984.

62. Bayley AC, Downing RG, et al: HTLV-III serology distinguishes atypical and endemic Kaposi's sarcoma in Africa. Lancet i:359–361, 1985.

63. Biggar RJ, Melbye M, Kestens L, et al: Kaposi's sarcoma in Zaire is not associated with HTLV-III infection. N Engl J Med 311:1051–1052, 1984.

64. Biggar RJ, Melbye M, Kestens L, De Feyter M, Saxinger C, Bodner AJ, Paluku L, Blattner WA, Gigase PL: The seropositivity of HTLV-III antibodies in a remote population of eastern Zaire. Br Med J 290:808–810, 1985.

65. Kestens L, Melbye M, Biggar RJ, Stevens WJ, Piot P, DeMuynck A, Taelman H, DeFeyter M, Paluku L, Gigase PL: Endemic African Kaposi's sarcoma is not associated with immunodeficiency. Int J Cancer 36:49–54, 1985.

66. Haverkos HW: Factors associated with the pathogenesis of AIDS. J Infect Dis 156:251–257, 1987.

67. Rubinstein P, Santiago RDC, Ostreicher R, Friedman-Kien AE: Immunogenetics and predisposition to Kaposi's sarcoma (EKS). *In* Gottlieb MS and Groopman JE (eds): Acquired Immune Deficiency Syndrome. New York, Alan R. Liss, Inc., 1984, pp 309–318.

68. Fenoglio CM, McDougall JK: The relationship of cytomegalovirus to Kaposi's sarcoma. *In* Friedman-Kien AE, Laubenstein LJ (eds): AIDS: The Epidemic of Kaposi's Sarcoma and Opportunistic Infections. New York, Masson Publishing USA, 1984, pp 329–336.

69. Giraldo G, Beth E, Coeur P, et al: Kaposi's sarcoma: A new model in the search for viruses associated with human malignancies. J Natl Cancer Inst 49:1495, 1972.

70. Drew WL, Mintz L, Miner RC, et al: Prevalence of cytomegalovirus infection in homosexual men. J Infect Dis 143:188–192, 1981.

71. Delli Bovi P, Donti E, Knowles DM II, Friedman-Kien AE, Luciw PA, Dina D, Dalla-Favera R, Basilico C: Presence of chromosomal abnormalities and lack of AIDS retrovirus DNA sequences in AIDs-associated Kaposi's sarcoma. Cancer Res 46:6333–6338, Dec. 1986.

72. Ambinder RF, Newman CL, Haywood GS, Biggar R, Gigase P, Quinn T, et al: Lack of cytomegalovirus in chronic African's Kaposi's Sarcoma. *In* Program of the International Conference on AIDS, Editions Scientifiques Elsevier, Paris, 1986.

73. Marmor M, Friedman-Kien AE, Zolla-Pazner S, et al: Kaposi's sarcoma in homosexual men: A seroepidemic case-control study. Ann Intern Med 100:809–815, June 1984.

74. Brooks JJ: Kaposi's sarcoma: A reversible hyperplasia. Lancet ii:1308, 1986.

75. Mortimer PP: Viral cause of Kaposi's sarcoma? Lancet i:280, 1987.

3

Clinical Simulators of the Lesions of Kaposi's Sarcoma

N. Patrick Hennessey
Alvin E. Friedman-Kien

The wide spectrum of clinical muco-cutaneous manifestations of Kaposi's sarcoma, especially as seen in association with the acquired immune deficiency syndrome (AIDS), can often mimic and may easily be mistaken for a number of totally unrelated dermatologic conditions.[1] The morphologic appearance of the lesion in patients with epidemic Kaposi's sarcoma is sometimes similar and often identical to the clinical appearance of lesions seen in patients with classical Kaposi's sarcoma.[2] The initial lesions in AIDS-related Kaposi's sarcoma may occur on the lower extremities, similar to the distribution most commonly observed in patients with the more indolent classical form of the disease, which is usually seen in older men between the fifth and the seventh decades of life. Since the recognition of the AIDS epidemic in the early 1980s, we have seen a few older male patients of homosexual or bisexual orientation, especially of Italian and Jewish extraction, who develop skin lesions of Kaposi's sarcoma. These cases can create a diagnostic dilemma for the clinician who may have problems in differentiating between the lesions of AIDS-related and classical forms of Kaposi's sarcoma, especially when they appear on the lower extremities in such individuals. A total evaluation of possible systemic disease and the patient's immunologic status may be helpful in making an accurate diagnosis.

The first chapter of this atlas emphasizes the high morphologic variability in lesions observed within the different clinical populations in whom Kaposi's sarcoma has been found, i.e., in patients with classical, endemic African, and epidemic AIDS-related Kaposi's sarcoma.

This chapter presents a variety of mucocutaneous lesions which are often seen as manifestations of totally unrelated conditions that can mimic and easily be confused with lesions of epidemic Kaposi's sarcoma and should be considered in the differential diagnosis of this devastating disease.

Vascular Simulators of Kaposi's Sarcoma
(Figures 3–1 to 3–12)

There are many dermatologic conditions characterized by lesions of a vascular nature that resemble the lesions of Kaposi's sarcoma. Vascular skin lesions in light-skinned individuals may be pink to red and sometimes have a purplish hue, whereas in darker-skinned individuals the same lesions tend to have a blue to deep brown color.

It is not surprising that the cutaneous lesions of purpura, due to intercellular extravasated red blood cells and the deposition of hemosiderin, are among the clinical simulators most often confused with epidemic Kaposi's sarcoma.[3] The subtle appearance of early pink lesions and the dark red and brown or purple patch-stage lesions of longer duration seen in the epidemic Kaposi's sarcoma can be mistaken easily for hemorrhagic phenomena such as petechiae or more extensive purpuric skin eruptions. In questionable cases, a tissue biopsy should be performed to provide the definitive histopathologic diagnosis when the clinical differentiation is uncertain. The occurrence of an idiopathic autoimmune-like thrombocytopenic purpura, a condition found to be associated with

AIDS, may further complicate the clinical distinction between purpuric skin lesions and those of epidemic Kaposi's sarcoma.[4] On rare occasions, idiopathic autoimmune-like thrombocytopenic purpura as well as Kaposi's sarcoma have been seen at different times during the course of the disease in a few patients with AIDS. Detailed assessment of the patient's platelet count and functional blood coagulation studies would confirm the diagnosis of idiopathic autoimmune-like thrombocytopenic purpura.

In addition to purpuric eruptions, there are a variety of other conditions, such as necrotizing vasculitis, which can resemble the lesions of epidemic Kaposi's sarcoma. Aside from a tissue biopsy, careful history and physical examination should elucidate the specific systemic manifestations associated with such a vascular disease and may help to establish the correct diagnosis.

The increasing awareness of the incidence of disseminated Kaposi's sarcoma associated with AIDS by both physicians and patients in "high-risk" groups has led to a heightened index of suspicion and more frequent misdiagnosis of some of the more common benign vascular lesions, such as angiomas and hemangiomas; these lesions can im-

itate some of the clinical lesions of Kaposi's sarcoma. The relatively common occurrence of multiple benign purple angiokeratomas (Fordyce spots) on the scrotum is an example of a benign vascular eruption that may resemble Kaposi's sarcoma. Other isolated, benign, vascular lesions such as a "venous lake" may be mistaken for Kaposi's sarcoma; the occurrence of a single skin or mucosal tumor lesion frequently has been observed to be the only presenting clinical manifestation of epidemic Kaposi's sarcoma.

The frequent incidence of multiple lesions occurring simultaneously or in tandem sequence at the same location or at multiple distant sites has been observed in patients with epidemic Kaposi's sarcoma. This observation may help to distinguish this AIDS-related neoplasm from other benign lesions of hemorrhagic or vasculitic origin. The duration of such lesions can be important in considering the clinical differential diagnosis. Most patients with one of the benign type of vascular lesions have usually been aware of their existence for a long time, and the size usually does not change. Lesions of erythema multiforme, hives, and urticaria pigmentosa may also on occasion be confused with epidemic Kaposi's sarcoma.

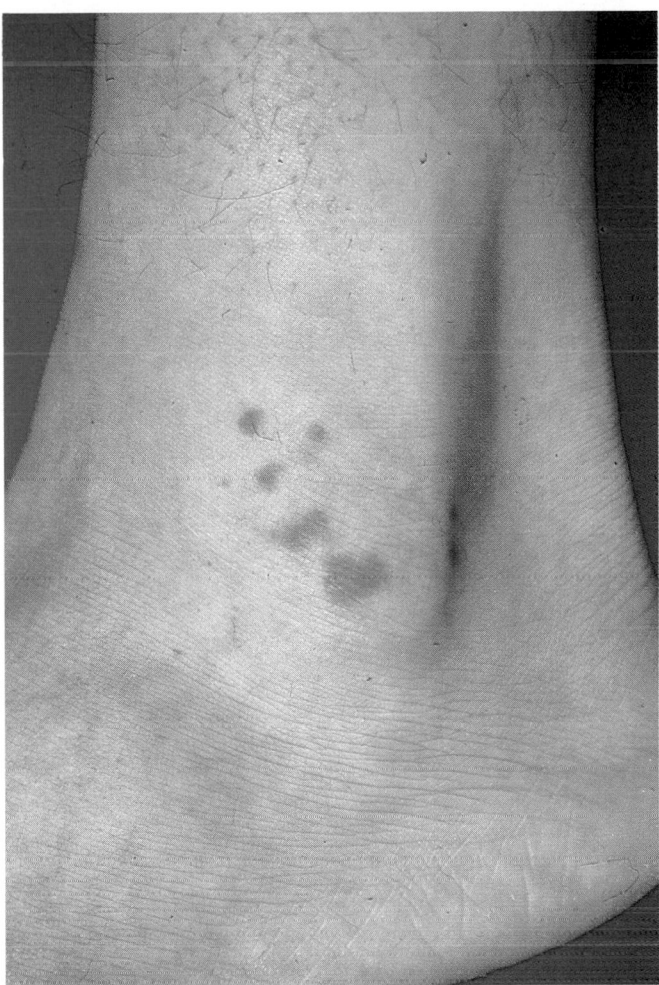

Figure 3–1. Multiple lesions of purpura.

The lesions on the skin of the ankle region mimic the morphologic appearance of Kaposi's sarcoma, and are located in an area in which lesions of both the epidemic and classical varieties of Kaposi's sarcoma are often seen.

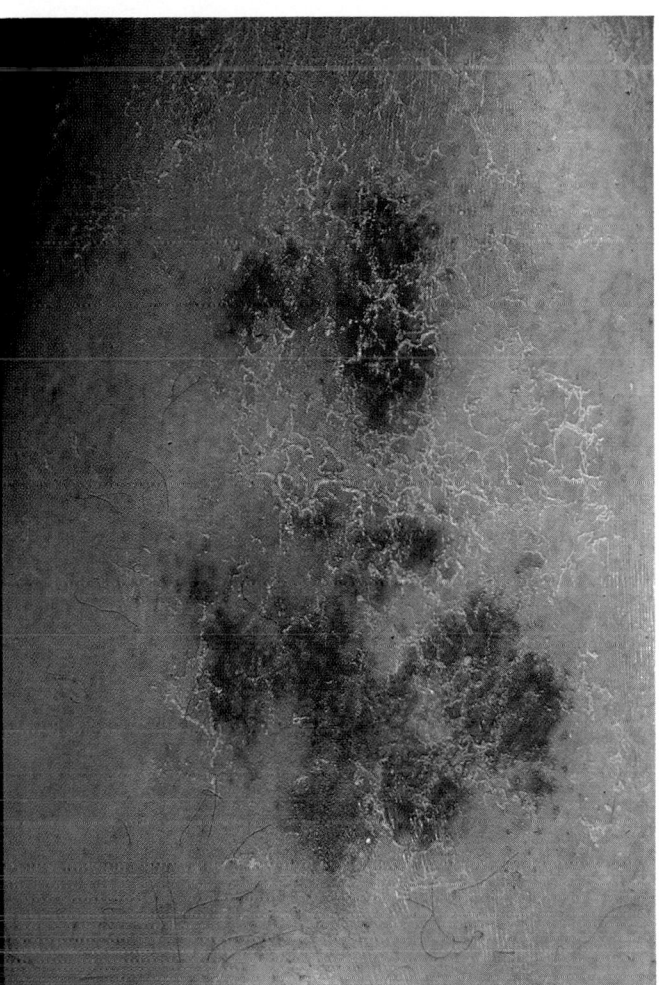

Figure 3–2. Older, hyperpigmented purpuric lesions.

A close-up view of a cluster of older, hyperpigmented purpuric lesions on the lower leg similar to lesions of epidemic Kaposi's sarcoma.

Figure 3–3. Faint erythematous patches of purpura.

These are similar to the early patch stage of epidemic Kaposi's sarcoma.

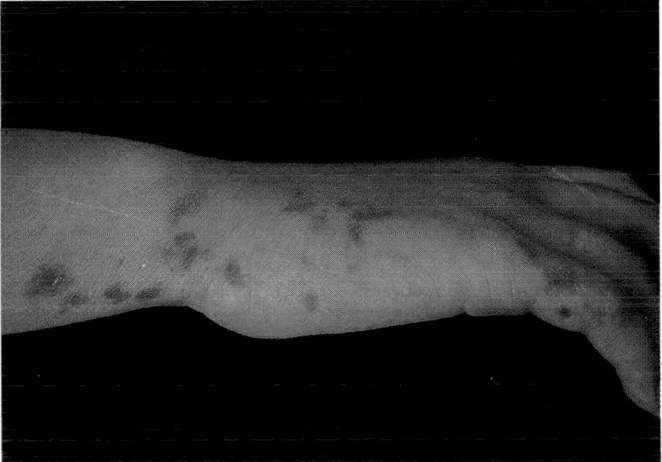

Figure 3–4. Multiple purpuric plaques.

The violaceous color of these lesions on the wrist is remarkably similar morphologically to the lesions of epidemic Kaposi's sarcoma.

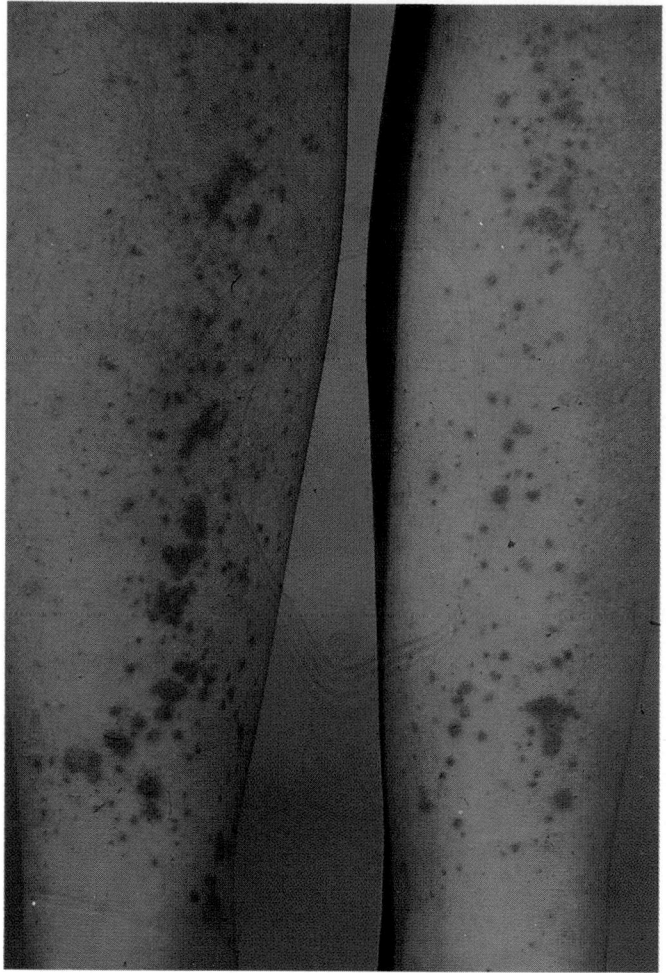

Figure 3–5. Pretibial lesions of purpura.

These lesions resemble lesions of both epidemic and classical Kaposi's sarcoma not only in location but also by the variations in the size of individual lesions.

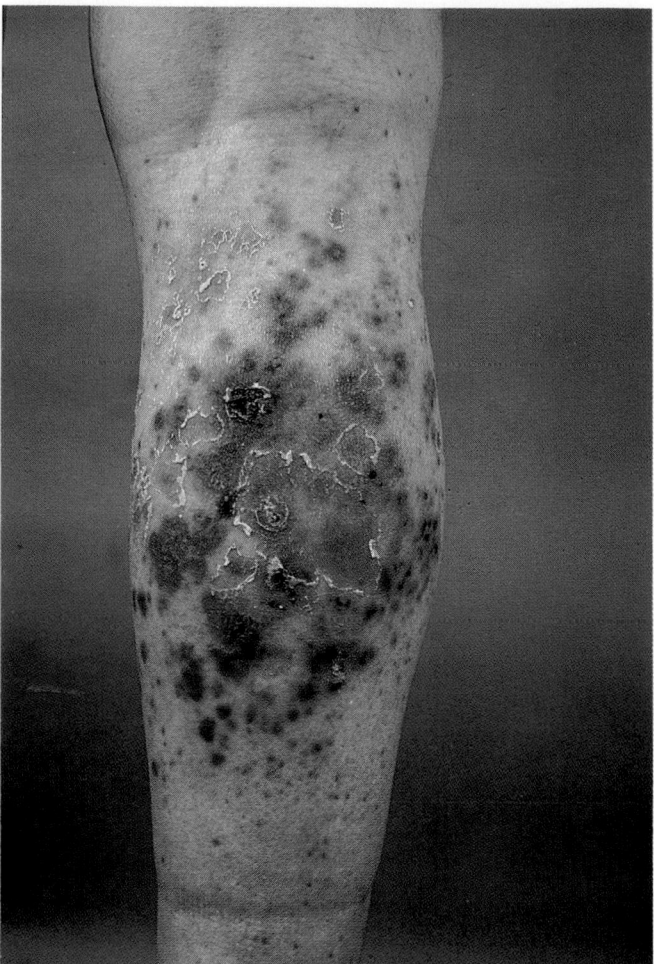

Figure 3–6. Necrotizing vasculitis.

This vasculitis involving the posterior calf of the leg is reminiscent of the extensive tissue involvement observed in some of the more advanced lesions of the classical and epidemic forms of Kaposi's sarcoma.

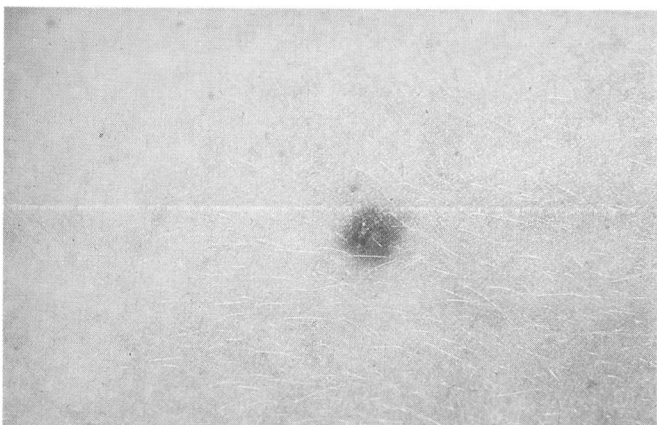

Figure 3–7. Solitary hemangioma.

The individual lesions of epidemic Kaposi's sarcoma can easily be confused with benign vascular lesions such as this solitary hemangioma. Note the patch and plaque morphologic appearance and the subtle variation in color.

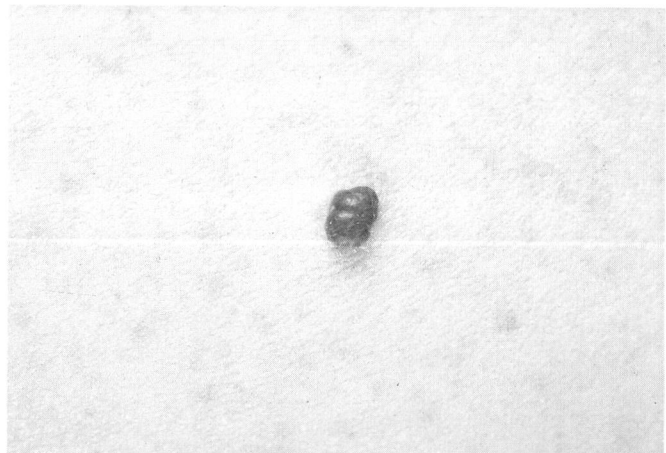

Figure 3–8. Solitary benign cutaneous hemangioma.

The nodular configuration and color of this solitary benign cutaneous hemangioma is reminiscent of some of the isolated nodules seen in epidemic Kaposi's sarcoma.

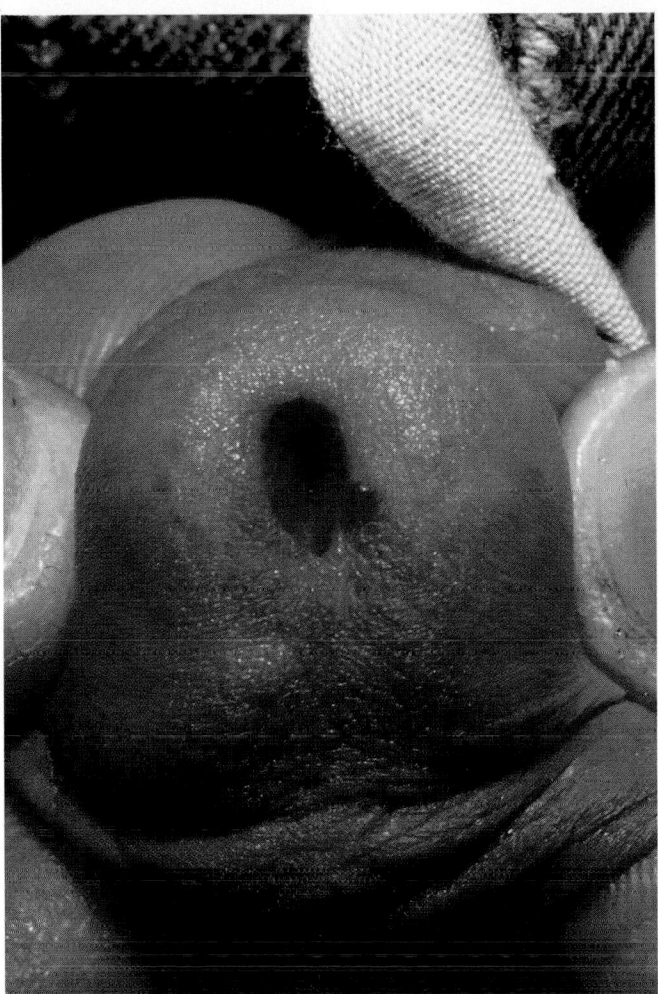

Figure 3–9. Hemangioma.

The sudden appearance of this purple nodule at the urethral meatus in a 30 year old homosexual male raised suspicion that he had epidemic Kaposi's sarcoma. Histologically, the lesion proved to be a hemangioma.

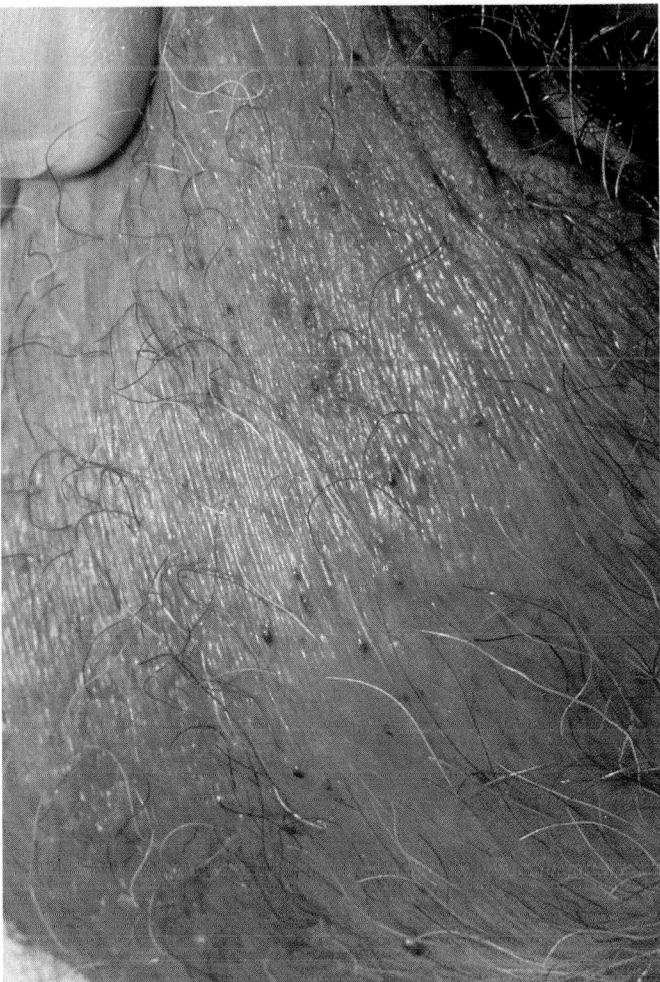

Figure 3–10. Multiple angiokeratomata.

Multiple, asymptomatic, purplish papules confined to the scrotum. Histologic examination revealed a diagnosis of multiple angiokeratomata.

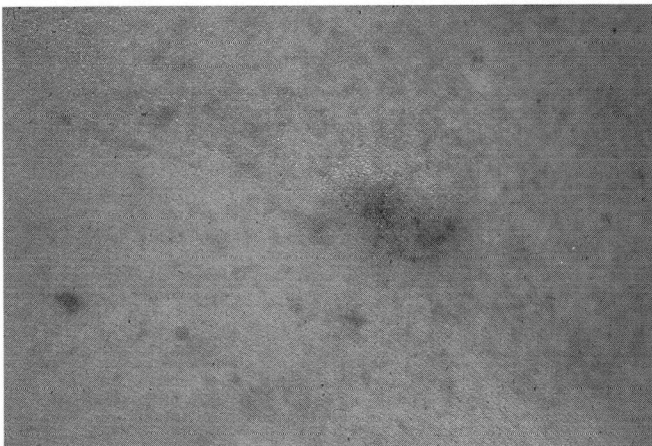

Figure 3–11. Hemangioma.

The violaceous color of this poorly defined faint hemangioma could be confused clinically with an early patch-stage lesion of epidemic Kaposi's sarcoma.

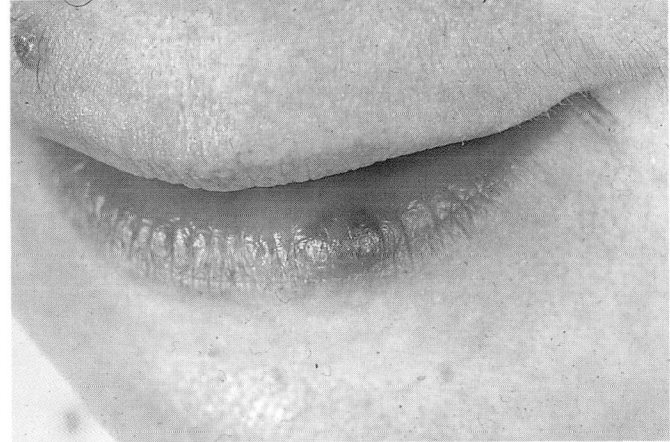

Figure 3–12. Venous lake.

This dark blue lesion on the lower lip represents a benign vascular lesion known as a venous lake, which could be mistaken for epidemic Kaposi's sarcoma.

Secondary Syphilis as a Simulator of Kaposi's Sarcoma
(Figures 3–13 to 3–19)

The chamelion-like mucocutaneous manifestations of secondary and tertiary syphilis have long been recognized by clinicians as eruptions that can mimic the lesions of a variety of other diseases. The morphologic features and distribution seen in syphilis lesions are often like those seen with disseminated Kaposi's sarcoma. Patch, plaques, and nodular lesions are commonly seen in both diseases and can sometimes be difficult to differentiate by clinical observation. One major consideration in the differential diagnosis between secondary syphilis and disseminated Kaposi's sarcoma is that syphilitic lesions will usually disappear, even without antibiotic therapy. Kaposi's sarcoma lesions persist and rarely, if ever, resolve spontaneously.

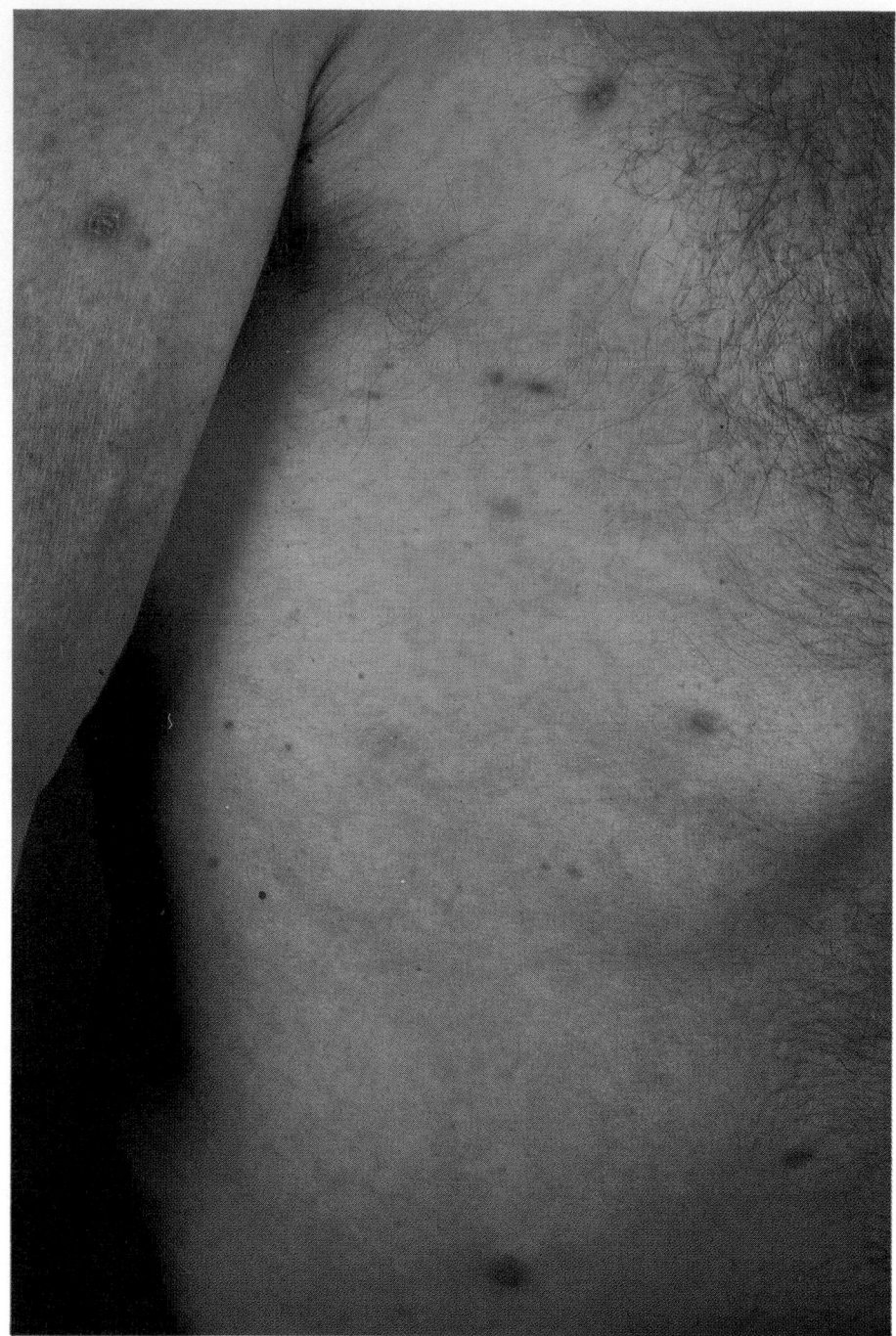

Figure 3–13. Secondary syphilis.

Multiple, discrete, asymptomatic reddish lesions were present in this patient with secondary syphilis. The color of the lesions and the symmetric distribution along the lines of Langer are similar to those often observed in pityriasis rosea and with epidemic Kaposi's sarcoma.

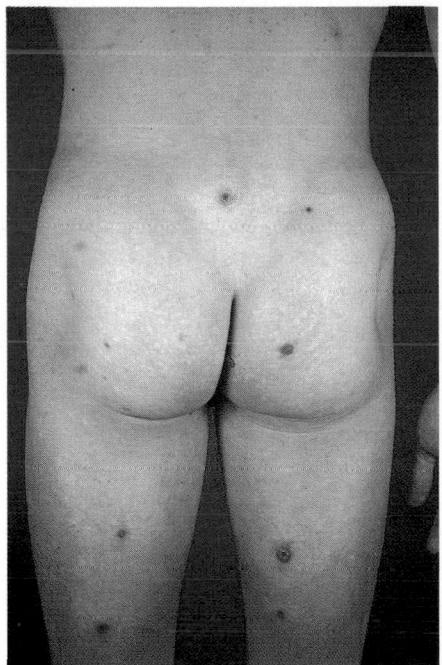

Figure 3–14. Secondary syphilis.

Another patient with secondary syphilis demonstrates a clinical similarity to the wide morphologic variation of skin lesions often seen with epidemic Kaposi's sarcoma.

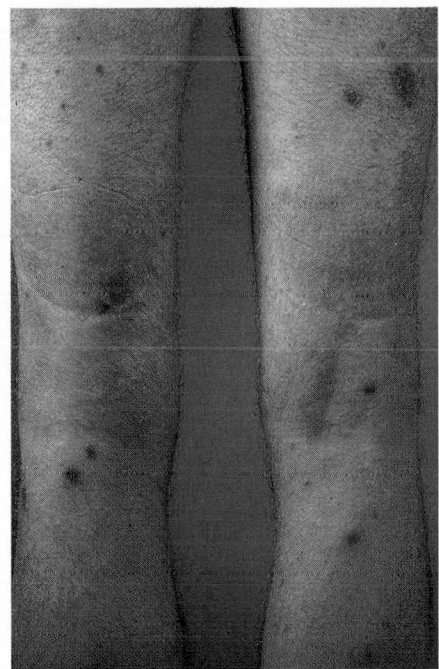

Figure 3–15. Skin lesions of secondary syphilis.

The plaque-like, brownish purple skin lesions of secondary syphilis seen in this patient made the clinical differentiation between secondary syphilis and epidemic Kaposi's sarcoma difficult.

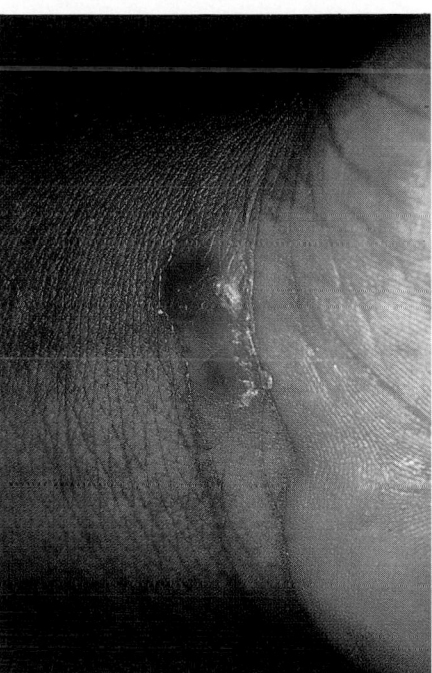

Figure 3–16. Secondary syphilis.

This black patient with secondary syphilis demonstrates the more pronounced morphologic appearance of syphilitic lesions frequently observed in dark-skinned individuals. Such lesions often resemble those of epidemic Kaposi's sarcoma.

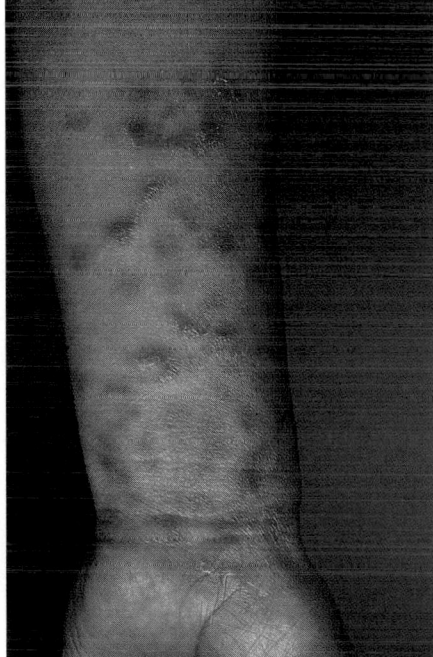

Figure 3–17. Patch and plaque lesions of secondary syphilis.

The patch and plaque lesions of secondary syphilis on this patient's forearm are comparable to some lesions seen with disseminated epidemic Kaposi's sarcoma.

Figure 3–18. Lesions of secondary syphilis.

These are frequently seen on the palms and soles of the feet. Lesions in this location are commonly observed in both the classical and epidemic varieties of Kaposi's sarcoma.

Figure 3–19. Condylomata lata.

These indurated bluish lesions of secondary syphilis located on the scrotum are known as condylomata lata and represent an uncommon genital manifestation of secondary syphilis, easily mistaken for epidemic Kaposi's sarcoma.

Inflammatory Lesions as Simulators of Kaposi's Sarcoma
(Figures 3–20 to 3–40)

Clinical differential diagnosis between Kaposi's sarcoma and various inflammatory lesions such as pityriasis rosea, granuloma annulare, and skin rashes associated with focal or systemic infections must often be considered by the clinician. Typically, inflammatory lesions may be numerous, and they may appear rapidly, often within a few days, and in some diseases, become generalized. The appearance of asymptomatic, multiple, erythematous skin patches and plaques developing over a relatively short period of time is characteristic of pityriasis rosea, which can imitate the disseminated form of epidemic Kaposi's sarcoma.[5] The tendency for pityriasis rosea to present

with lesions along the lines of skin cleavage (Langer's lines) is similar to that distribution frequently observed with widespread lesions of epidemic Kaposi's sarcoma.

Granuloma annulare is another example of an inflammatory condition that can mimic the lesions of epidemic Kaposi's sarcoma. Most inflammatory eruptions are, however, commonly associated with varying degrees of pruritus, unlike those of Kaposi's sarcoma, which are typically asymptomatic. The inflammatory papulosquamous skin eruptions characteristic of lichen planus can often be difficult to differentiate clinically from some of the lesions seen in epidemic Kaposi's sarcoma. Lichen planus may be manifest by variability in the numbers and locations of lesions, and they can often have a remarkably similar appearance to the plaque-stage lesions of Kaposi's sarcoma.

The differential diagnosis between various benign inflammatory skin diseases and the lesions of Kaposi's sarcoma can be difficult to differentiate, especially in dark-skinned individuals, because of a common tendency toward the development of postinflammatory, secondary hyperpigmentation of the lesions or the deposition of hemosiderin.[6] Such lesions may be confused with primarily pigmented lesions such as nevi or melanomas, for example. Other single inflammatory lesions that mimic epidemic Kaposi's sarcoma include prurigo nodularis and chronically inflamed insect bites.[7] Pyogenic granulomas and dermatofibromas are among the more common solitary inflammatory skin conditions that can also resemble the individual lesions of Kaposi's sarcoma.

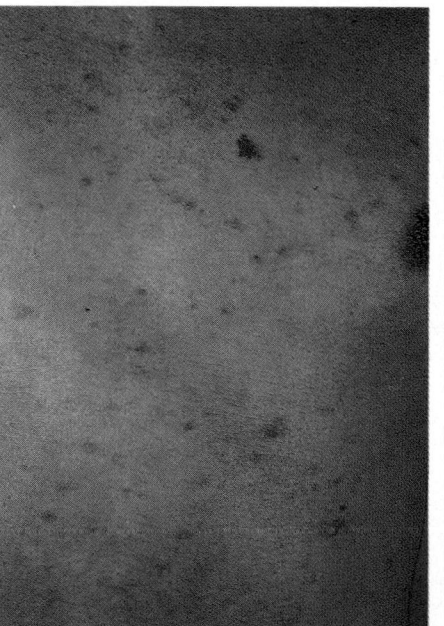

Figure 3–20. Pityriasis rosea.
These typical fawn-colored ovoid patches of pityriasis rosea located on the trunk in widespread symmetric distribution could be difficult to differentiate from disseminated lesions found in epidemic Kaposi's sarcoma.

Figure 3–21. Pityriasis rosea.
Similarities between the faint patches seen in early cases of epidemic Kaposi's sarcoma and pityriasis rosea.

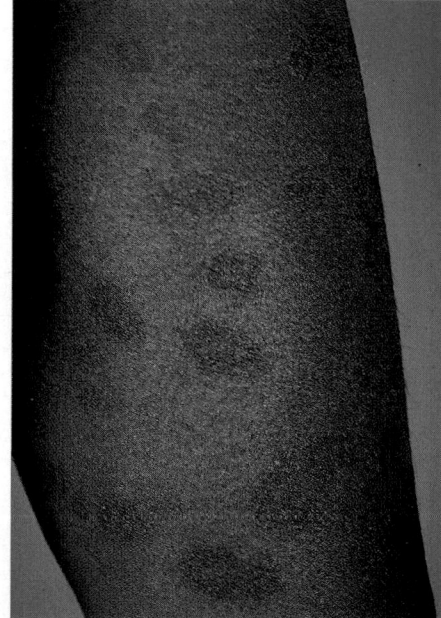

Figure 3–22. Dark lesions of pityriasis rosea.
The dark lesions of pityriasis rosea seen on the forearm of this black patient demonstrate the marked degree of hyperpigmentation that often occurs in dark-skinned individuals with this self-limited, benign skin disease. Such a clinical picture mimics the multifocal pattern of lesions seen with epidemic Kaposi's sarcoma.

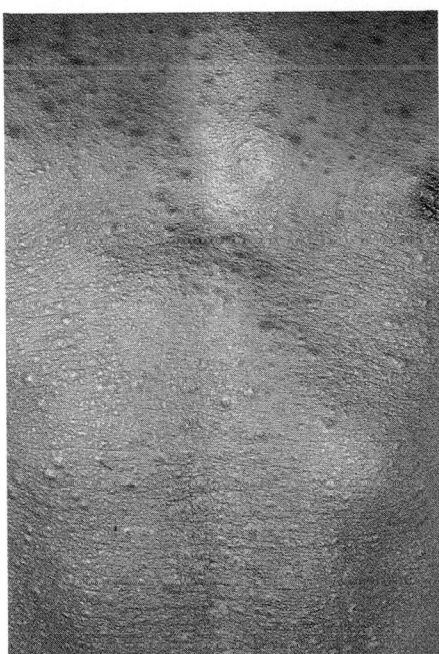

Figure 3–23. Pityriasis rosea.

The widespread symmetric and hyperpigmented skin eruptions characteristic of pityriasis rosea as seen on the torso of this black patient resemble disseminated epidemic Kaposi's sarcoma.

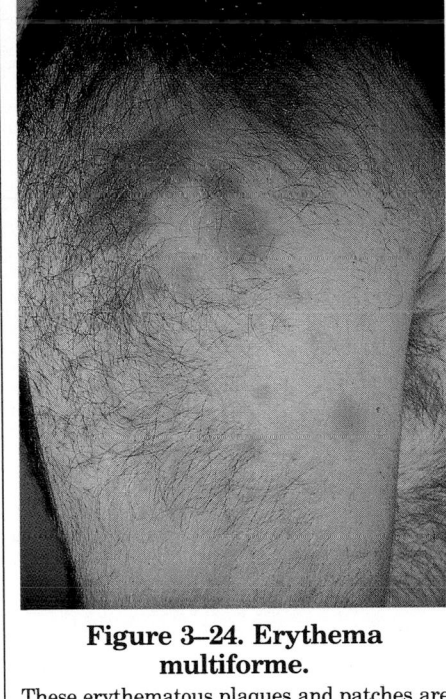

Figure 3–24. Erythema multiforme.

These erythematous plaques and patches are examples of erythema multiforme seen in the shoulder area and could be confused with AIDS-related Kaposi's sarcoma.

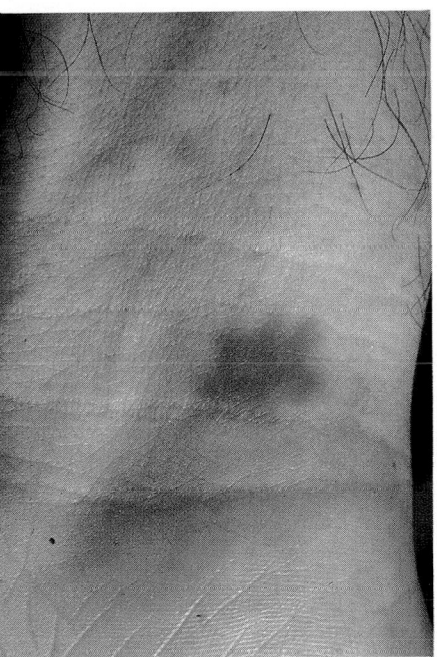

Figure 3–25. Granuloma annulare.

This asymptomatic plaque of granuloma annulare was one of several widespread lesions seen on the skin of this patient. The morphologic appearance and variegated color are strikingly similar to some of the lesions of epidemic Kaposi's sarcoma.

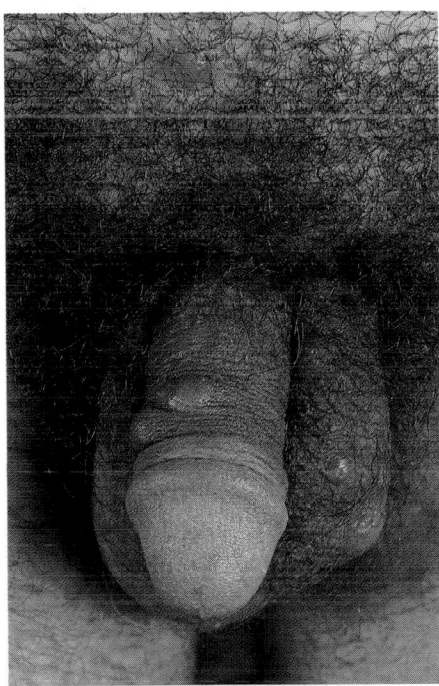

Figure 3–26. Host immune reaction to scabies.

These multiple nodular lesions resembling Kaposi's sarcoma seen in the genital region proved to be due to a marked host immune reaction due to chronic infestation with scabies.

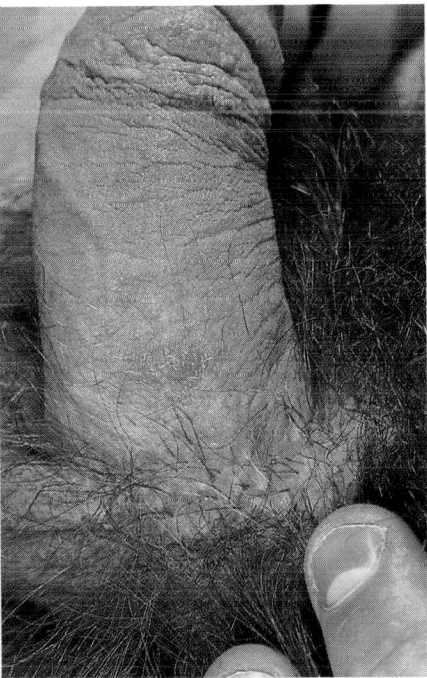

Figure 3–27. Scabies.

This pale pink patch lesion of the penile shaft was due to scabies. It is reminiscent of some of the early lesions seen in epidemic Kaposi's sarcoma.

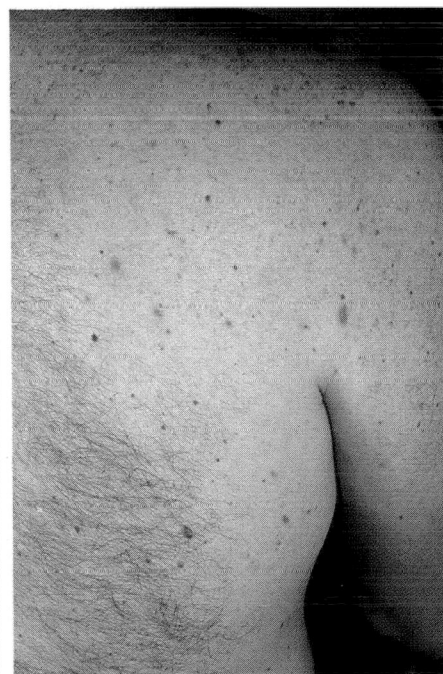

Figure 3–28. Urticaria pigmentosa.

These disseminated erythematous skin lesions proved to be urticaria pigmentosa by histologic examination. They look very much like Kaposi's sarcoma.

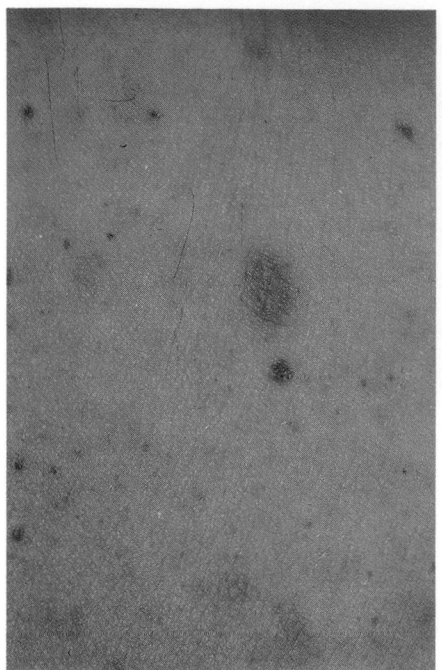

Figure 3–29. Urticaria pigmentosa.

This close-up view of urticaria pigmentosa emphasizes the clinical similarity to faint patch-stage lesions of epidemic Kaposi's sarcoma.

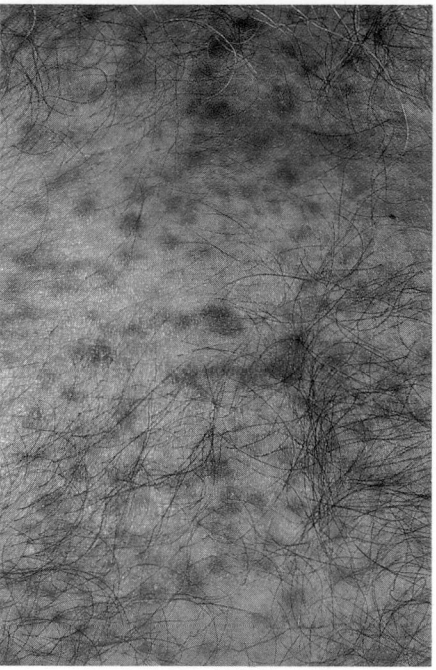

Figure 3–30. Urticaria pigmentosa.

This unusual disseminated case of generalized urticaria pigmentosa could resemble the widespread eruptions occasionally seen with advanced Kaposi's sarcoma associated with AIDS.

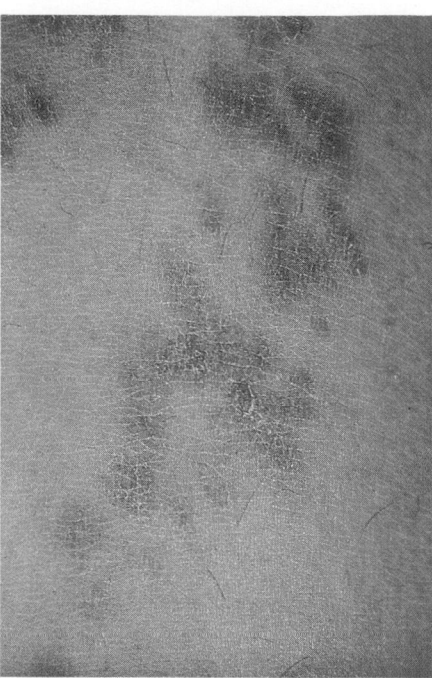

Figure 3–31. Lichen planus.

These violaceous to brownish skin plaque lesions represent lichen planus. They are reminiscent of some of the lesions seen in patients with either purpura or epidemic Kaposi's sarcoma.

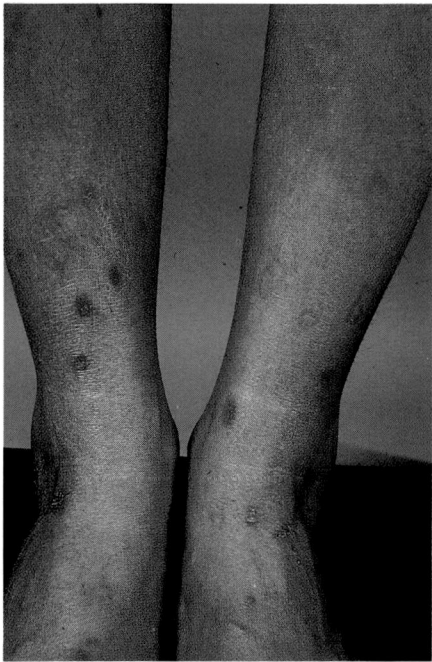

Figure 3–32. Lichen planus.

These multiple pigmented discrete lesions of lichen planus located on the lower legs are similar in appearance to the patches and plaques often observed with epidemic Kaposi's sarcoma.

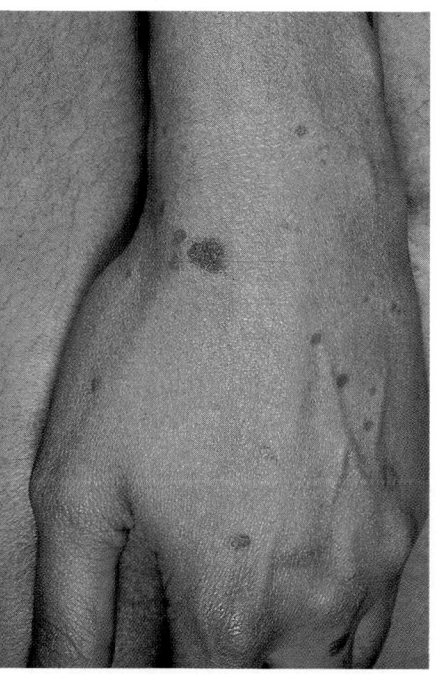

Figure 3–33. Lichen planus.

These are typically hyperpigmented polygonal flat papules of lichen planus seen in a dark-skinned individual. These lesions could easily be confused with those of epidemic Kaposi's sarcoma.

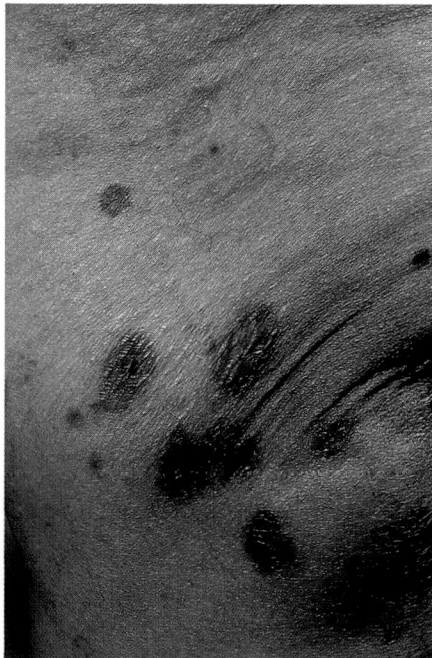

Figure 3–34. Lichen planus.

These deep brown plaque lesions represent an uncommon, long-standing hypertrophic variety of lichen planus, not unlike lesions seen in epidemic Kaposi's sarcoma.

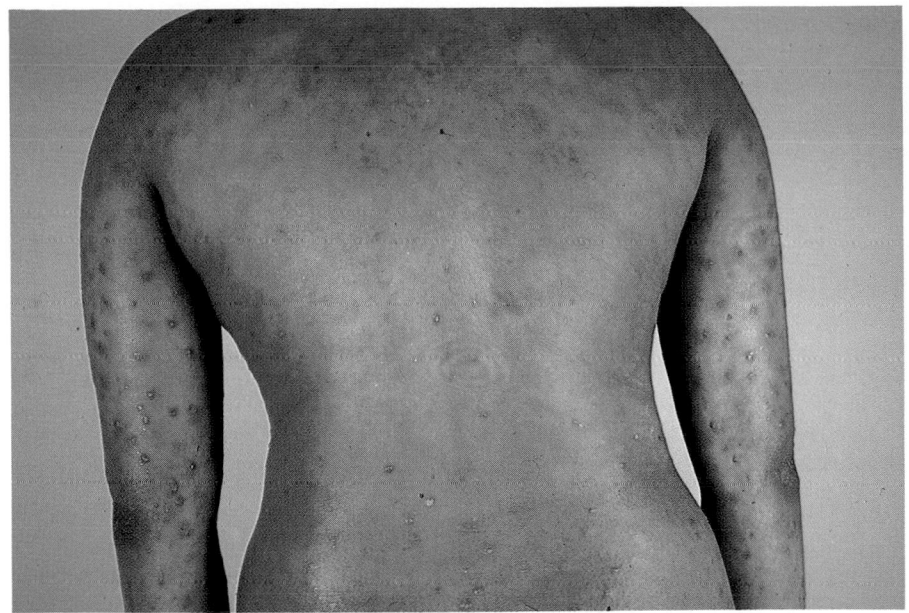

Figure 3–35. Prurigo nodularis.

Generalized lesions of prurigo nodularis can look very much like the disseminated late stage of epidemic Kaposi's sarcoma.

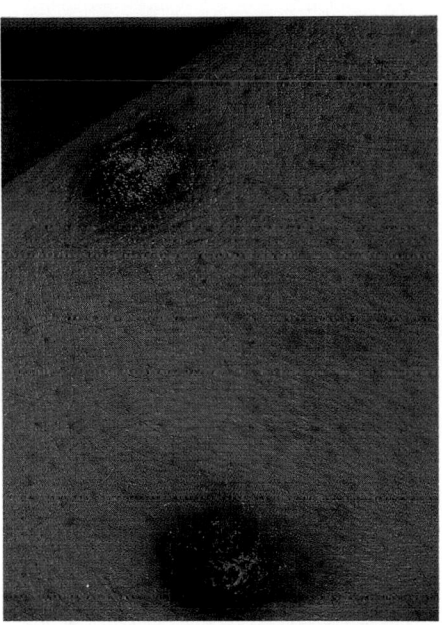

Figure 3–36. Chronic prurigo nodularis.

The dark nodular lesions seen in this patient's forearm represent the lesions of chronic prurigo nodularis, which could easily be mistaken for a nodular form of epidemic Kaposi's sarcoma.

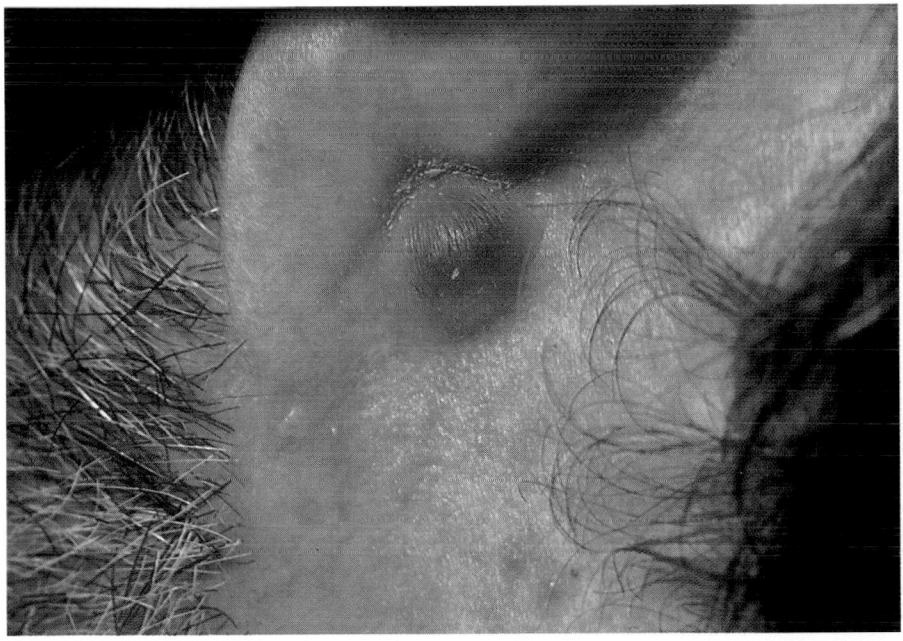

Figure 3–37. Granulomatous dermatitis.

This postauricular nodule represents a benign nodular granulomatous dermatitis. It is located in a site common to lesions of epidemic Kaposi's sarcoma.

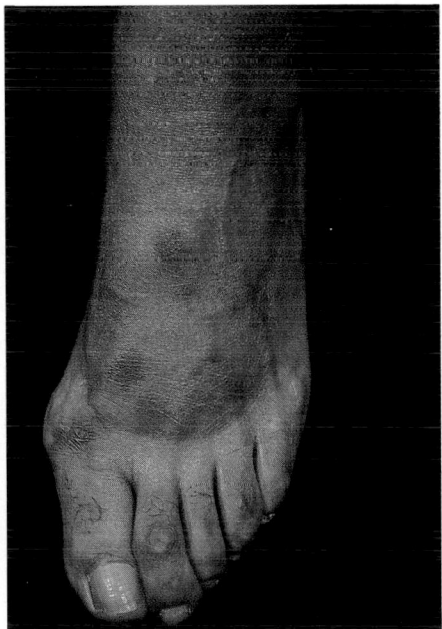

Figure 3–38. Postinflammatory hyperpigmentation.

The multiple dark plaques seen on the dorsum of the foot are a result of postinflammatory hyperpigmentation. Lesions of epidemic Kaposi's sarcoma often present a similar picture.

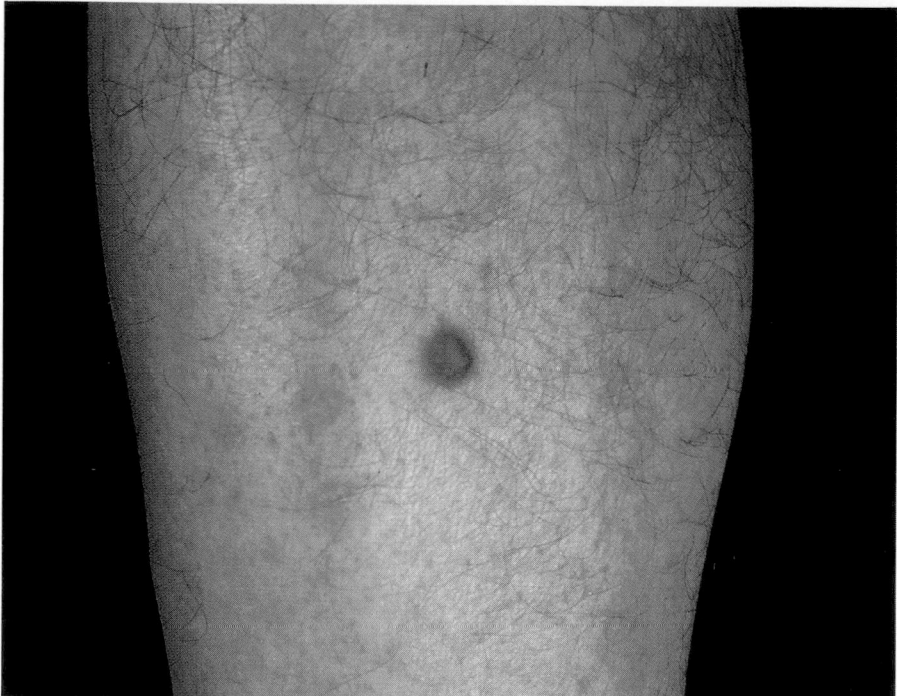

Figure 3–39. Dermatofibroma.

This benign red-brown nodule on the lower leg is a dermatofibroma. Such lesions are often confused with lesions of epidemic Kaposi's sarcoma.

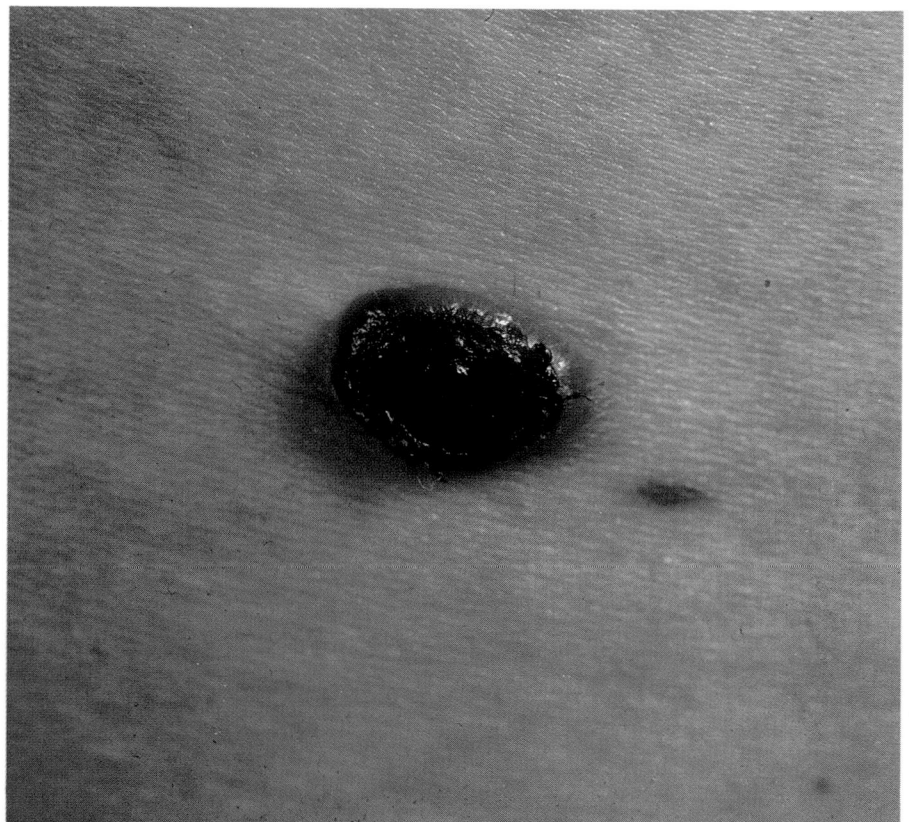

Figure 3–40. Pyogenic granulomas.

These can present as a dark hemorrhagic, eroded, nodular lesion clinically resembling a malignant melanoma as well as advanced nodular tumors of epidemic Kaposi's sarcoma.

Nevi and Malignant Melanomas as Simulators of Kaposi's Sarcoma
(Figures 3–41 to 3–46)

Many pigmented mucocutaneous lesions simulate Kaposi's sarcoma. Benign intradermal and junctional nevi, as well as dysplastic nevi and malignant melanomas,[8] may resemble lesions of epidemic Kaposi's sarcoma. The discrete and often solitary nature of the common, benign pigmented skin lesions makes them clinically difficult to differentiate from some of the dark lesions of Kaposi's sarcoma. The invasive and metastatic behavior of cutaneous malignant melanomas may simulate widely disseminated eruptions seen with epidemic Kaposi's sarcoma.

Another cutaneous tumor that simulates Kaposi's sarcoma is the basal cell carcinoma, especially the pigmented variety, which may provide a clinical picture that can be confused with either primary pigmented nevi, melanomas, or an isolated lesion of epidemic Kaposi's sarcoma. In such cases, a biopsy and histopathologic examination are the only means of confirming the diagnosis.

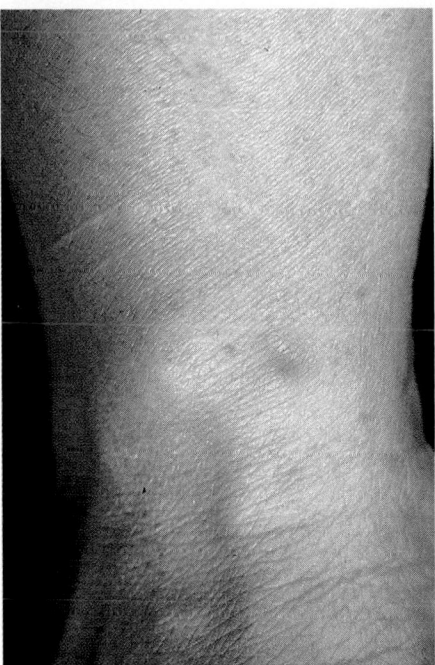

Figure 3–41. Interdermal blue nevus.

The distinct bluish color seen in this benign deeply situated interdermal blue nevus is the result of the Tyndall effect. Such lesions may simulate those seen in epidemic Kaposi's sarcoma.

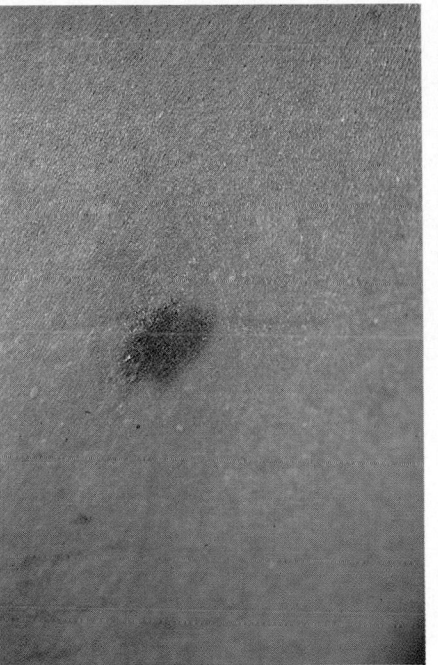

Figure 3–42. Solitary pigmented junctional nevus.

This could easily be mistaken for a lesion of epidemic Kaposi's sarcoma.

Figure 3–43. Malignant melanoma in situ.

This localized deeply pigmented lesion represents a malignant melanoma in situ, which could resemble some of the lesions seen in epidemic Kaposi's sarcoma.

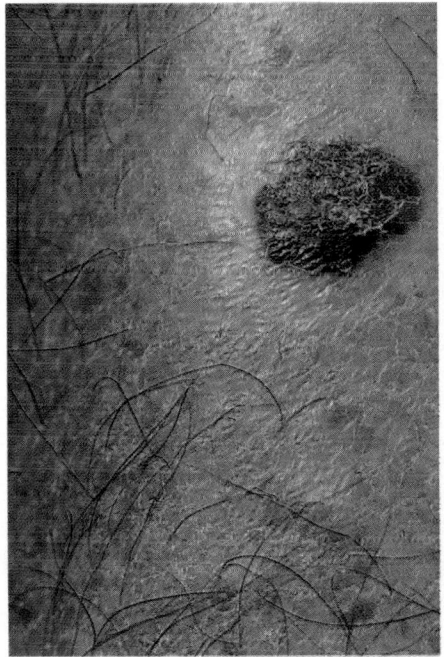

Figure 3–44. Malignant melanoma.

The marked pigmentation and irregular borders of this malignant melanoma clinically look similar to some of the lesions seen in epidemic Kaposi's sarcoma lesions.

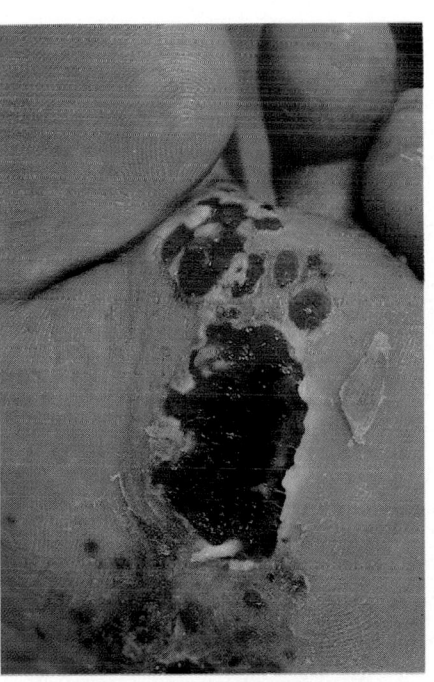

Figure 3–45. Malignant melanoma.

A cluster of invasive nodules surrounding the original tumor lesion on the plantar surface in a patient with malignant melanoma. Patients with both the classical and epidemic forms of Kaposi's sarcoma may develop multiple nodular lesions on the soles of the feet.

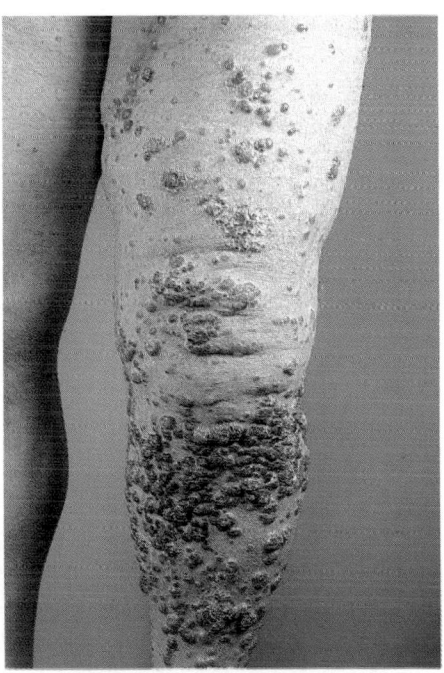

Figure 3–46. Metastatic melanoma.

This case represents extensive cutaneous metastatic melanoma on the lower extremity. The variations in color and clusters of multiple tumor lesions on the legs can also be seen in advanced cases of classical as well as epidemic forms of Kaposi's sarcoma.

Other Cutaneous Tumors as Simulators of Kaposi's Sarcoma
(Figures 3–47 to 3–60)

Cutaneous malignancies which may resemble the lesions of epidemic Kaposi's sarcoma are not confined to melanomas and pigmented basal cell carcinomas. Lymphoreticular malignancies which may occur on the skin can sometimes look like Kaposi's sarcoma; these tumors may be as varied in their morphologic appearance as the lesions of epidemic Kaposi's sarcoma are in their broad clinical appearance.[9, 10] Lymphoid malignancies frequently present with similar patch, plaque, and nodular lesion configurations seen with Kaposi's sarcoma. Nonmalignant pseudolymphomas of the skin can also be confused clinically with epidemic Kaposi's sarcoma and other malignancies of lymphoreticular origin. The frequent occurrence of epidemic Kaposi's sarcoma lesions in the posterior auricular and cervical regions can render a difficult clinical differentiation between pseudolymphoma and other entities which are also found in these areas. Perhaps the most difficult differential diagnosis among the clinical simulators of epidemic Kaposi's sarcoma are found among the cutaneous lesions of the more malignant sarcomas. Both the discrete and more diffuse plaques and nodules seen in angiosarcoma and reticulum cell sarcomas can readily mimic some of the lesions of epidemic Kaposi's sarcoma. They can be distinguished definitively only by histopathologic examination. Rare tumor lesions including leiomyomas, glomus tumors, and cutaneous metastases of adenocarcinoma from the breast or visceral organs can be remarkably similar to Kaposi's sarcoma. Conditions such as eruptive xanthomas and keloids may also be mistaken for this AIDS-associated neoplasm.

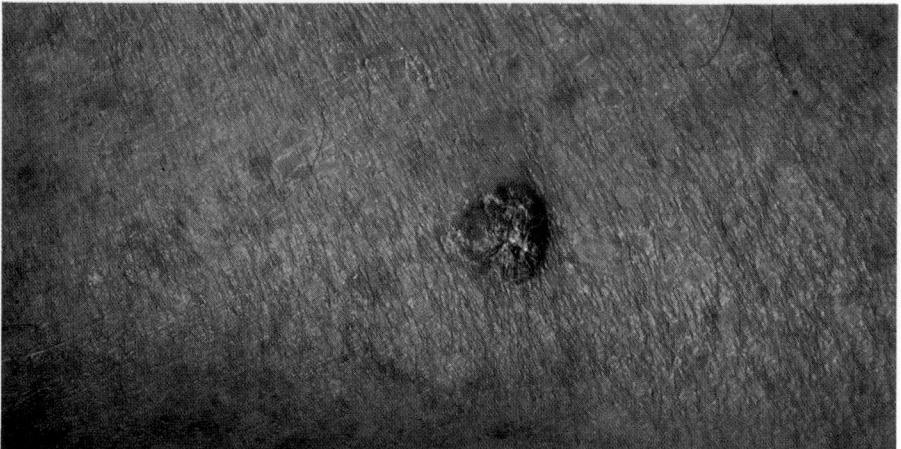

Figure 3–47. Basal cell carcinoma.
The violaceous color and hyperpigmentation of this basal cell carcinoma could easily be confused with a nodule of epidemic Kaposi's sarcoma.

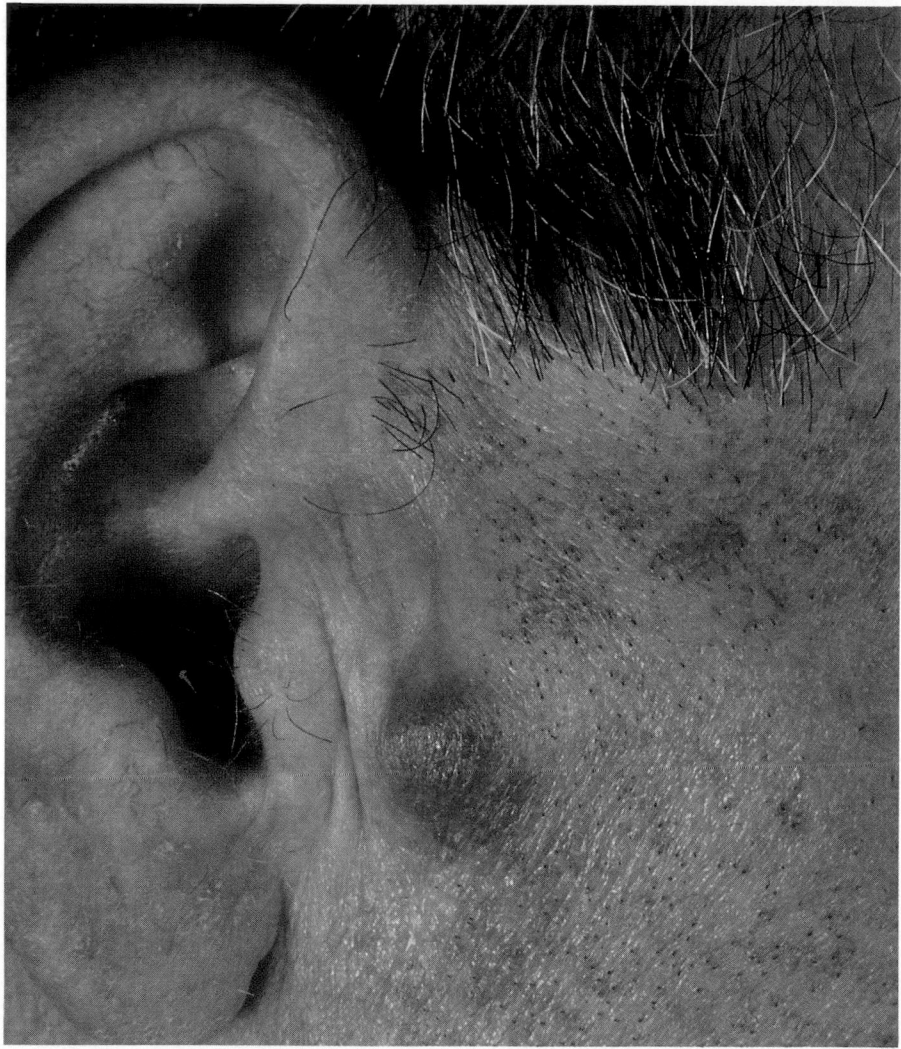

Figure 3–48. Pseudolymphoma.
The nodular lesions of pseudolymphoma often resemble those seen in epidemic Kaposi's sarcoma.

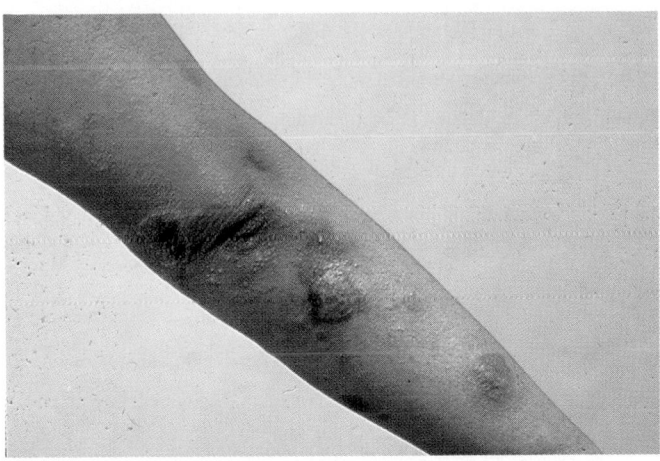

Figure 3–49. Cutaneous lymphoma.
Multiple large plaques of cutaneous lymphoma are seen on the forearm. The morphologic features and color of these plaques are similar to those of epidemic Kaposi's sarcoma seen in dark skin.

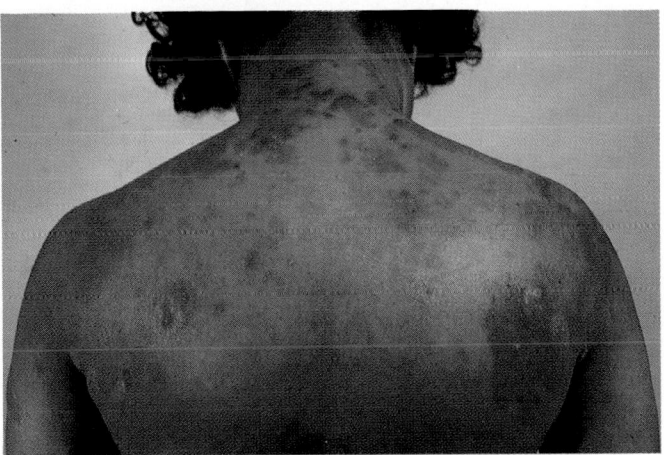

Figure 3–50. Cutaneous lymphoma.
Cutaneous lymphoma with multiple patches and plaques extending over the skin surface. These lesions are similar to those seen in epidemic Kaposi's sarcoma.

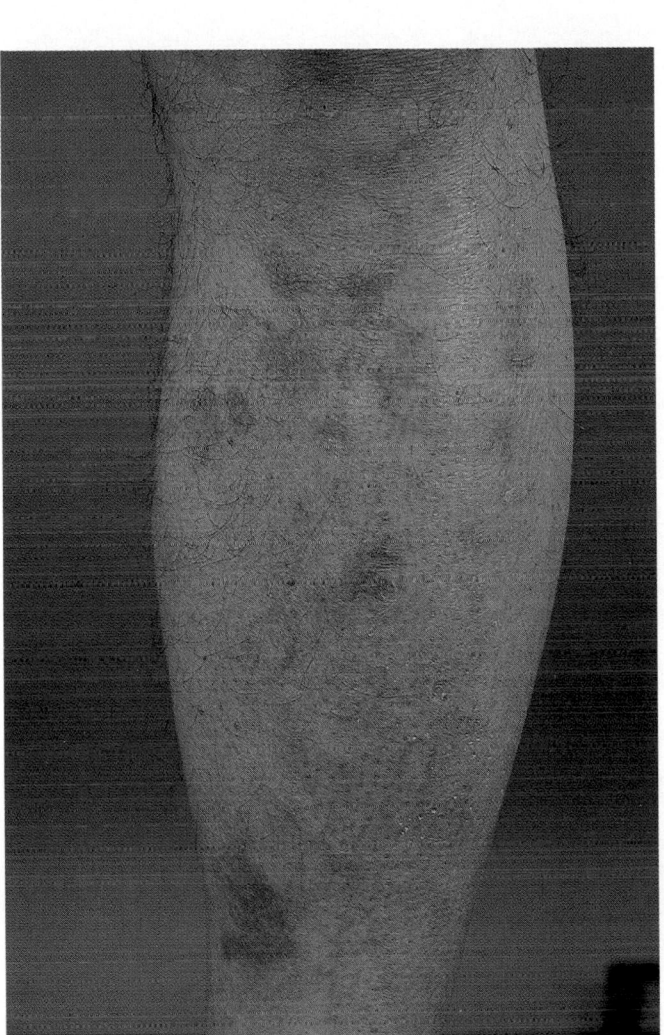

Figure 3–51. Mycosis fungoides.
The subtle lesions of early mycosis fungoides (cutaneous T cell lymphoma) seen on the leg mimic the early skin patches often observed in epidemic Kaposi's sarcoma.

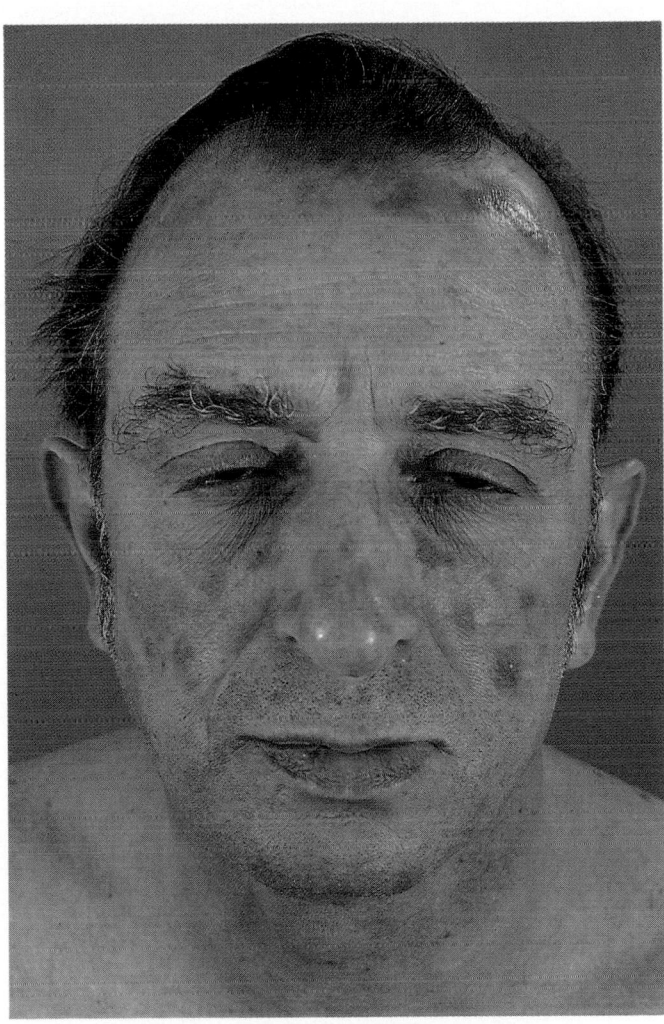

Figure 3–52. Mycosis fungoides.
Extensive facial involvement with plaques caused by mycosis fungoides resemble some advanced lesions seen with epidemic Kaposi's sarcoma.

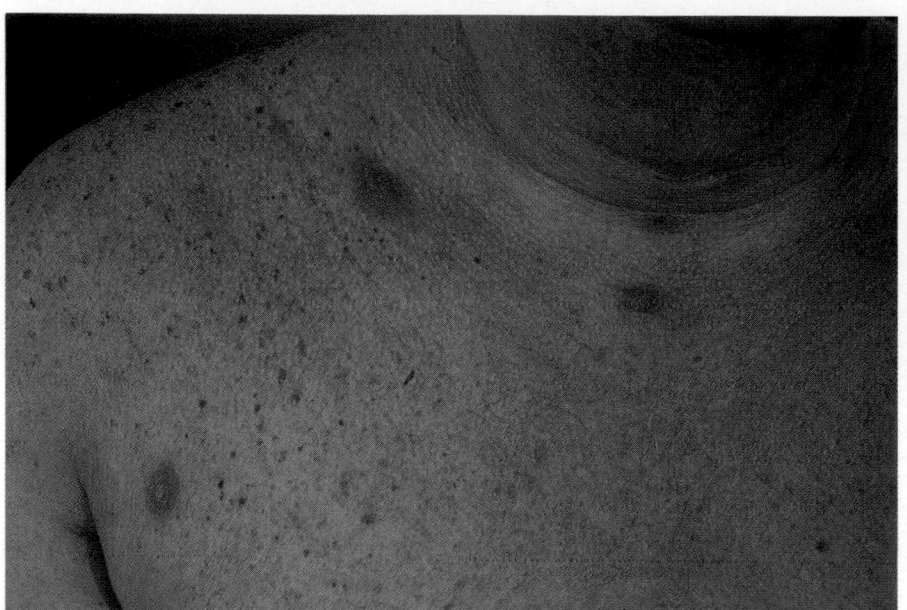

Figure 3–53. Reticulum cell sarcoma.

Both the distribution and morphologic appearance of these multiple erythematous plaques of reticulum cell sarcoma are clinically indistinguishable from certain lesions found in epidemic Kaposi's sarcoma.

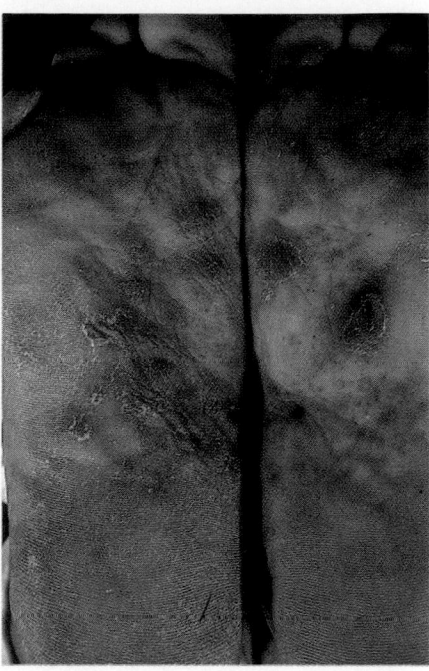

Figure 3–54. Reticulum cell sarcoma.

Extensive infiltrative plaques of reticulum cell sarcoma are seen on the soles of this patient's feet. This clinical presentation can mimic lesions seen in either the classical or epidemic form of Kaposi's sarcoma.

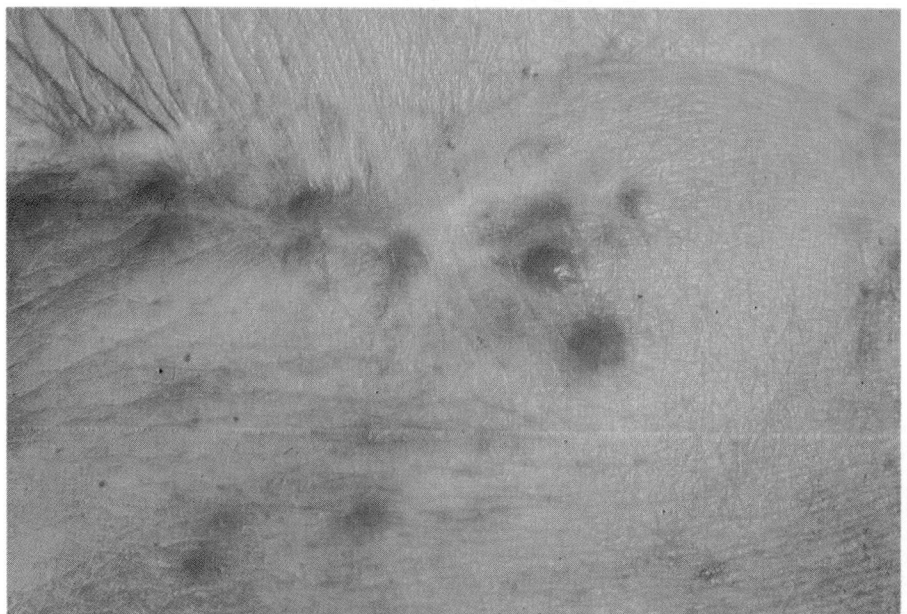

Figure 3–55. Adenocarcinoma.

The nodules of cutaneous metastatic lesions of adenocarcinoma of the breast seen adjacent to the surgical scar could be difficult to differentiate clinically from some of the tumors seen in epidemic Kaposi's sarcoma.

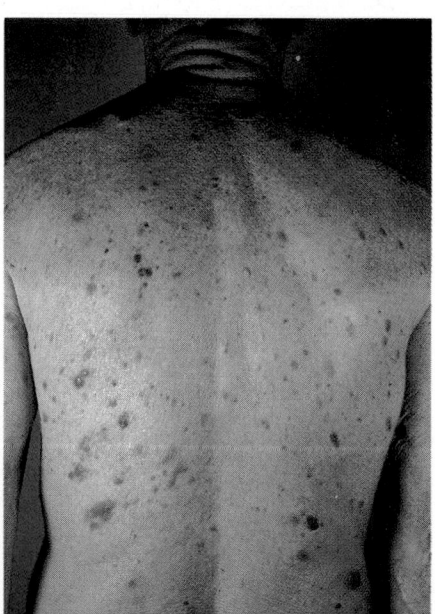

Figure 3–56. Eruptive xanthomata.

Multiple plaques and nodules found on the back of this individual represent eruptive xanthomata. The dark purplish hue of these lesions is reminiscent of the clinical appearance of epidemic Kaposi's sarcoma.

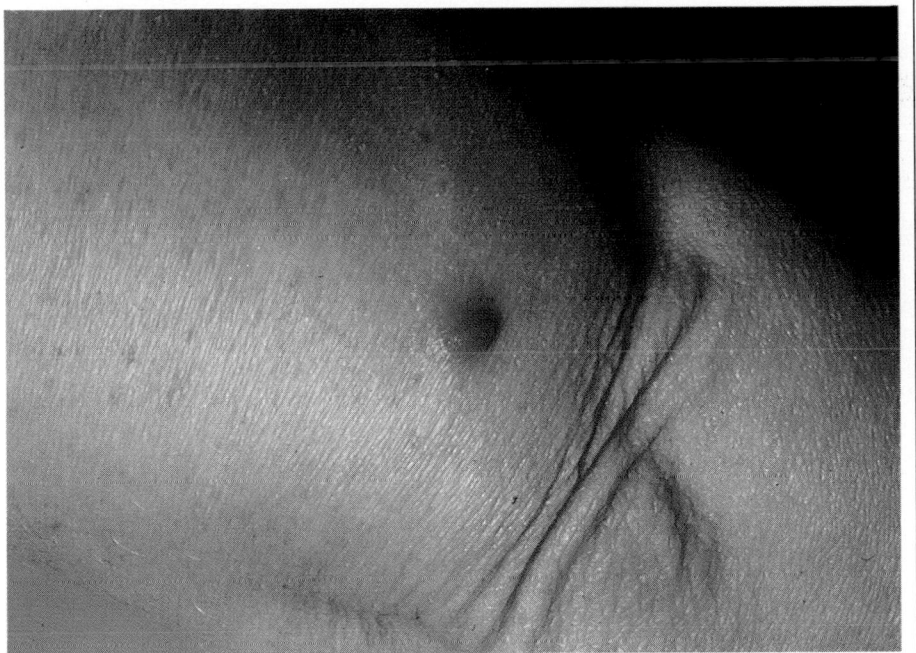

Figure 3–57. Glomus tumor.

This solitary skin nodule is a glomus tumor, resembling a nodular lesion of epidemic Kaposi's sarcoma.

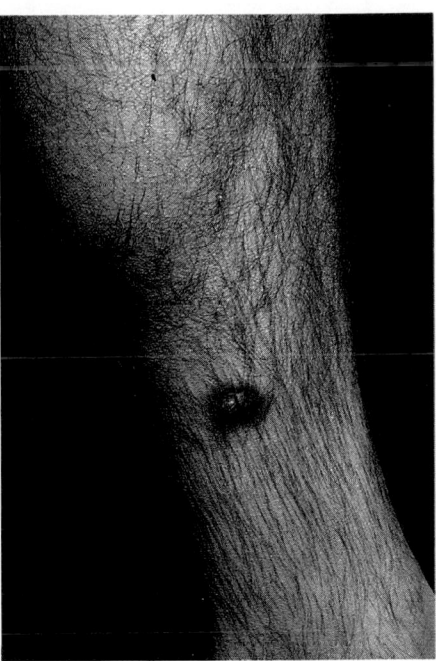

Figure 3–58. Leiomyoma.

This single leiomyoma on the lower leg simulates the lesions of either classical or epidemic Kaposi's sarcoma in both color and location.

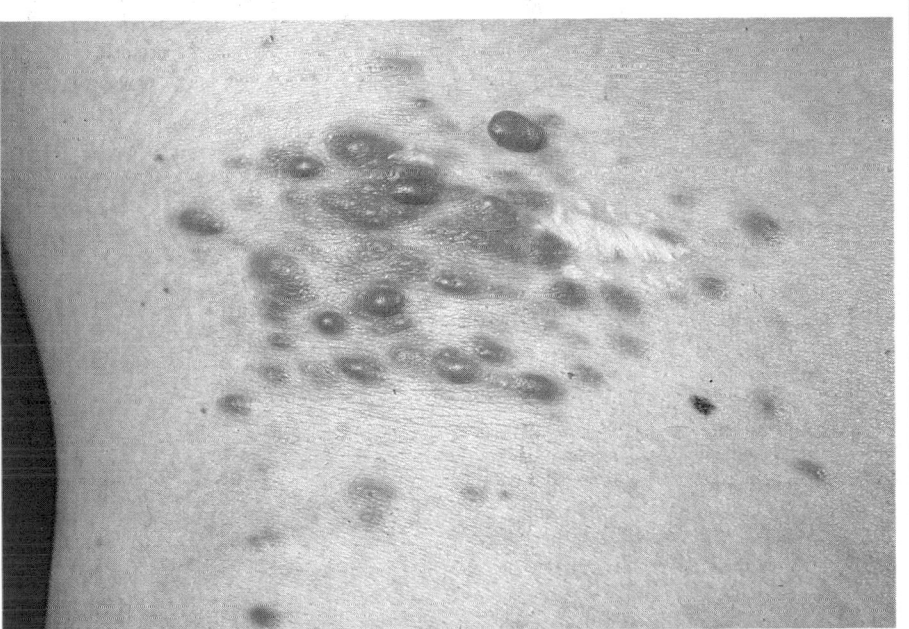

Figure 3–59. Leiomyomas.

Leiomyomas can also be clustered. The red color of these lesions is similar to that observed in some lesions of epidemic Kaposi's sarcoma.

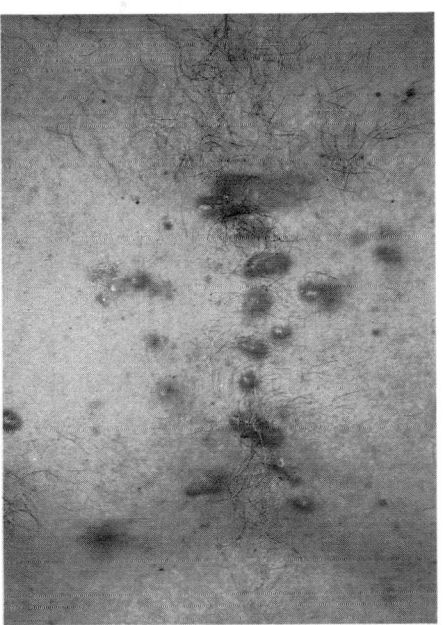

Figure 3–60. Keloids.

These keloids on the anterior area of the chest are similar to lesions observed in patients with epidemic Kaposi's sarcoma.

Sarcoidosis as a Simulator of Kaposi's Sarcoma
(Figures 3–61 to 3–66)

Among granulomatous diseases, the skin lesions of sarcoid deserve special attention as a simulator of epidemic Kaposi's sarcoma.[11] The variations in the clinical manifestations of cutaneous sarcoid lesions parallel the variation in color and lesion configuration observed with epidemic Kaposi's sarcoma.

Although the majority of clinical simulators of lesions of epidemic Kaposi's sarcoma so far discussed are found among the lesions of vascular, inflammatory, pigmentary, malignant, lymphoreticular, and granulomatous diseases, there are still other clinical entities that can cause confusion. It is apparent that there are large numbers of other "look alike" cutaneous lesions which must be considered in the differential diagnosis of Kaposi's sarcoma, especially those tumor lesions seen with the epidemic variety of this tumor associated with AIDS.

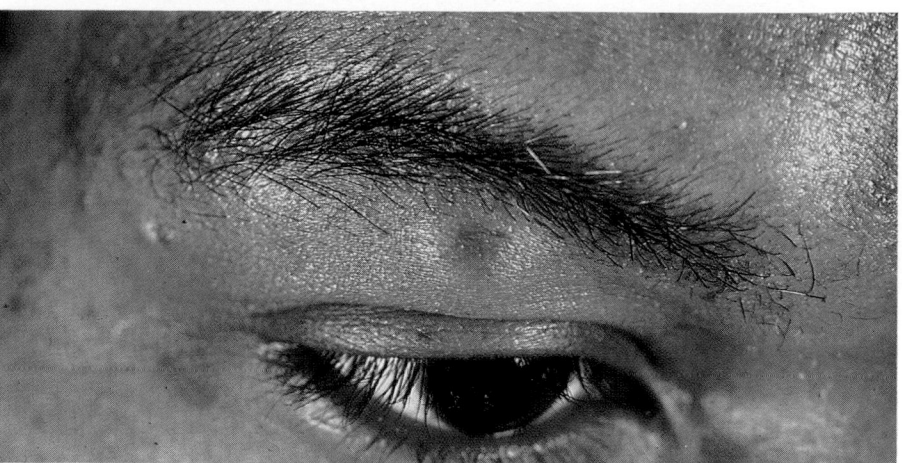

Figure 3–61. Sarcoidosis.
The hyperpigmented patches and plaques on the face of this individual are typical of sarcoidosis. They resemble the dark-colored lesions seen in dark-skinned patients with epidemic Kaposi's sarcoma.

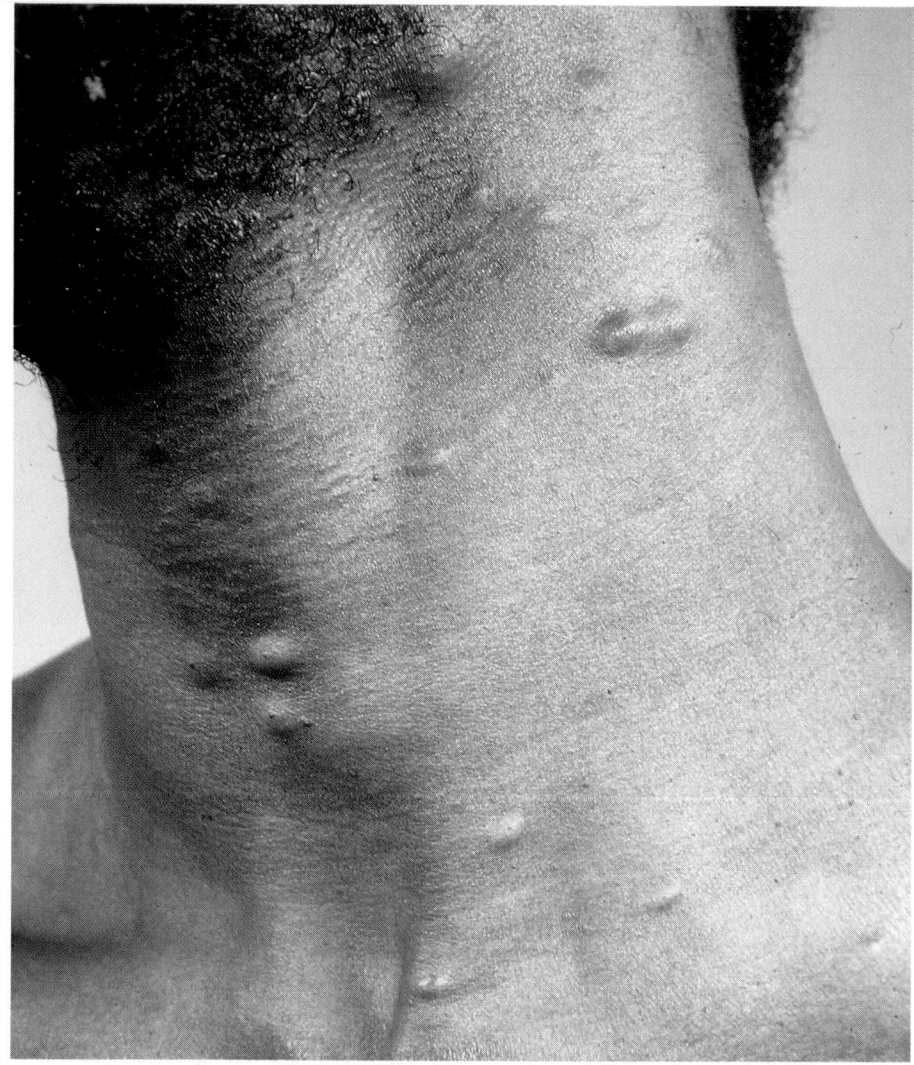

Figure 3–62. Sarcoid plaques.
These plaques of sarcoid located on the neck could be confused with lesions of epidemic Kaposi's sarcoma.

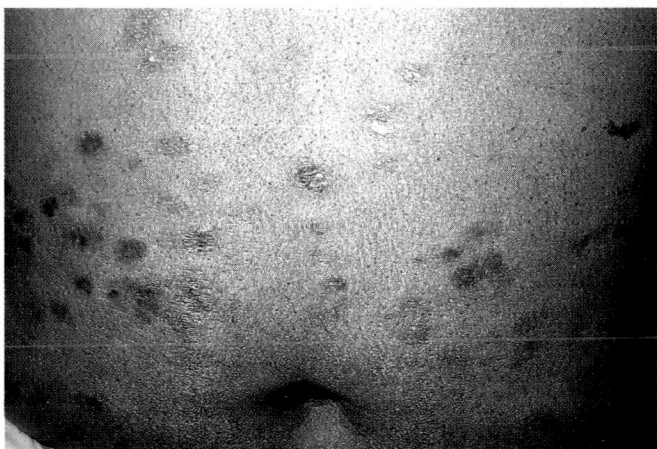

Figure 3–63. Sarcoidosis.
Diffuse cutaneous patch and plaque lesions of sarcoidosis appeared on the abdomen of this dark-skinned patient, simulating the disseminated lesions observed with AIDS-associated Kaposi's sarcoma.

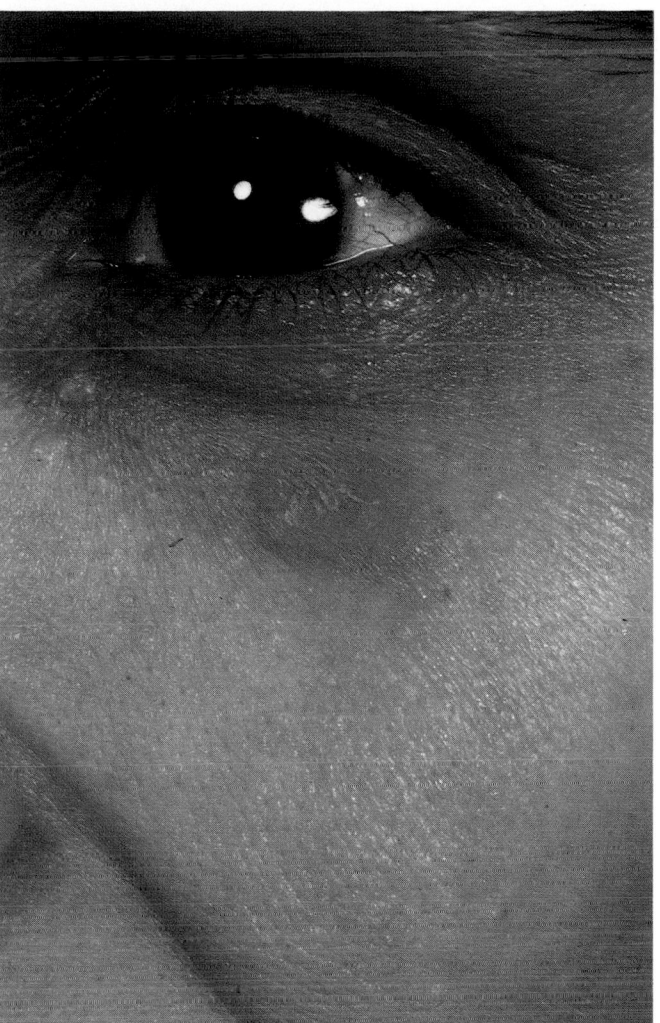

Figure 3–64. Sarcoid lesion.
The differential diagnosis of this erythematous sarcoid lesion located on the cheek should include epidemic Kaposi's sarcoma.

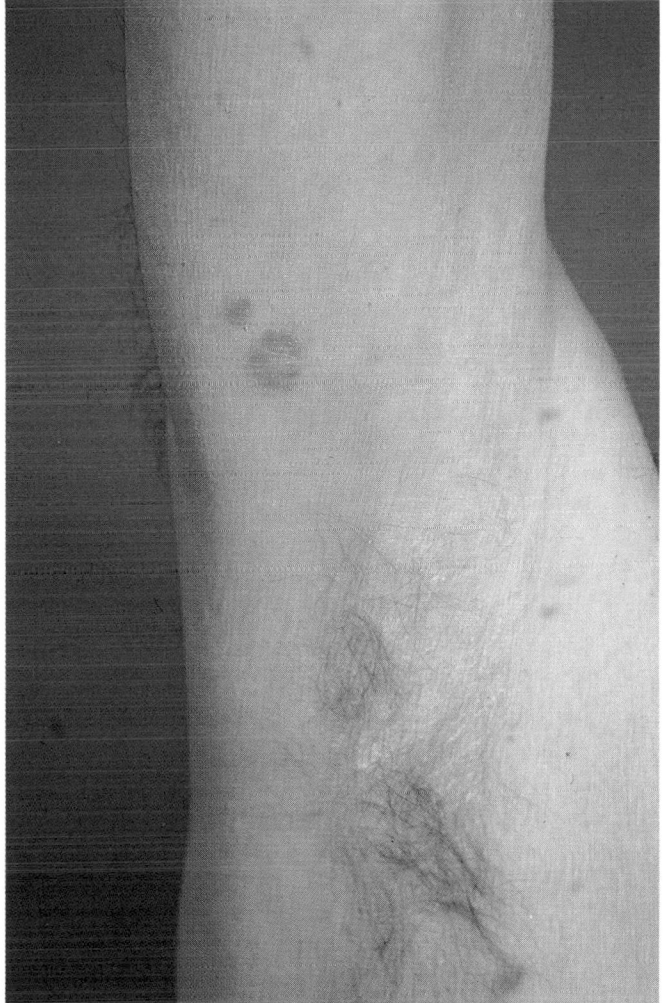

Figure 3–65. Sarcoid plaques.
Erythematous plaques of sarcoid on the arm resemble some of the cutaneous lesions of epidemic Kaposi's sarcoma seen in light-skinned individuals.

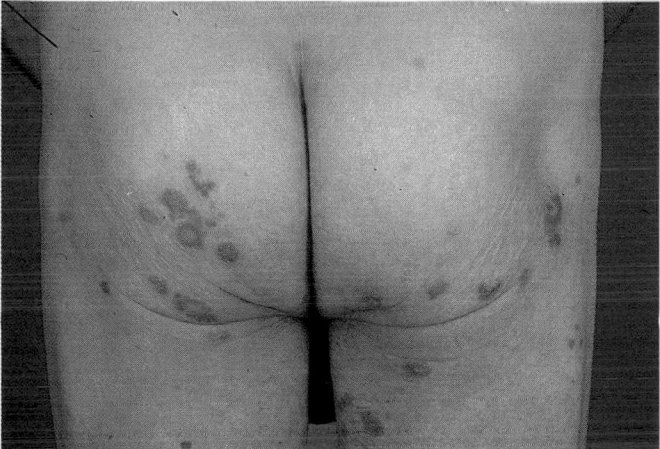

Figure 3–66. Sarcoid lesions.
These lesions involve the buttocks and upper thigh, demonstrating the widespread distribution commonly seen in sarcoidosis that are morphologically reminiscent of the disseminated lesions of epidemic Kaposi's sarcoma.

References

1. Friedman-Kien AE, Ostreicher R: Overview of classical and epidemic Kaposi's sarcoma. *In* Friedman-Kien AE, Laubenstein LJ (eds): AIDS: The Epidemic of Kaposi's Sarcoma and Opportunistic Infections. New York, Masson Publishing USA, 1984, pp 28–29.
2. Templeton AE: Kaposi's sarcoma. *In* Andrade R, Gumport SL, et al (eds): Cancer of the Skin: Biology, Diagnosis and Management. Philadelphia, W. B. Saunders Co., 1976, p 1183.
3. Champion RH: Purpura. *In* Rook A, Wilkinson D, Ebling F (eds): Textbook of Dermatology. London, Blackwell Scientific Publications, 1979, pp 981–990.
4. Karpatkin S: Idiopathic thrombocytopenic purpura in homosexual men. *In* Friedman-Kien AE, Laubenstein LJ (eds): AIDS: The Epidemic of Kaposi's Sarcoma and Opportunistic Infections. New York, Masson Publishing USA, 1984, pp 207–210.
5. Ostrow DG: Differential diagnosis of secondary syphillis. *In* Sexually Transmitted Diseases in Homosexual Men. New York, Plenum Medical Books, 1983, pp 44–46.
6. Rosen T, Martin S: Atlas of Black Dermatology. Boston, Little, Brown and Company, 1981, pp 66, 78.
7. Hoepuch PD (ed): Infectious Diseases. Philadelphia, Harper & Row, 1983, p 1017.
8. Kopf AE: Clinical diagnosis of cutaneous malignant melanoma. *In* Kopf AE, Bart RS, Rodriguez-Sains RS, and Ackerman AB (eds): Malignant Melanoma. New York, Masson Publishing USA, 1979, pp 15–23.
9. Zutzner MA, Zugler JL: Kaposi's sarcoma. *In* Fitzpatrick TB, et al (eds): Dermatology in General Medicine. New York, McGraw Hill Book Co., 1979, p 747.
10. Braverman IM: Lymphomas and allied disorders. *In* Skin Signs of Systemic Disease. Philadelphia, W. B. Saunders Co., 1981, pp 109–167.
11. Braverman IM: Sarcoidosis. *In* Braverman IM (ed): Skin Signs of Systemic Disease. Philadelphia, W. B. Saunders Co., 1981, pp 516–530.

4

The Microscopic Diagnosis of Classical and Epidemic Kaposi's Sarcoma

David N. Silvers

Lesions of classic Kaposi's sarcoma and of AIDS-related or epidemic Kaposi's sarcoma are conventionally described as patch, plaque, or nodular. A given lesion may show combined features—for example, a nodule arising within a patch. Not all nodular lesions have a clinically demonstrable patch or plaque precursor phase. Nevertheless, it is likely that every nodular lesion has gone through a patch phase and a plaque phase, although these developmental phases may be fleeting and may go unrecognized clinically.

The histologic features of classic Kaposi's sarcoma parallel the clinical appearance of the lesion. Patch-type lesions contain ectatic vascular spaces, a perivascular infiltrate, but a relatively sparse number of tumor cells. Plaque-type lesions show a greater number of tumor cells, and these cells characteristically form a fascicle-like pattern around vascular spaces. Nodular lesions of classic Kaposi's sarcoma show well-circumscribed, densely packed aggregates of tumor cells, which replace the collagen.

In contrast, the histologic findings in AIDS-related lesions of Kaposi's sarcoma do not necessarily correlate well with the clinical appearance of the lesions. It is not unusual to see very subtle histologic features in a violaceous nodule of epidemic Kaposi's sarcoma, whereas a barely palpable plaque may show diagnostic histologic features. When a clinical diagnosis of epidemic Kaposi's sarcoma is suspected and the patient has multiple lesions, biopsies from at least three lesions should be taken because it is difficult to pre-dict which lesion will show the most diagnostic features.

The histologic features of classical Kaposi's sarcoma, except for some patch-stage lesions, are sufficiently distinctive to be diagnostic. The histologic features of a given lesion of epidemic Kaposi's sarcoma, however, may be similar to a number of relatively common conditions such as dermatofibromas, scars, and syphilis, making clinical correlation mandatory. Although it is important for the pathologist to be aware of the more subtle histologic features of lesions of epidemic Kaposi's sarcoma so as not to overlook this condition, especially when it has not been suspected clinically, it is likely that histologic "overdiagnosis" has occurred in persons belonging to "high-risk" groups for development of AIDS.

Histologic Features

Classical Kaposi's Sarcoma

The patch and plaque stages of classic Kaposi's sarcoma are characterized by a proliferation of spindle-shaped cells which aggregate around ectatic endothelium-lined vascular spaces in the dermis (Figures 4–1 to 4–6). The spindle cells, like the vascular spaces, are predominantly oriented parallel to the epidermis (Figures 4–1 and 4–4). Extravasated erythrocytes are scattered between the spindle cells (Figure 4–3). Hemosiderin is variably present (Figure 4–5). A perivascular arrangement of plasma cells is a relatively consistent feature in this stage of classical Kaposi's sarcoma (Figures 4–1 and 4–6).

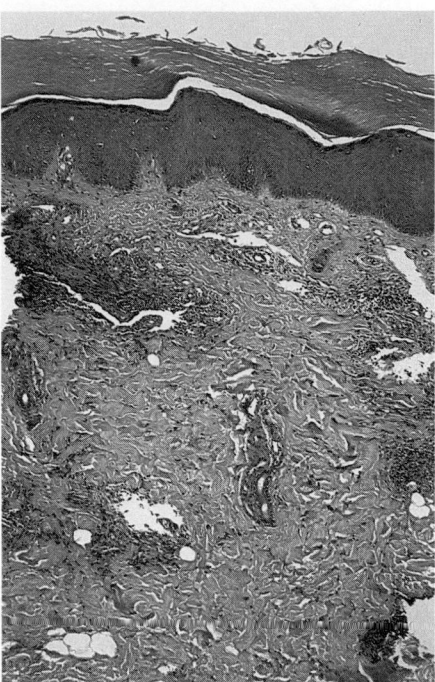

Figure 4–1. Classical Kaposi's sarcoma, patch and plaque lesions.

There are ectatic vascular spaces oriented parallel to the epidermis and surrounded by an infiltrate.

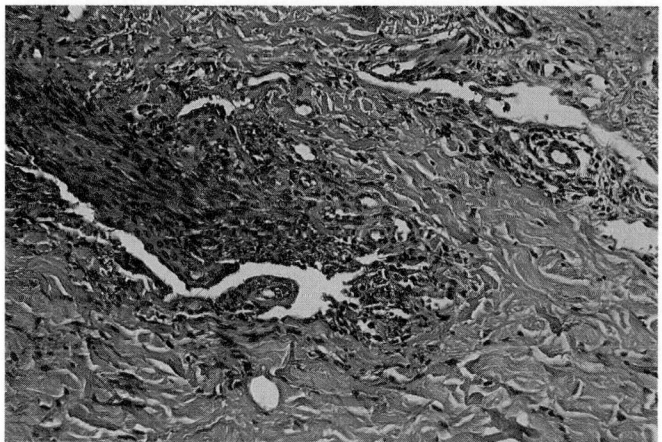

Figure 4–2. Classical Kaposi's sarcoma, patch and plaque lesion.
Spindle cells are concentrically arranged around an ectatic vessel.

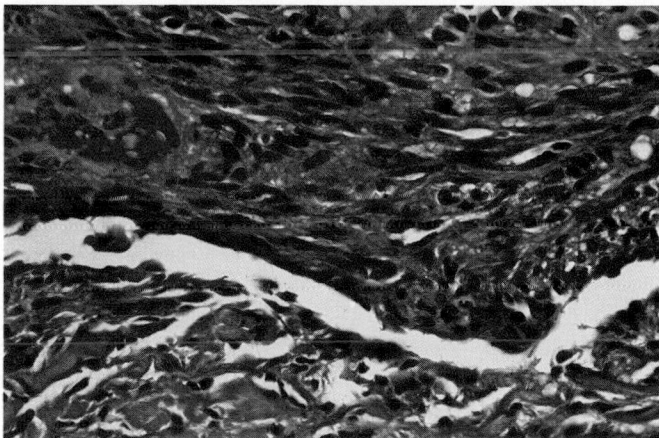

Figure 4–3. Classical Kaposi's sarcoma, patch and plaque lesion.
Spindle cells form a vascular-slit pattern with erythrocytes.

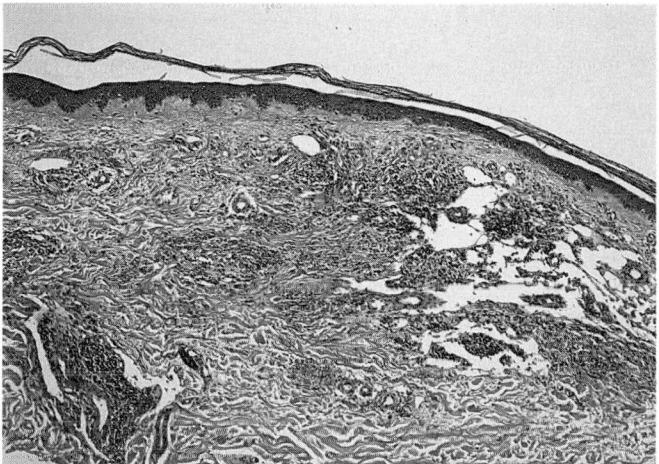

Figure 4–4. Classical Kaposi's sarcoma, patch and plaque lesion.
Anastomosing, ectatic, vascular spaces form a large cistern. There is prominent hemorrhage.

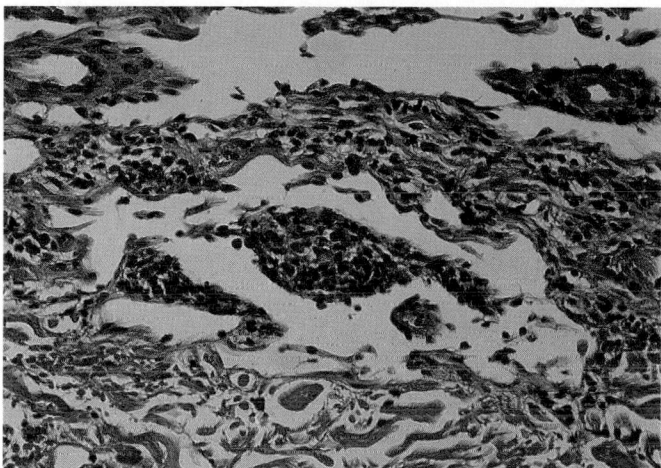

Figure 4–5. Classical Kaposi's sarcoma, patch and plaque lesion.
Hemosiderin is present around vascular spaces. There is an infiltrate of plasma cells.

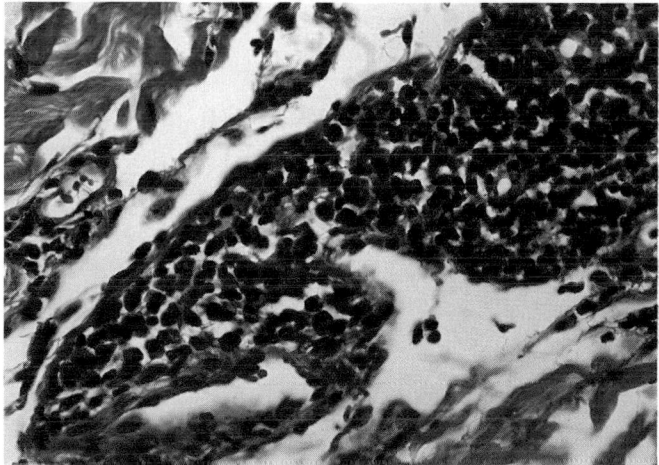

Figure 4–6. Classical Kaposi's sarcoma, patch and plaque lesion.
Plasma cells "cuff" a vessel in the dermis.

The nodular stage of classical Kaposi's sarcoma shows a well-circumscribed, nonencapsulated nodule composed of tightly packed spindle cells which form a vascular-slit pattern with extravasated erythrocytes (Figures 4–7 to 4–10). The epidermis is often flattened and attenuated, presumably by compression from the tumor below (Figure 4–7). The spindle cells may vary in configuration, size and shape of the nucleus, prominence of the nucleolus, and number of mitoses (Figure 4–10). However, within a given nodule, these cytologic features are usually consistent from one area to another. There may be a small increase in the number of vascular spaces at the periphery of a nodule, but true endothelium-lined vascular spaces are rare to absent within the nodule itself. Unlike the patch and plaque stages, plasma cells are not a principal feature of the nodular stage of classic Kaposi's sarcoma.

AIDS-Related Epidemic Kaposi's Sarcoma

Is classical Kaposi's sarcoma histologically distinguishable from epidemic Kaposi's sarcoma? All the microscopic features described in classical Kaposi's sarcoma may be present in epidemic Kaposi's sarcoma. However, there are microscopic features consistently seen in the majority of lesions of epidemic Kaposi's sarcoma, especially lesions of the patch and plaque stages, which enable the pathologist to deduce correctly the appropriate clinical setting. Whether or not these histologic features are significant in terms of the etiology of epidemic Kaposi's sarcoma is problematic, but their recognition is important in order to avoid misdiagnosis, for a number of conditions, including an-

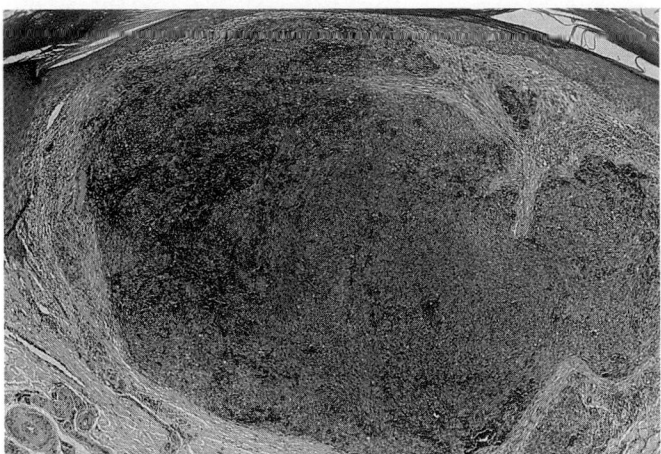

Figure 4–7. Classical Kaposi's sarcoma, nodular lesion.

The well-circumscribed nonencapsulated nodule composed of spindle cells in a fascicle-like arrangement effaces the overlying epidermis.

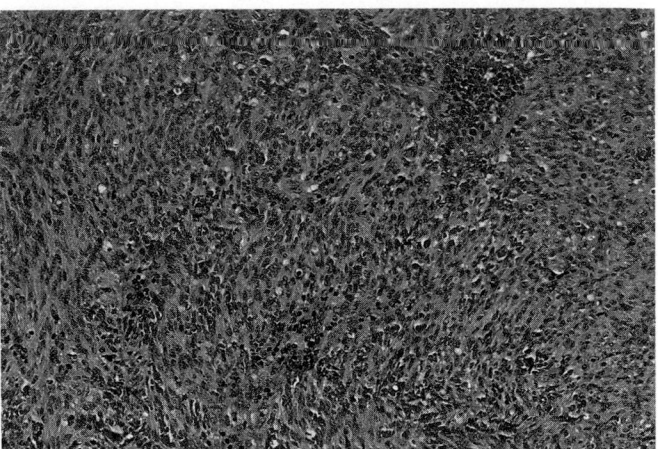

Figure 4–8. Classical Kaposi's sarcoma, nodular lesion.

There are densely packed spindle cells and erythrocytes but no evidence of endothelium-lined vascular spaces.

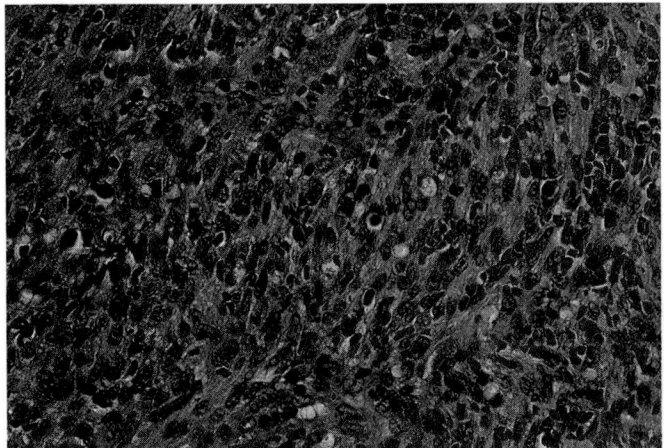

Figure 4–9. Classical Kaposi's sarcoma, nodular lesion.

Spindle cells form a vascular-slit pattern with extravasated erythrocytes.

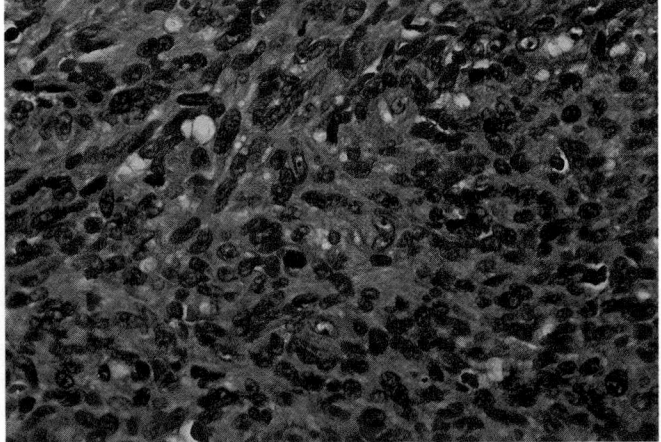

Figure 4–10. Classical Kaposi's sarcoma, nodular lesion.

There is variation in the size and shape of the tumor cells. A mitotic figure is present.

giosarcoma, dermatofibroma, keloid, and secondary syphilis, can histologically simulate epidemic Kaposi's sarcoma.

In the AIDS-related form of Kaposi's sarcoma, patch- and plaque-type lesions typically show spindle-shaped cells forming cleft-like arrangements between collagen bundles at all levels of the dermis (Figures 4–11 to 4–14). The spindle cells appear to form anastomosing spaces between the intertwining layers of collagen (Figures 4–12 and 4–14). These clefts resemble vascular lumen, although they do not contain crythrocytes (Figure 4–13). Several layers of spindle cells may surround arterioles in cross section, and plasma cells may be present (Figure 4–14). However, a pallisaded arrangement of spindle cells and extravasated erythrocytes forming a vascular-slit pattern is uncommon.

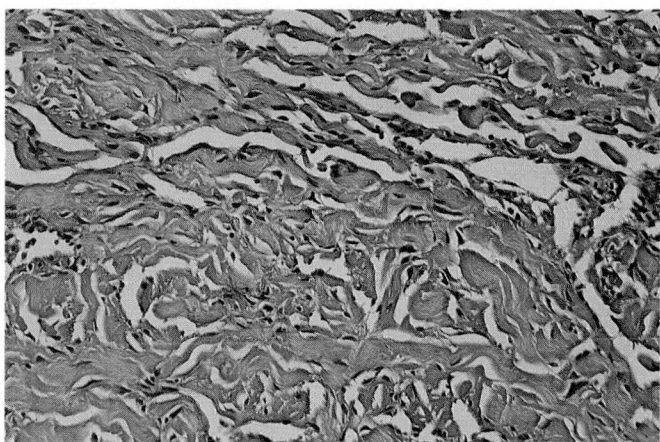

Figure 4–12. Epidemic Kaposi's sarcoma, patch and plaque lesion.

Spindle cells line empty clefts between collagen bundles.

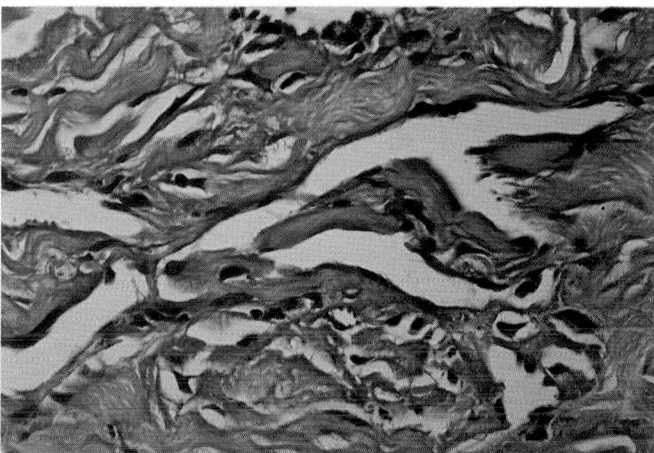

Figure 4–13. Epidemic Kaposi's sarcoma, patch and plaque lesion.

The cleft-like spaces lined by spindle cells form a complex anastomosing pattern.

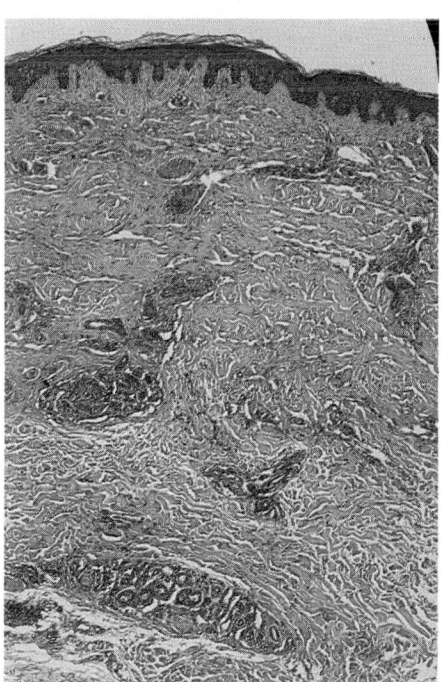

Figure 4–11. Epidemic Kaposi's sarcoma, patch and plaque lesion.

This lesion simulates angiosarcoma (head and neck type).

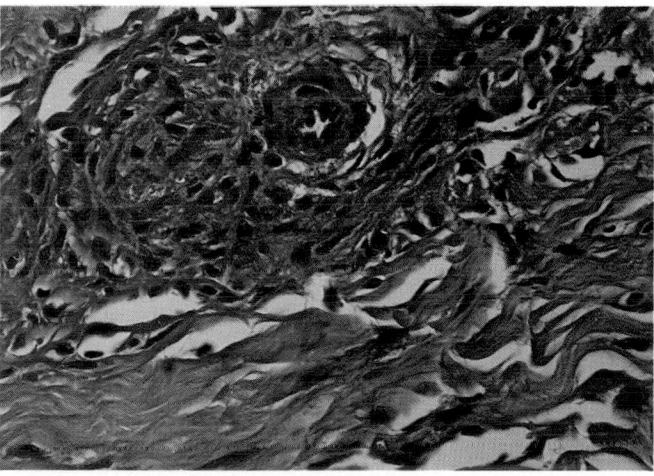

Figure 4–14. Epidemic Kaposi's sarcoma, patch and plaque lesion.

Spindle cells form a concentric arrangement around an arteriole. A few plasma cells are present.

The patch and plaque stages of epidemic Kaposi's sarcoma demonstrate histologic features closely resembling angiosarcoma of the head and neck (Figures 4–15 to 4–18). Epidemic Kaposi's sarcoma may also present a histologic appearance resembling dermatofibroma. In dermatofibroma-like lesions of epidemic Kaposi's sarcoma, spindle cells proliferate between thick bundles of collagen, and numerous plasma cells are present around blood vessels in the superficial and deep dermis (Figures 4–19 to 4–21). Extravasated erythrocytes rarely are numerous.

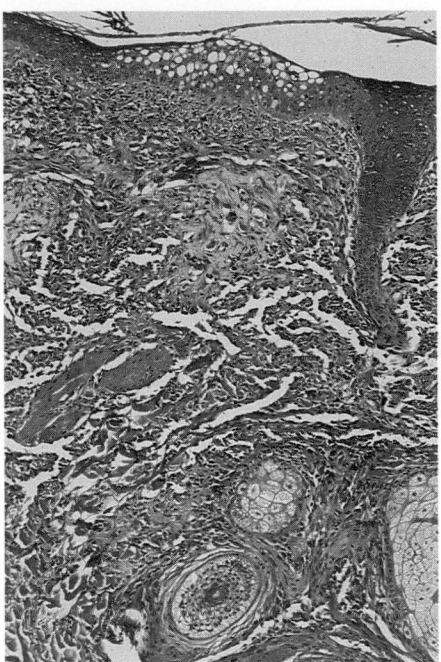

Figure 4–15. Angiosarcoma of the scalp.

Cleft-like spaces lined by spindle cells forming a pattern similar to that seen in the patch and plaque lesion of epidemic Kaposi's sarcoma.

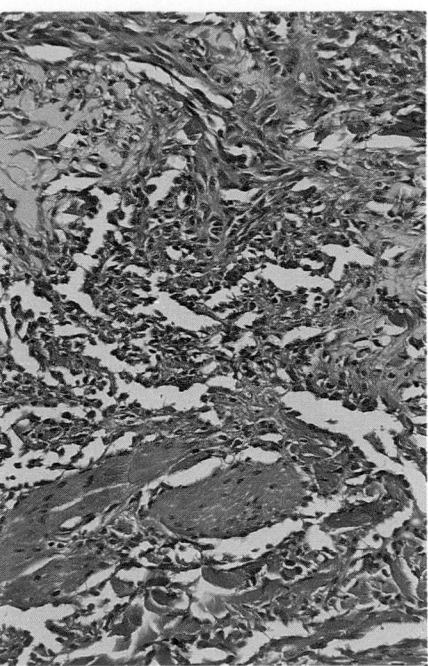

Figure 4–16. Angiosarcoma of the scalp.

The spindle cells lining the clefts are more numerous and perhaps more plump than those in lesions of epidemic Kaposi's sarcoma.

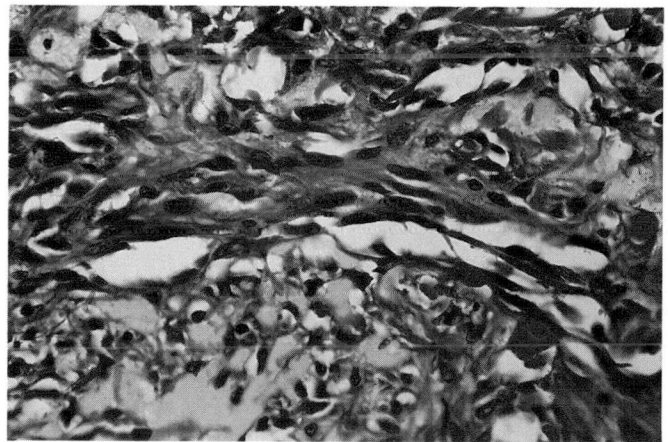

Figure 4–17. Angiosarcoma of the scalp.

Plasma cells are not typically present in nonulcerated lesions of angiosarcoma, whereas they are a constant feature in epidemic Kaposi's sarcoma lesions.

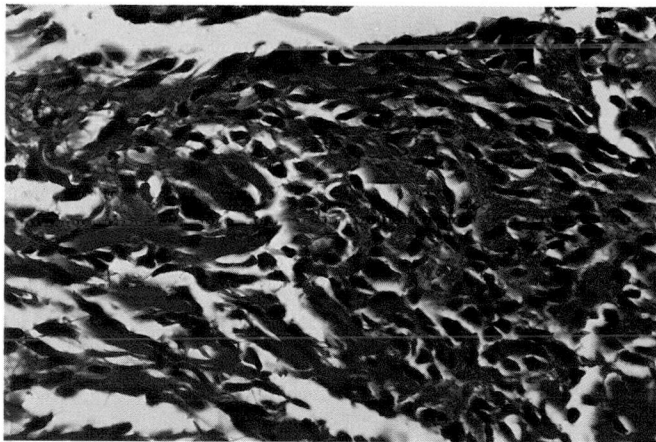

Figure 4–18. Angiosarcoma of the scalp.

The cleft-like spaces in both epidemic Kaposi's sarcoma and angiosarcoma do not contain erythrocytes.

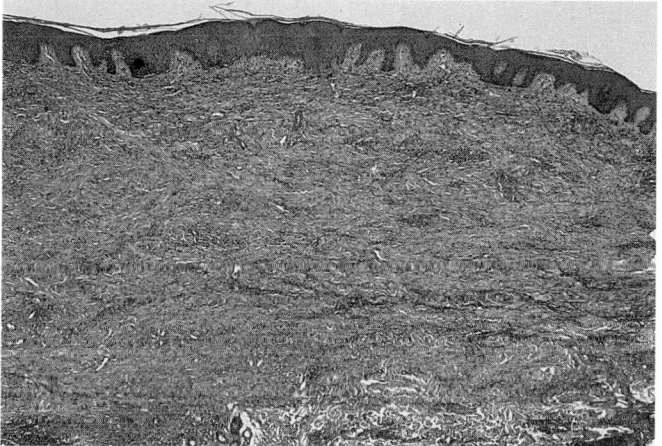

Figure 4–19. Epidemic Kaposi's sarcoma, patch and plaque lesion.

This lesion simulates dermatofibroma.

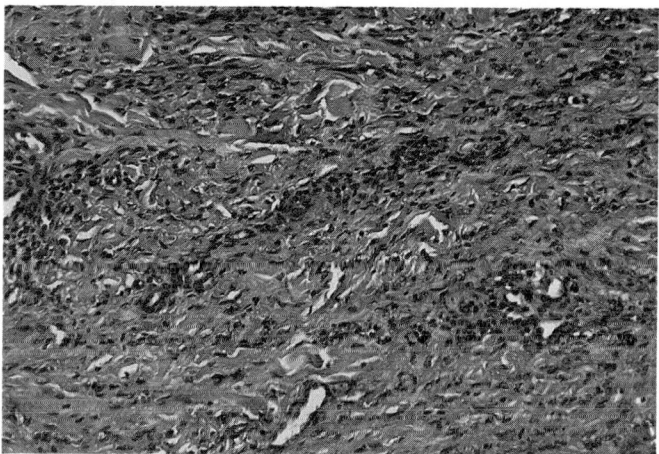

Figure 4–20. Epidemic Kaposi's sarcoma, patch and plaque lesion.

Spindle cells insinuate between thick collagen bundles. A few cleft-like spaces can be seen, and there is a perivascular round cell infiltrate.

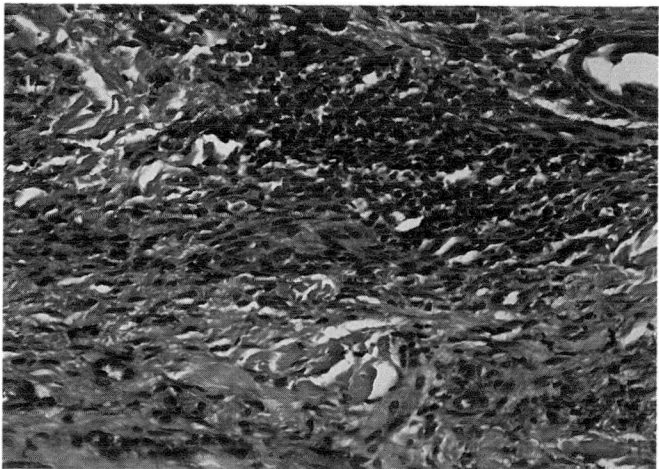

Figure 4–21. Epidemic Kaposi's sarcoma, patch and plaque lesion.

The perivascular infiltrate is composed almost exclusively of plasma cells.

Dermatofibromas, particularly those of the so-called "sclerosing hemangioma" type, can be distinguished from lesions of epidemic Kaposi's sarcoma by the presence of a histiocytic component, including xanthoma-like cells and multinucleated giant cells (Figures 4–22 to 4–24).

Scars, including keloids may histologically resemble lesions of AIDS-related Kaposi's sarcoma (Figures 4–25 to 4–28). Extravasated erythrocytes may be found in scars, and together with the increased number of fibrocytes, they can give the appearance of vascular slits (Figures 4–26 and 4–27). However, when cleft-like spaces are formed, they are not lined by spindle cells, as is typically the case in lesions of the patch and plaque type of epidemic Kaposi's sarcoma (Figure 4–28).

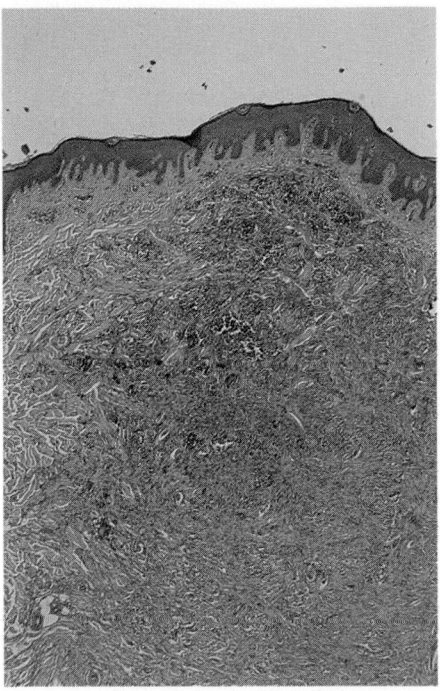

Figure 4–22. Dermatofibroma.
Sclerosing hemangioma type.

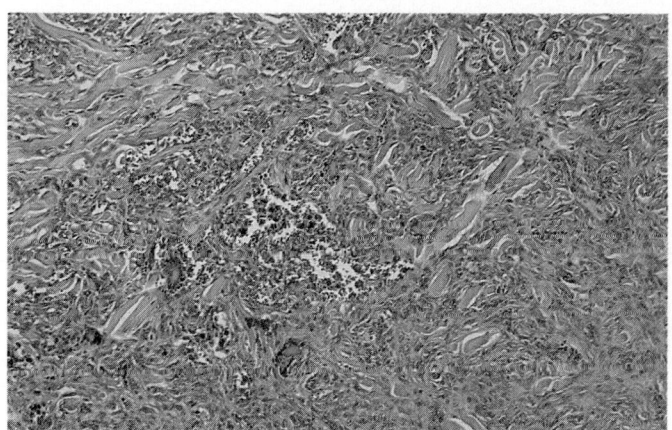

Figure 4–23. Dermatofibroma.

Sclerosing hemangioma type. There are collections of spindle cells associated with a swirling arrangement of collagen. Extravasated erythrocytes form "pools" between collagen bundles.

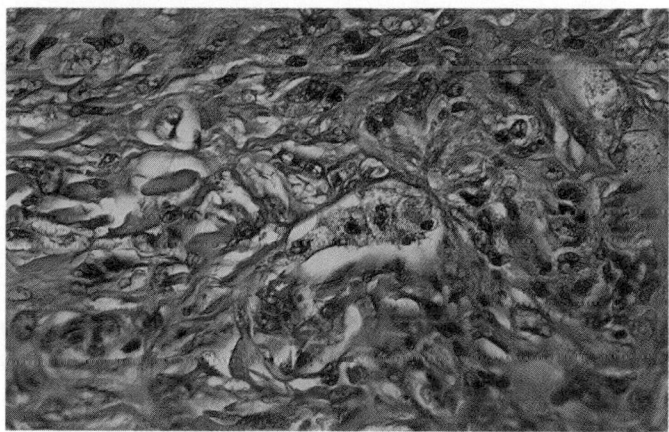

Figure 4–24. Dermatofibroma.

Sclerosing hemangioma type. There are foamy histiocytes, some of which contain hemosiderin, and multinucleate giant cells.

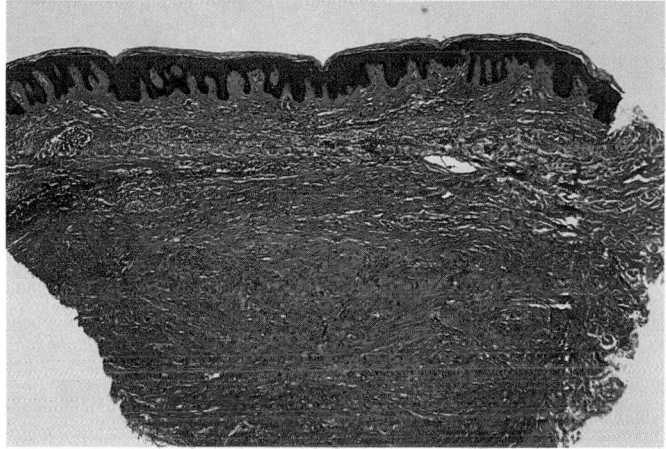

Figure 4–25. Scar.

There is a proliferation of spindle cells oriented parallel to the overlying epidermis.

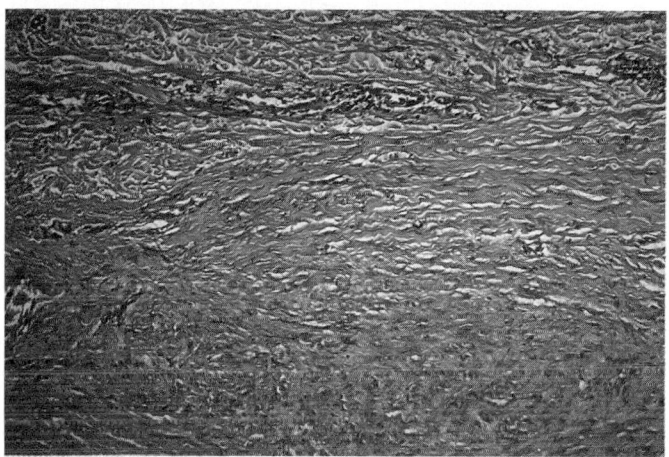

Figure 4–26. Scar.

Collagen bundles are thickened.

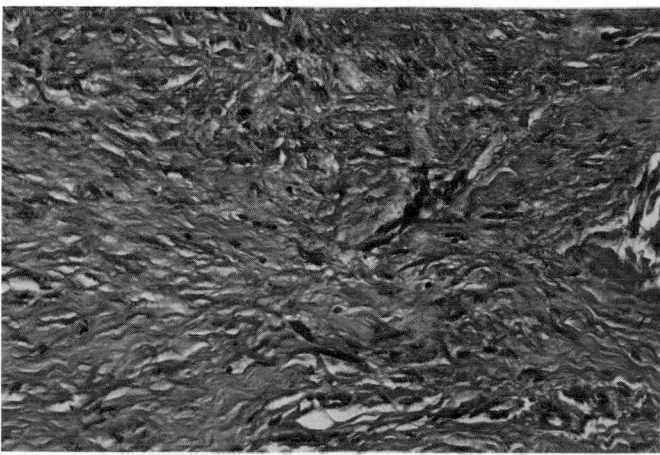

Figure 4–27. Scar.

The hemorrhage together with the numerous spindle cells simulates the vascular-slit pattern of both the classical and epidemic forms of Kaposi's sarcoma.

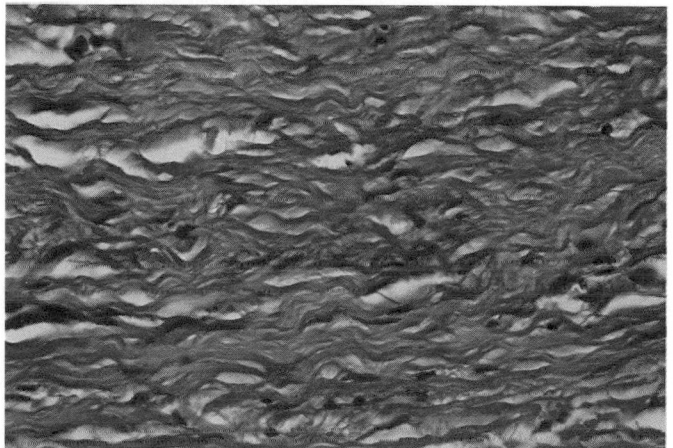

Figure 4–28. Scar.

The fibrocytes in this scar are cytologically more wispy than are the spindle cells of a lesion of epidemic Kaposi's sarcoma. Spaces between fascicles of collagen bundles are not lined by the spindle cells.

Early lesions of epidemic Kaposi's sarcoma which contain a relatively small number of spindle cells but a conspicuous perivascular infiltrate of plasma cells can easily be confused with lesions of secondary syphilis (Figures 4–29 to 4–31). Clinical distinction between these conditions may require correlation with serologic titers and whether or not the lesions resolve following administration of penicillin.

Nodular lesions of AIDS-related Kaposi's sarcoma are histologically indistinguishable from nodules of the classical form of Kaposi's sarcoma (Figures 4–32 to 4–34). However, the dermis surrounding the nodule in lesions of epidemic Kaposi's sarcoma may contain an increased number of spindle cells, forming an arrangement similar to the pattern described in patch and plaque lesions of epidemic Kaposi's sarcoma (Figure 4–34). Whether this feature is consistent enough to be useful in distinguishing nodular lesions of the classical variety from those of epidemic Kaposi's sarcoma will require confirmation in a large series of cases.

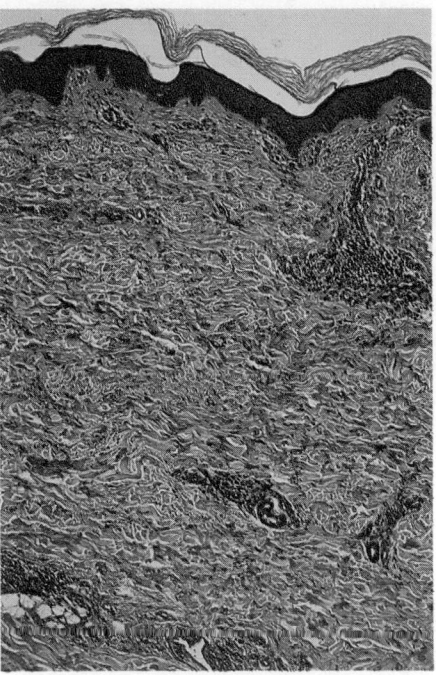

Figure 4–29. Epidemic Kaposi's sarcoma, patch and plaque lesion.

This lesion resembles secondary syphilis. There is a perivascular round cell infiltrate.

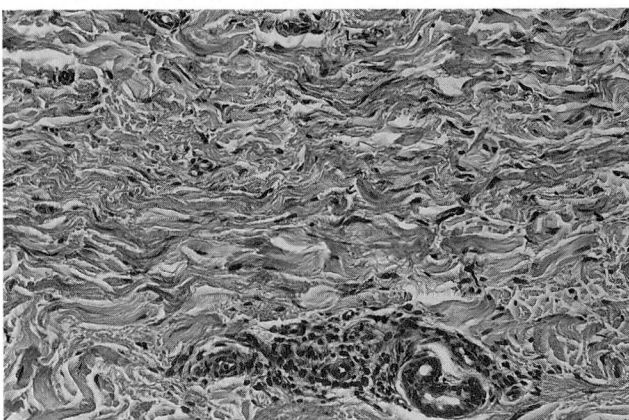

Figure 4–30. Epidemic Kaposi's sarcoma, patch and plaque lesion.

The increased number of spindle cells is noted within the stroma.

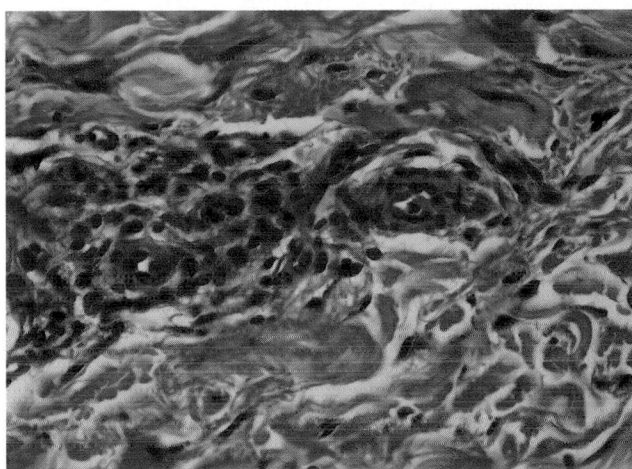

Figure 4–31. Epidemic Kaposi's sarcoma, patch and plaque lesion.

The infiltrate around the blood vessel is composed of plasma cells.

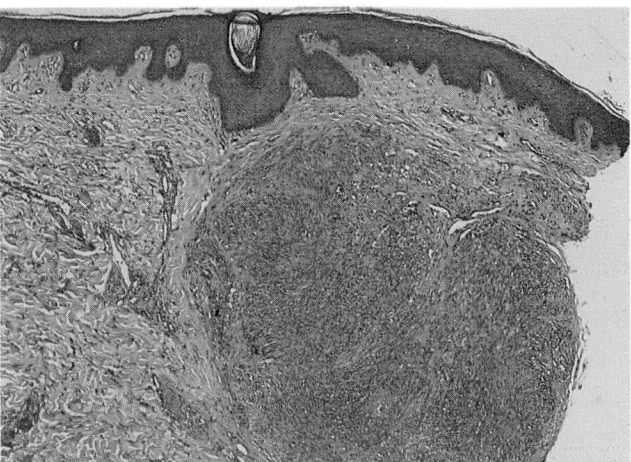

Figure 4–32. Epidemic Kaposi's sarcoma, nodular lesion.

The lesion is very similar to a nodular lesion of classical Kaposi's sarcoma.

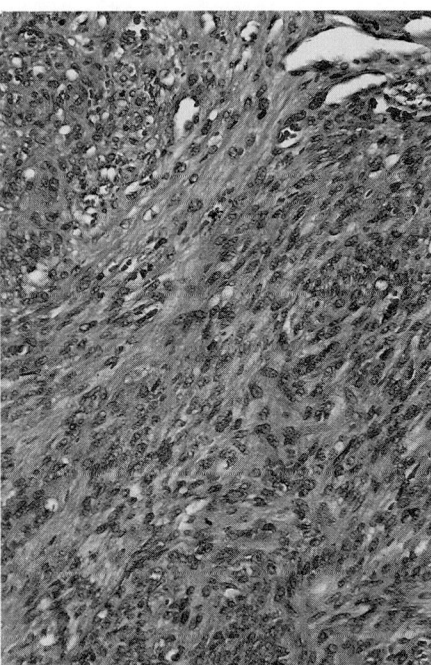

Figure 4–33. Epidemic Kaposi's sarcoma, nodular lesion.

The spindle cells form dense fascicles, and there are erythrocytes between some of the spindle cells.

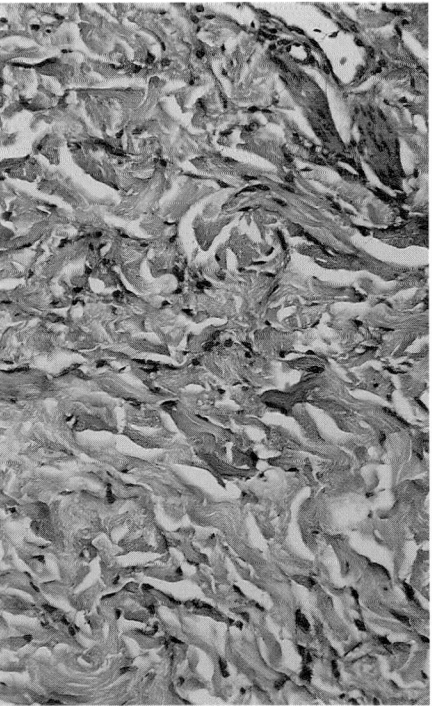

Figure 4–34. Epidemic Kaposi's sarcoma, nodular lesion.

The dermis immediately adjacent to the nodule contains an increased number of spindle cells, a feature which may help to distinguish the nodular phase of epidemic Kaposi's sarcoma from that of the classical form of the disease.

References

1. Ackerman AB: Subtle clues to diagnosis by conventional microscopy: The patch stage of Kaposi's sarcoma. Am J Dermatopathol *1*:164, 1979.
2. Cox FH, Helwig EB: Kaposi's sarcoma. Cancer *12*:289, 1979.
3. Gottlieb GJ, Ackerman AB: Kaposi's sarcoma: An extensively disseminated form in young homosexual men. Hum Pathol *13*:882, 1982.
4. Lever WF, Schaumberg-Lever G: Kaposi's sarcoma. *In* Histopathology of the Skin. 6th ed. Philadelphia, J. B. Lippincott Co., 1983, p 636.
5. Murray JF, Lothe F: The histopathology of Kaposi's sarcoma. Acta Un Int Cancer *18*:413, 1962.
6. O'Connell KM: Kaposi's sarcoma: Histopathological study of 159 cases from Malawi. J Clin Pathol *30*:687, 1977.
7. Reynolds WA, Winkelmann RK, Soule EH: Kaposi's sarcoma: A clinicopathologic study with particular reference to its relationship to the reticuloendothelial system. Medicine *44*:419, 1965.
8. Slavin G, Cameron HM, Forbes C, et al: Kaposi's sarcoma in East African children: A report of 51 cases. J Pathol *100*:187, 1970.
9. Taylor JF, Templeton AC, Vogel CL, et al: Kaposi's sarcoma in Uganda: A clinicopathological study. Int J Cancer *8*:122, 1971.
10. Templeton AC: Kaposi's sarcoma. *In* Andrade R, Gumport SL, Popkin GL, et al (eds): Cancer of the Skin: Biology, Diagnosis, and Management. Philadelphia, W. B. Saunders Co., 1976, p 1183.

5

Ultrastructural Features of Kaposi's Sarcoma and Other Biopsy Findings Relevant to AIDS

Dorothea Zucker-Franklin

At the very outset of this chapter, it should be stated that electron microscopy is not necessary to establish the diagnosis of Kaposi's sarcoma or the acquired immune deficiency syndrome (AIDS). However, ultrastructural analysis of biopsy specimens has become a routine procedure in many institutions, including those in areas where only few patients with Kaposi's sarcoma or AIDS are seen. Therefore, the intent of the illustrations provided in these pages is to help answer questions which invariably arise when tissues of these patients are examined by pathologists who are not familiar with this material.

Ultrastructural Features

In general, the ultrastructural features of Kaposi's sarcoma parallel those seen on light microscopy. When the lesions are fully developed, the cells have a monotonous appearance with prominent nucleoli, as is the case with other neoplasms (Figure 5–1). It should be appreciated that in thin section (600 to 800 Å), the spindle-shaped configuration of the cells may not be appreciated unless the plane of section runs parallel to their long axis (Figure 5–2). The same applies to the peculiar clefts which form between the cells. These cleft-like spaces may appear round on cross section. Because of the higher resolution afforded by electron microscopy, cleft formation is seen earlier in its development. Here it is particularly noteworthy that the process is unrelated to blood vessels (Figure 5–2). When the clefts are larger (Figures 5–3 and 5–4), their "emptiness" becomes even more striking. Presumably, *in vivo,* such spaces are filled with fluid that is lost during the preparatory procedures used for light or electron microscopy. Alternatively, the clefts are artifacts which result from an unusual state of dehydration of the lining cells. In

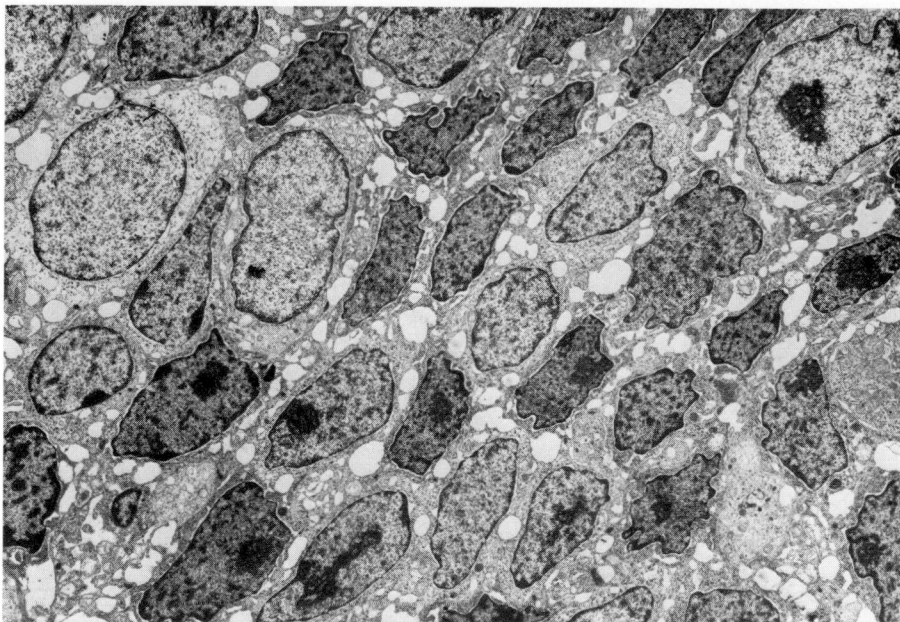

Figure 5–1. Kaposi's sarcoma plaque.

Survey electron micrograph of a cross section of spindle-shaped cells seen in a Kaposi's sarcoma plaque. (×5000)

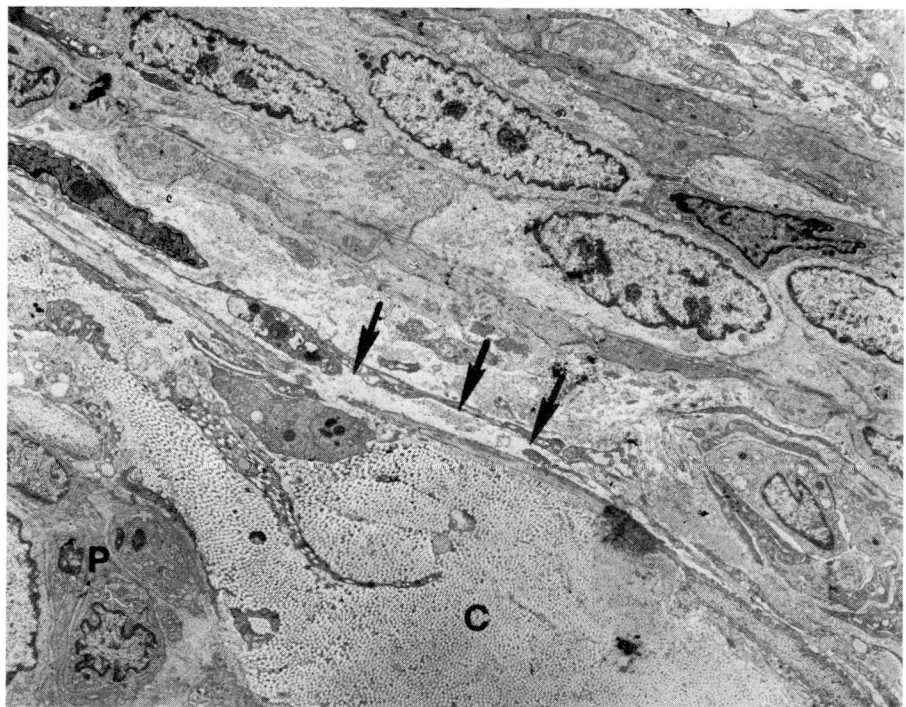

Figure 5–2. Kaposi's sarcoma plaque.

This micrograph shows the spindle-shaped cells with oval nuclei to good advantage. The development of a narrow, cleft-like space is seen *(arrows).* A large amount of collagen (C) has already infiltrated this lesion. P, a cluster of plasma cells. (×4200)

either case, one would have to assume that the cells lining the clefts elaborate a large amount of water-soluble substance(s) which cannot be preserved by currently available techniques. Furthermore, it is likely that the rigidity of the collagen mesh, which is characteristic for Kaposi's sarcoma, prevents the collapse of the clefts during the dehydration and embedding procedures.

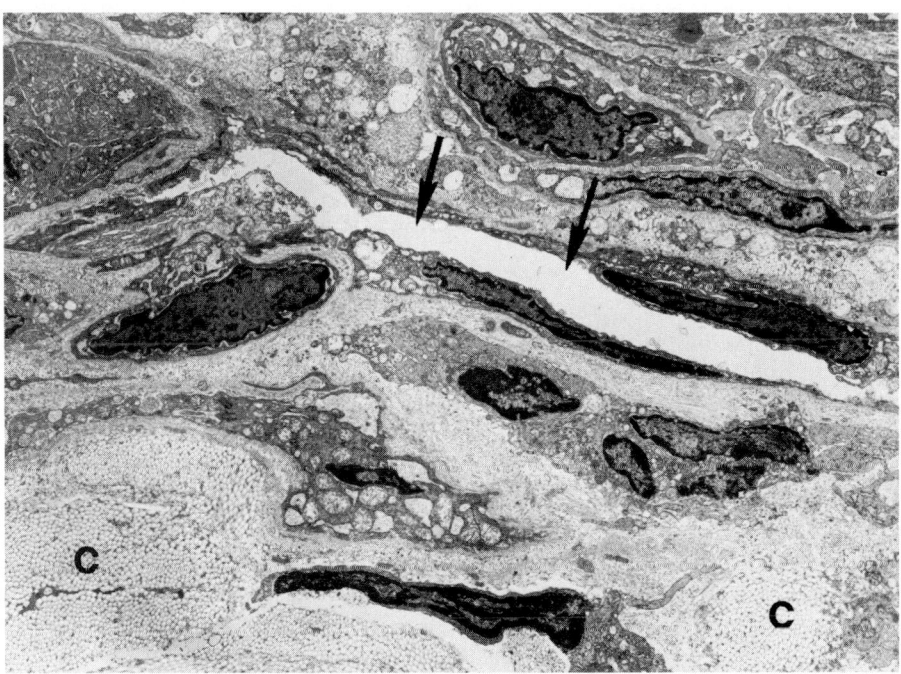

Figure 5–3. Kaposi's sarcoma plaque.

Cleft-like space lined by spindle-shaped cells has an "empty" appearance *(arrows)*. Distorted cells with an abundance of rough endoplasmic reticulum could represent plasma cells or fibroblasts (see text). C, collagen. (×5000)

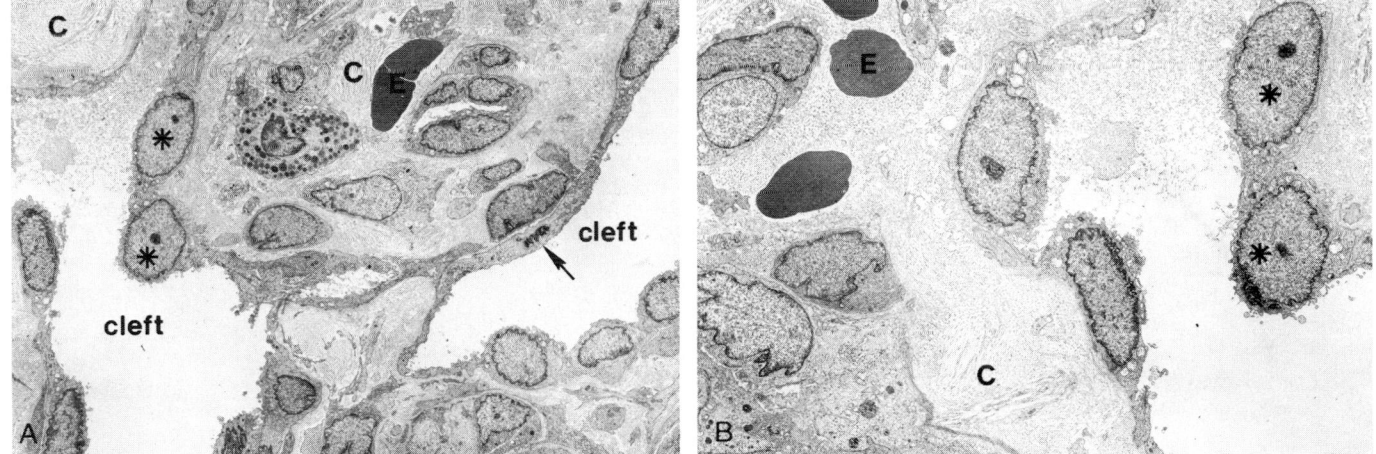

Figure 5–4. Kaposi's sarcoma plaque.

A, Thin section of a Kaposi's sarcoma plaque illustrates two "empty"-appearing clefts. The erythrocytes (E) are surrounded by collagen (C), remote from any blood vessel. The granulated cell is a tissue mast cell. The area to the left of the cells indicated by asterisks is seen at higher magnification in *B*. The arrow indicates a cell that contains tubuloreticular structures shown at higher magnification in Figure 5–7. C, collagen. (×1900)

B, Higher magnification of the cells indicated with an asterisk in *A* and the area adjacent to them. The cells lining the cleft seem to be retracted. Three erythrocytes (E) are located among collagen fibrils. (×3000)

Ultrastructural analysis also confirms that red blood cells have extravasated into extravascular tissue, sometimes into areas which seem remote from any blood vessel (Figure 5–4A and B). Because erythrocytes are not migratory, one can only wonder how the cells have arrived at these sites. It is conceivable that extravasation occurred before fibrosis developed, i.e., that the collagen fibrils seen contiguous to erythrocytes were actually synthesized after disintegration of the blood tissue barrier had occurred. Early lesions show some infiltration with inflammatory cells and mononuclear leukocytes, among which plasma cells are prominent (Figure 5–5). Regarding the last-named cell, it should be realized that fibroblasts are also basophilic on light microscopy, that both cell types have large amounts of rough endoplasmic reticulum on electron microscopy, and that both plasma cells and fibroblasts may have a distorted surface configuration in neoplastic tissues. Therefore, one may, at times, be hard put to tell the cells apart in lesions of Kaposi's sarcoma (Figure 5–5). Immunohistochemistry or fluorescence microscopy utilizing antisera to immunoglobulin or collagen can settle the dilemma. In some lesions, even those limited to the plaque stage, the bulk of the biopsy specimen may consist of collagen. Distorted tumor cells, fibroblasts as well as plasma cells, lymphocytes, and phagocytic histiocytes are then seen dispersed among thick bundles of collagen fibrils (Figures 5–6A and B).

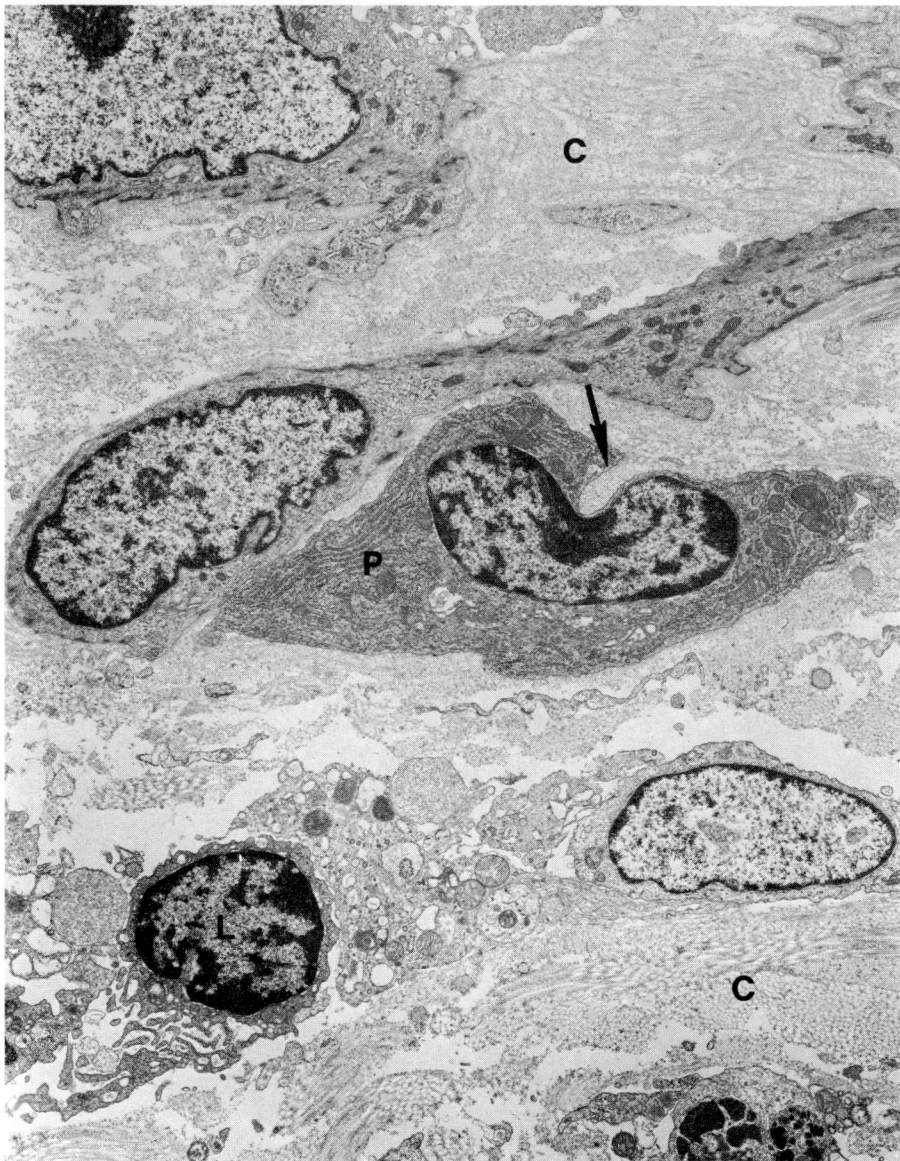

Figure 5–5. Kaposi's sarcoma lesion.

Survey of Kaposi's sarcoma lesion. The cell in the center (P) could be a plasma cell because its cytoplasm is replete with rough endoplasmic reticulum. However, it is invaginated by collagen fibrils *(arrow)*, raising the possibility that it is a fibroblast which may have been responsible for the synthesis of the collagen. Only immunohistochemistry could resolve this question. The cell labeled L is probably a B lymphocyte showing villous processes. At the bottom, right, a portion of a phagocytic cell containing debris is evident. C, collagen. (×7700)

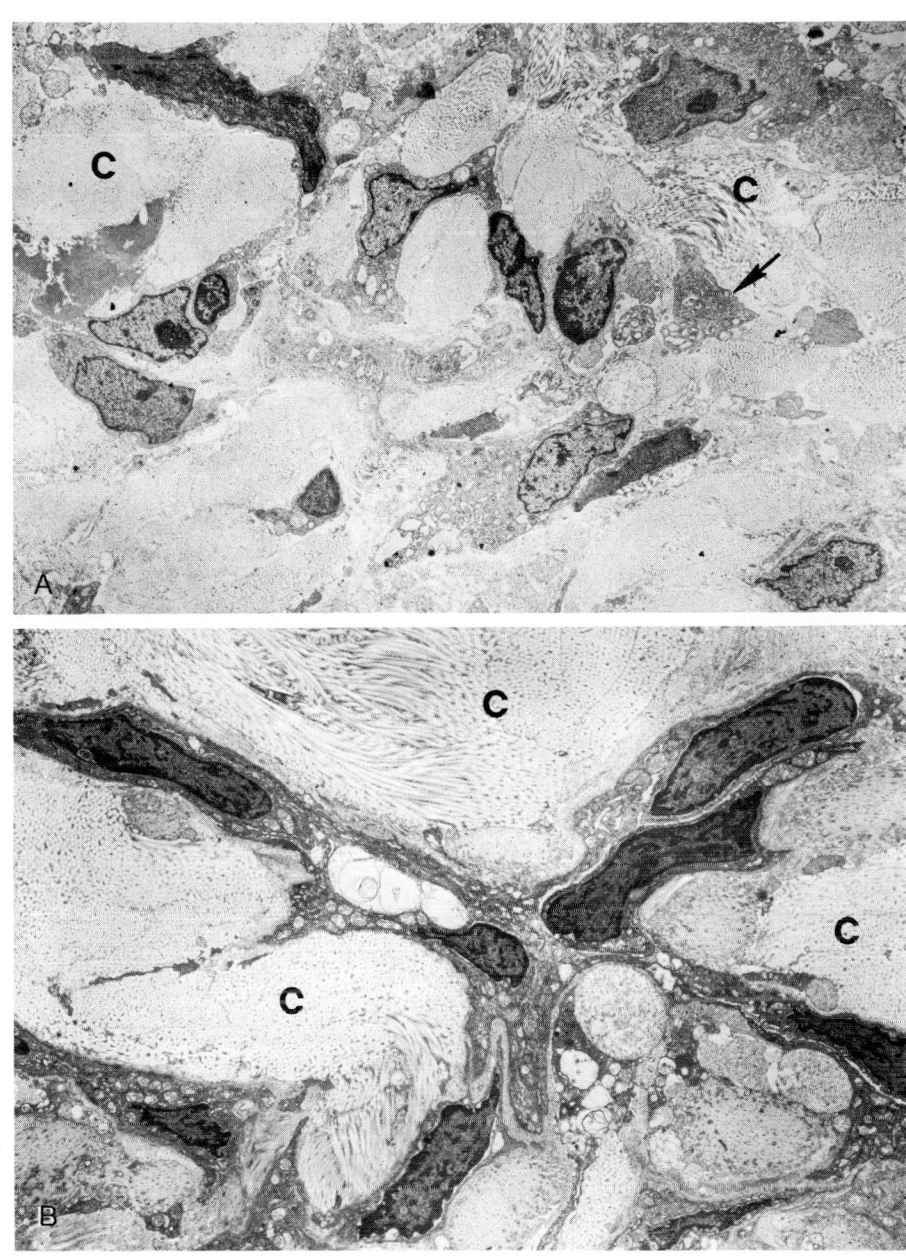

Figure 5–6. Kaposi's sarcoma lesion.

A, Different areas in the same Kaposi's sarcoma lesion illustrate the extent of fibrosis which frequently develops *(B)*. Distorted fibroblasts, plasma cells, and tumor cells are scattered among thick bundles of collagen *(C)*. Arrow indicates portion of a plasma cell. (*A*, ×3200; *B*, ×4700)

Tubuloreticular Structures

On a subcellular level, there are two types of inclusions which will be observed sooner or later by anyone who subjects Kaposi's sarcoma or other biopsy material obtained from patients with AIDS to electron microscopy. The most prevalent of these inclusions is the tubuloreticular structure. This consists of a system of undulating tubules which measure 25 to 30 nm in diameter and appear to arise from the endoplasmic reticulum (Figures 5–7 and 5–8). The structures were first described by Sinkovics et al.[1] and have since been seen in numerous diseases. The highest frequency of tubuloreticular structures is found in patients with connective tissue disorders, particularly systemic lupus erythematosus, but the structures are also seen in patients with cancer and in a large variety of virus infections.[2] Although, morphologically, tubuloreticular structures may look like measles viruses or the nucleocapsids of some paramyxoviruses, they cannot be digested with RNase or DNase, an observation which puts their viral nature in question. In addition, it has been reported that the structures can be induced by treating cultured lymphocytes with 5-bromodeoxyuridine.[3] However, this maneuver does not help to settle the question as to their viral identity either, because it is known that halogenated pyrimidines activate tumor viruses. More recently, several investigators have reported that alpha and beta interferons, but not gamma interferon, causes the development of tubuloreticular structures.[4] Cancer patients who are treated with interferon appear to develop the structures. Therefore, a relationship between the tubuloreticular structures and viral infections or interferon production is likely. In any event, for these reasons, it is not surprising that the structures are seen in all patients with AIDS and probably in all Kaposi's sarcoma biopsies.

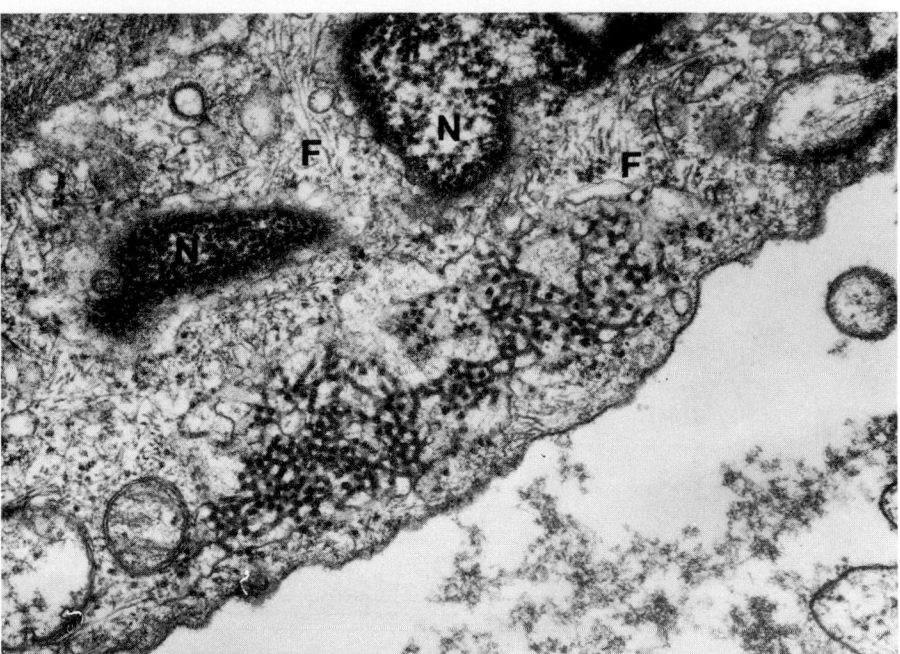

Figure 5–7. Kaposi's sarcoma lesion.
Detail of the cell indicated by the arrow in Figure 5–4A shows tubuloreticular structure. The tubules arise from smooth endoplasmic reticulum. Also note that the cytoplasm of this cell is replete with microfilaments (F). N, nucleus. ($\times$45,000)

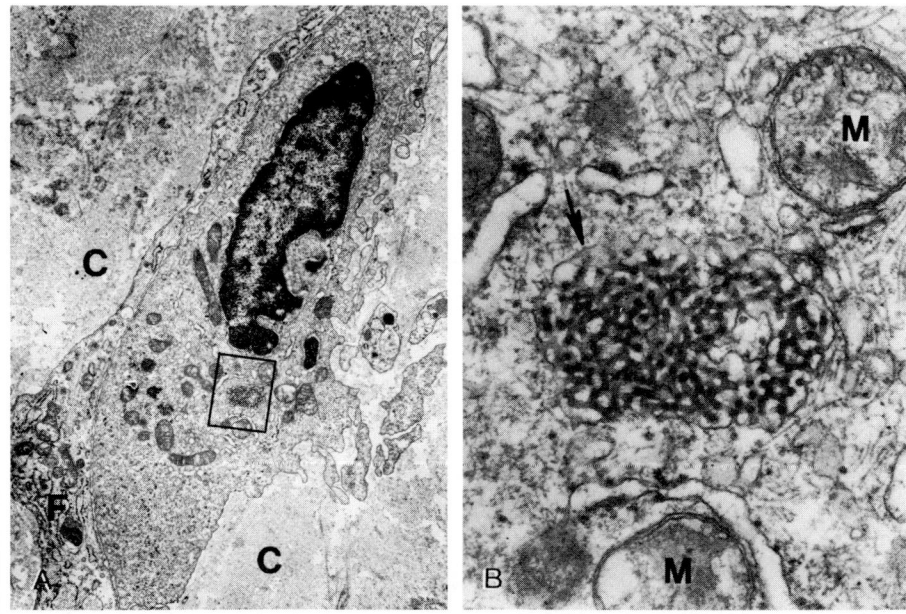

Figure 5–8. Kaposi's sarcoma lesion.
A, A spindle-shaped cell in Kaposi's sarcoma lesion chosen to show tubuloreticular structure in area demarcated by rectangle. C, collagen. The cell at left bottom is believed to be a fibroblast because of the abundance of rough endoplasmic reticulum. The area within the rectangle is shown at higher magnification in B. ($\times$7000)
B, Tubuloreticular structure demarcated by rectangle in A shown at higher resolution. The tubular nature of the inclusion is clearly seen (see text). M, mitochondrion. Arrow indicates smooth endoplasmic reticulum. ($\times$51,000)

Confronting Cisternae

The second structure that warrants brief discussion is the so-called confronting cisterna. This is seen in only 20 to 30 per cent of patients with AIDS and in a much smaller percentage of Kaposi's sarcoma lesions.[5] One of the earliest descriptions dealt with the development of confronting cisternae in herpesvirus-infected tissue culture cells. Since that time, they have been observed in rat hepatomas, fibrosarcoma, rhabdomyosarcoma, giant cell tumor of bone, and multiple sclerosis (for review, see Chadially[6]). Perhaps significant in relation to AIDS is the observation that confronting cisternae are seen in hepatocytes of chimpanzees inoculated with serum from patients with non-A, non-B hepatitis.[7] It is likely that many patients with this syndrome carry the virus. In our material, confronting cisternae have been observed in hepatocytes, lymphocytes, monocytes, and plasma cells as well as in the cells constituting Kaposi's sarcoma (Figures 5–9 and 5–10).

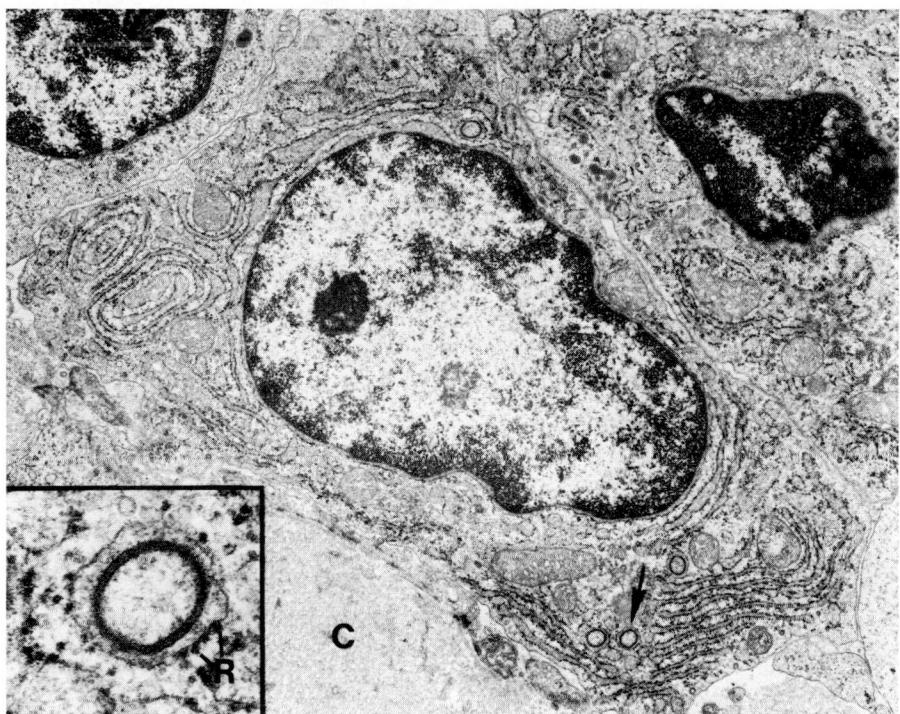

Figure 5–9. Plasma cell.

Plasma cell in a hypertrophic lymph node from a patient with AIDS. Four confronting cisternae are seen. The one indicated by the arrow is shown at higher magnification in the inset. The structure consists of two membranes which enclose electron-opaque material. It occupies a cistern of rough endoplasmic reticulum, as evidenced by the attached ribosomes (R). C, collagen. The cell at upper right is also a plasma cell, whereas the cell on the left appears to be a lymphocyte. (×11,500; inset, ×76,000)

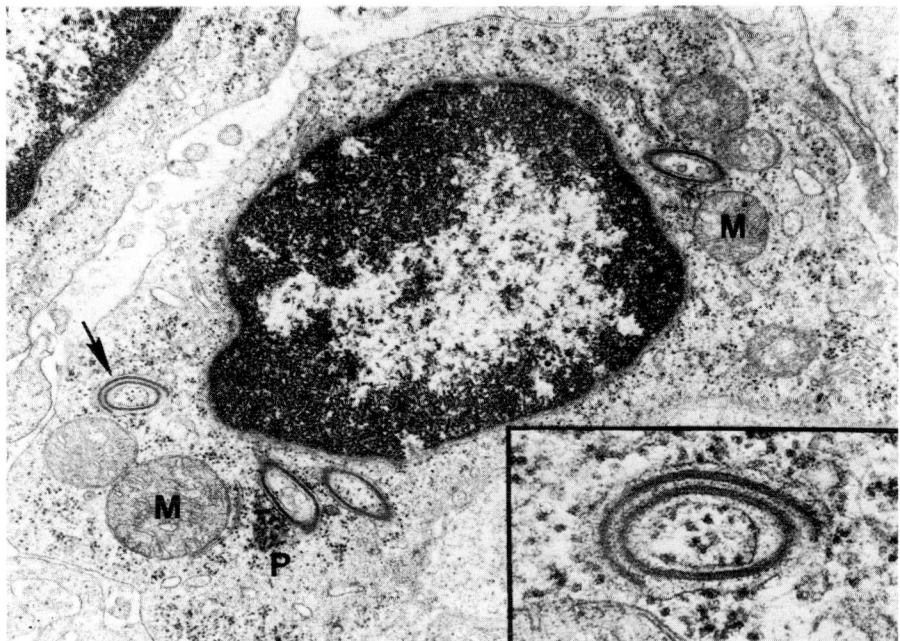

Figure 5–10. Lymphocyte.

Lymphocyte in a lymph node biopsy from a patient with AIDS shows four confronting cisternae. The one indicated by the arrow is shown at higher magnification in the inset. Such reduplication of confronting cisternae is rare. M, mitochondria; P, unidentified particles. (×22,000; inset, ×71,000)

Other Findings at Biopsy

Many unusual, less well defined inclusions seen in the tissues of patients afflicted with AIDS are secondary to infections with a large variety of viruses, fungi, and other opportunistic microorganisms. This is particularly confusing in lymph node biopsies and bronchial aspirates. The lymph nodes undergo a dynamic process which commences with follicular hyperplasia as well as hyperplasia of the paracortical area. Initially, there are no features which distinguish these hypertrophic nodes from those associated with benign infections or inflammatory processes. Gradually, however, the intense proliferation of lymphocytes and plasma cells obliterates normal nodal architecture. Terminally, there is involution and fibrosis. These changes are not entirely symmetric, i.e., within the same node, one area may still be hyperplastic while a contiguous area may already show fibrosis. The inclusions described before are also seen in the lymph nodes. With some search, sporadic virus and virus-like particles are also found in fresh tissue isolates, but with the exception of the cytomegalovirus, culture of specimens is necessary for virus identification. Therefore, a description of viruses will be omitted here.

On the other hand, the protean morphologic aspects of *Pneumocystis carinii* are illustrated lest they be mistaken for microorganisms of etiologic significance in the diseases under discussion (Figures 5–11 and 5–12). The life cycle of *Pneumocystis carinii* is incompletely understood, and its ultrastructural characteristics have been only partially described. Yet, this organism harbors particles that are reminiscent of phage, and the outer wall of the mature cysts tend to "bud" like viruses off mammalian cell membranes (Figure 5–12). Familiarity with these structures may facilitate interpretation of bronchial aspirates or biopsies obtained from these patients.

To all the above must be added that under the best of circumstances, the ultrastructure of biopsy specimens obtained from desperately ill patients is difficult to preserve, even when fixation of such tissues is performed at the bedside. Besides the tissue destruction which is part and parcel of the underlying disease, the infiltration with local anesthetics, pressure of surgical instruments, and the almost inevitable delay in laboratory processing introduce alterations which may arouse the curiosity of the investigator, but which, in the end, prove to be of little significance.[8]

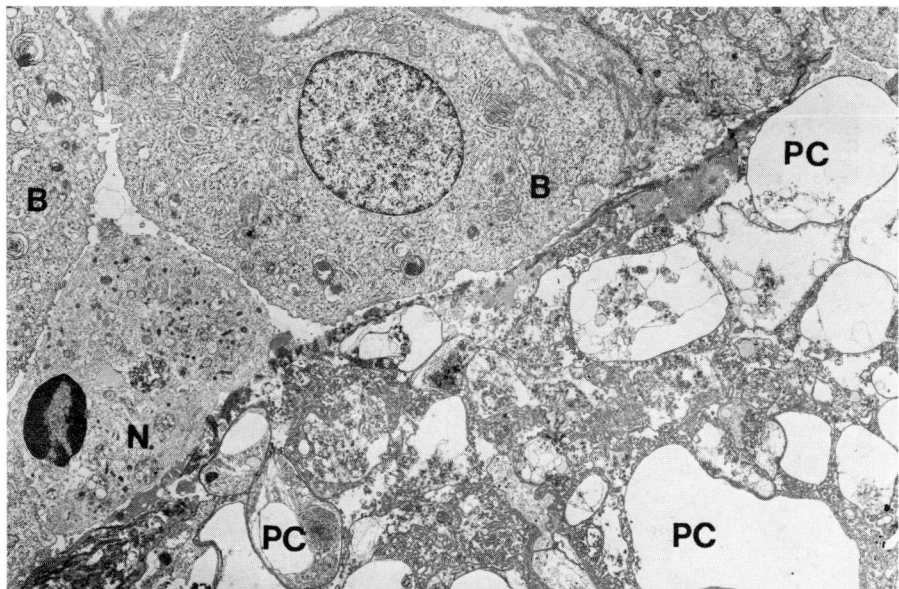

Figure 5–11. Bronchial biopsy.

Bronchial biopsy obtained from a patient with AIDS and *Pneumocystis carinii* (PC) infection. The microorganism, (seen in various phases of development and disintegration) is surrounded by debris. B, bronchial epithelial cells. N, polymorphonuclear leukocyte. (×5700)

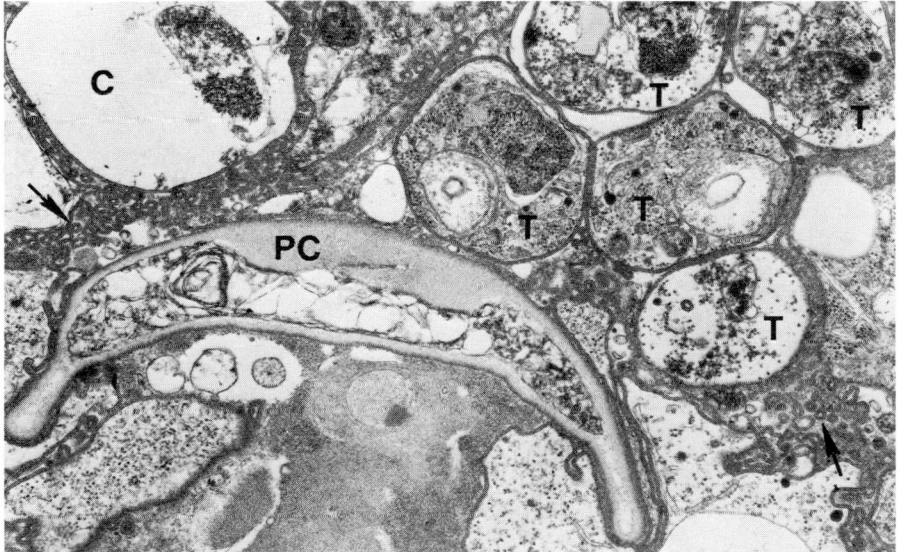

Figure 5–12. Cyst of *Pneumocystis carinii.*

Longitudinal section through a collapsed *Pneumocystis carinii* cyst (PC). Note the thickness of the wall. Developing trophozoites, T. Arrows indicate particles with virus-like morphologic appearance that seem to pinch off cyst walls. (×23,000)

Acknowledgment

The studies were supported in part by grant AM 012274 from the National Institutes of Health.
The help of George Gusky and Susan Dittmar is gratefully acknowledged.

References

1. Sinkovics JG, Gyorkey F, Thoma GW: A rapidly fatal case of systemic lupus erythematosus: Structures resembling viral nucleoprotein strands in the kidney and activities of lymphocytes in culture. Tex Rep Biol Med 27:887–908, 1969.
2. Schaff Z, Barry DW, Grimley PM: Cytochemistry of tubuloreticular structures in lymphocytes from patients with systemic lupus erythematosus and in cultured human lymphoid cells: Comparison to a paramyxovirus. Lab Invest 29:577–586, 1973.
3. Grimley PM, Barry DW, Schaff Z: Induction of tubular structures in the endoplasmic reticulum of human lymphoid cells by treatment with 5-bromo-2′=deoxyuridine. J Natl Cancer Inst 51:1751–1760, 1973.
4. Rich SA, Owens TR, Bartholomew LE, Gutterman JU: Immune interferon does not stimulate formation of alpha or beta interferon induced human lupus-type inclusions. Lancet 1:127–128, 1983.
5. Sidhu G: Ultrastructural markers of AIDS. Lancet 1(8331):990–991, 1983.
6. Ghadially FN: Ultrastructural Pathology of the Cell and Matrix. Boston, Butterworths, 1982, pp 372–377.
7. Jackson D, Tabor E, Gerety RJ: Acute non-A, non-B hepatitis: Specific ultrastructural alterations in endoplasmic reticulum of infected hepatocytes. Lancet 1:1249–1250, 1979.
8. Zucker-Franklin D: "Looking" for the cause of AIDS. N Engl J Med 308:837–838, 1983.

6

Cutaneous Signs of AIDS
Other Than Kaposi's Sarcoma

Clay J. Cockerell

The acquired immune deficiency syndrome (AIDS) may be manifest in many different ways. Patients may suffer from serious internal illnesses, or they may show only innocuous external signs. Because of the grave nature of this ailment, it is of utmost importance that the clinician be cognizant of the early and subtle cutaneous features of this disease. Once the diagnosis has been made, treatment should be instituted as soon as possible. Many clinical signs of AIDS are manifest in the skin. The astute physician should suspect and diagnose this syndrome using the most basic tool of physical diagnosis, namely, visual inspection.

Certain cutaneous symptoms may reflect an opportunistic infectious disease with a profound underlying immunodeficiency. The infectious diseases may be due to viral, bacterial, fungal, or protozoan organisms. Cutaneous manifestations of noninfectious disorders also associated with AIDS may be induced by an external agent, such as a drug (i.e., drug eruptions or hives), or they may be endogenous (i.e., nonspecific pruritus or intracutaneous hemorrhages such as petechiae or ecchymoses related to thrombocytopenia). The occurrence of Kaposi's sarcoma lesions present on the skin or oral mucosa in high-risk individuals may be sufficient to make the diagnosis of AIDS. In other instances, the physician may be able only to suspect that a given patient may later develop the syndrome.

In this chapter we describe the various cutaneous and mucocutaneous signs other than Kaposi's sarcoma which are frequently associated with AIDS. First, the infectious diseases that affect the skin of patients with the syndrome will be described. Then, the noninfectious skin disorders that may lead one to suspect a diagnosis of AIDS will be discussed.

Infectious Skin Diseases

Cytomegalovirus Infection
(Figures 6–1 to 6–4)

The cytomegalovirus is a common pathogen in immunosuppressed patients, those with AIDS notwithstanding. The most common manifestations of cytomegalovirus (CMV) inclusion disease are systemic rather than cutaneous; however, the skin may be involved. Petechiae and purpura sometimes related to thrombocytopenia induced by CMV are common cutaneous signs of this systemic viral infection. Although vesicular or bullous eruptions are rarely seen, a generalized morbilliform skin eruption involving the trunk and extremities is more associated with CMV infection.[1] Occasionally, hyperpigmented indurated cutaneous plaques have been reported as heralding a disseminated cytomegalovirus infection.[2] There is one case report of a generalized bullous toxic epidermal necrolysis-like eruption described in association with cytomegalovirus hepatitis in a patient with AIDS.[3] Bluish red cutaneous papules and nodules have been reported in association with pediatric AIDS during the neonatal period which, when biopsied, consisted of foci of extramedullary hematopoietic tissue.[4]

An additional cutaneous manifestation of cytomegalovirus infection is that of persistent perianal ulcerations which resemble the perianal ulcerations seen with anogenital herpes simplex.[5] Unlike herpetic ulcerations, ulcers due to cytomegalovirus do not respond to topical treatments such as sitz baths and compresses. All patients we examined who had ulcers such as these also had coexistent intractable proctitis or colitis with diarrhea that was caused by enteric CMV infection. The CMV ulcers most likely represent a continuous spread of the infection to the skin from the gastrointestinal tract. Patients with CMV ulcerations are usually thought to have persistent herpes simplex infection.

Biopsy, light microscopic, and electron microscopic examination of biopsy specimen or virus isolation are required to confirm the diagnosis and pathogenesis. The finding of CMV-induced perianal ulcers confers a grave prognosis. Although experimental new treatment with dihydroxypropoxylguanine (DHPG) has been shown to be effective in AIDS patients who developed this infectious complication, most patients died within two months following the diagnosis. Persistent ulceration of the perianal area not responsive to the conventional therapy for ulcers should be biopsied in search of the characteristic intranuclear inclusions of CMV.

It should also be remembered that occasionally ulcerations may be caused by more than one infectious agent. It is not uncommon to find cells containing inclusions of CMV along with characteristic multinucleated giant cells of herpes simplex. In addition, one case has been reported in which skin lesions were found to contain acid-fast bacilli as well as cells infected with CMV and herpesvirus.[6] Thus, it is important to identify all infectious agents in a patient with AIDS because therapy for each disease differs dramatically.

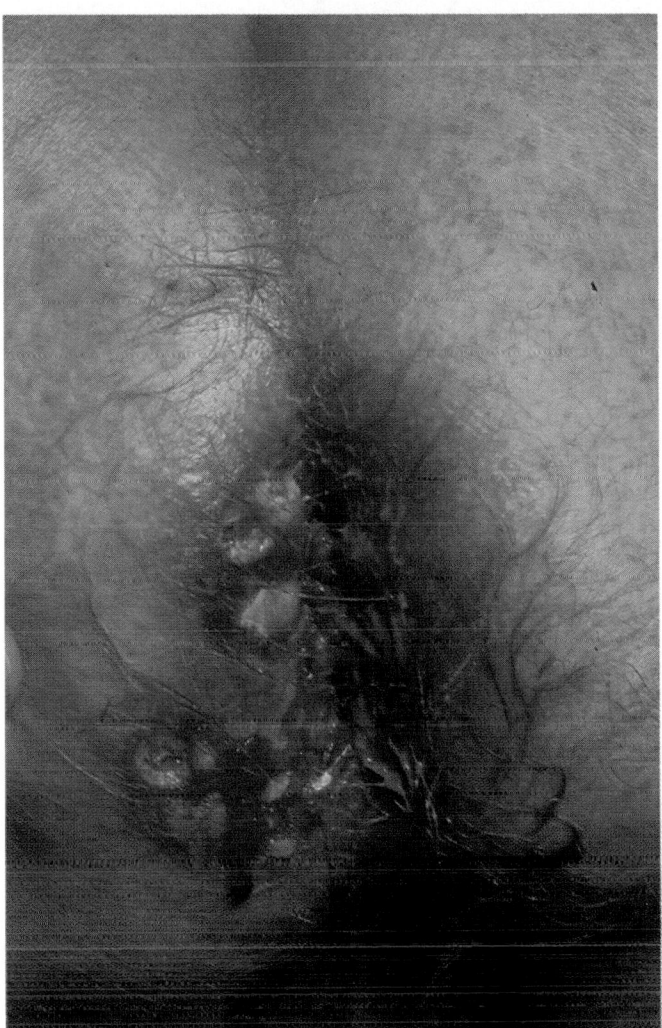

Figure 6–1. Cytomegalovirus ulcerations.

Necrotizing nonhealing perianal ulcerations due to cytomegalovirus in a patient with AIDS. This is the most common cutaneous manifestation of cytomegalovirus infection.

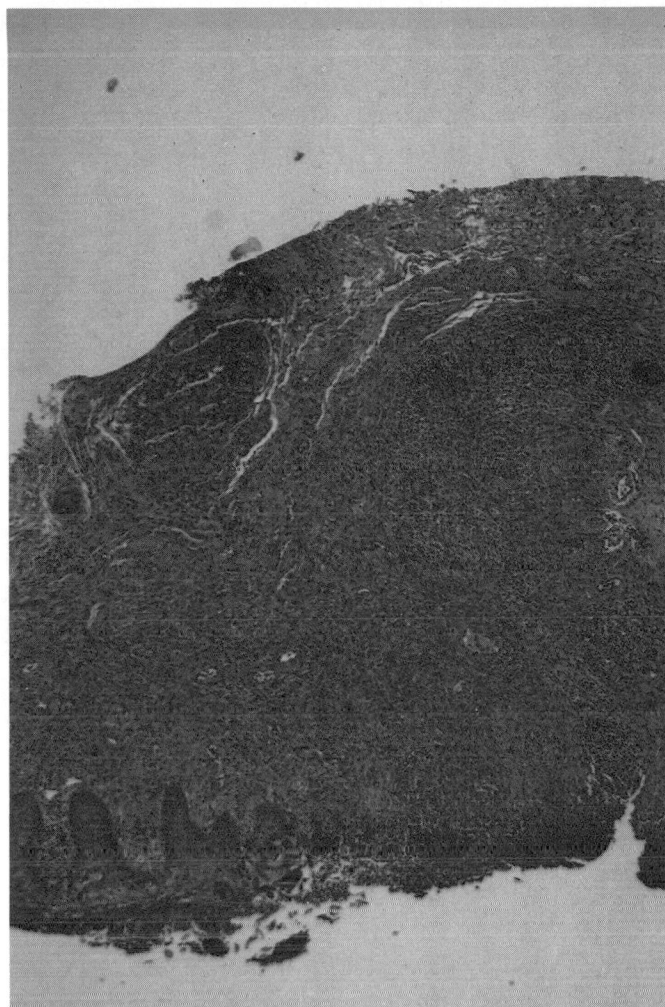

Figure 6–2. Cytomegalovirus ulceration.

This punch biopsy taken from near a mucous membrane shows an ulceration with a dense inflammatory cell infiltrate.

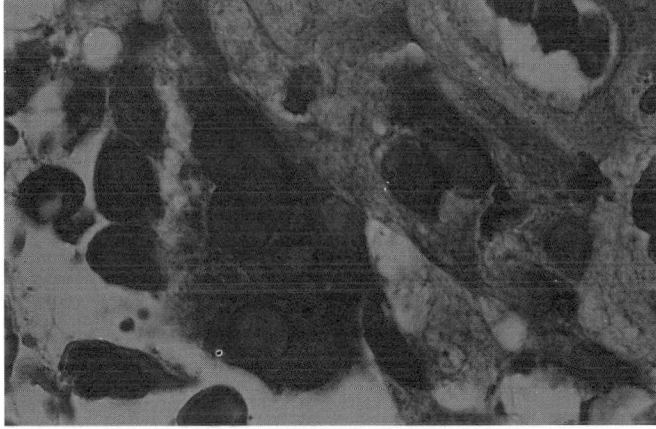

Figure 6–3. Herpes simplex ulcer.

Higher magnification at the surface of the ulcer shows multinucleated giant cells of herpes simplex virus infection.

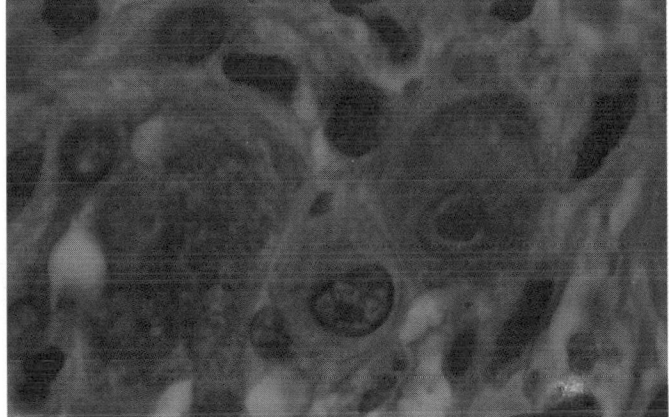

Figure 6–4. Cytomegalovirus ulceration.

Another area taken from beneath the ulceration shows giant fibroblasts with intranuclear and intracytoplasmic purplish inclusion bodies of cytomegalovirus. Thus, perianal ulcerations may be caused by more than one infectious agent.

Herpes Zoster and Herpes Simplex
(Figures 6–5 to 6–8)

Herpes zoster infection is thought to result from reactivation of a latent varicella-zoster virus infection in the dorsal root ganglion of patients with previous varicella infection, and it is usually manifested by painful clusters of vesicles in a localized neurodermatomal distribution. The vesicles often lie on a patch of erythema. In AIDS patients the initially localized zoster infection often becomes generalized with widely disseminated vesicles appearing at distant sites from the original dermatome involved. In some cases of disseminated zoster, lung and central nervous system involvement occurs. Often the patient may require hospitalization. The severe zoster infections seen in patients with AIDS or AIDS-related complex tend to leave residual scars more often than is usually found in other patients; however, the incidence of postherpetic neuralgia does not appear to be greater in AIDS patients despite the severity of the acute zoster infection. Herpes zoster, *Candida albicans,* and herpes simplex infections are found to occur with greater frequency in patients with AIDS. It is known that herpes zoster infections occur in other individuals with defects in their cell-mediated immunity, such as patients with Hodgkin's disease, those with chronic lymphocytic leukemia, and in iatrogenically immunosuppressed organ transplant recipients. Even otherwise "healthy" zoster patients have a diminished *in vitro* cell-mediated response to the varicella-zoster viral antigen during acute disease. The occurrence of herpes zoster infection in a patient from a high-risk group for developing AIDS should alert the physician to the possibility of the impending development of AIDS-related diseases.[7]

Patients with AIDS, as well as those with other immunodeficiency disorders, are often plagued by severe recurrent herpes simplex infections. These infections are often more extensive, last longer, and are less responsive to antiviral therapy with acyclovir than herpes simplex infections occurring in healthy hosts.

Although uncommon, when herpes simplex infection is disseminated, as in some AIDS patients, the entire skin surface may be studded with individual lesions and clusters of erythematous papules and vesicles. Anogenital herpetic infections in the immunocompromised host can be prolonged and painful, often with extensive perianal ulcerations and erosions which may become superinfected with bacterial organisms as a result of secondary contamination. Patients with this degree of involvement require stool softeners and careful attention to maintenance of cleanliness in the infected area. These persistent herpetic infections are best treated with intravenous acyclovir when they are severe; prophylaxis with oral acyclovir may be beneficial in some patients to lessen the number and frequency of recurrent attacks.

Molluscum Contagiosum
(Figure 6–9)

Molluscum contagiosum is an infection of the skin characterized by pearly, yellowish, waxy papular lesions often with a central umbilication caused by a poxvirus which is often spread by close contact. Mollusca contagiosa papules are commonly seen any place on the skin of children. In sexually active young adults, the pubic and inner thigh areas are frequently involved. In patients with AIDS, cutaneous infections with molluscum contagiosum are widely disseminated; the lesions are more numerous and can be several times larger than those usually seen in children. Occasionally, the lesions may be confused with basal cell carcinomas or ordinary nevi. In general, molluscum papules are easily eradicated by simple curettage or cryosurgery with the topical application of liquid nitrogen; lesions found in AIDS patients, however, are often refractory to treatment and tend to recur and spread with greater frequency.

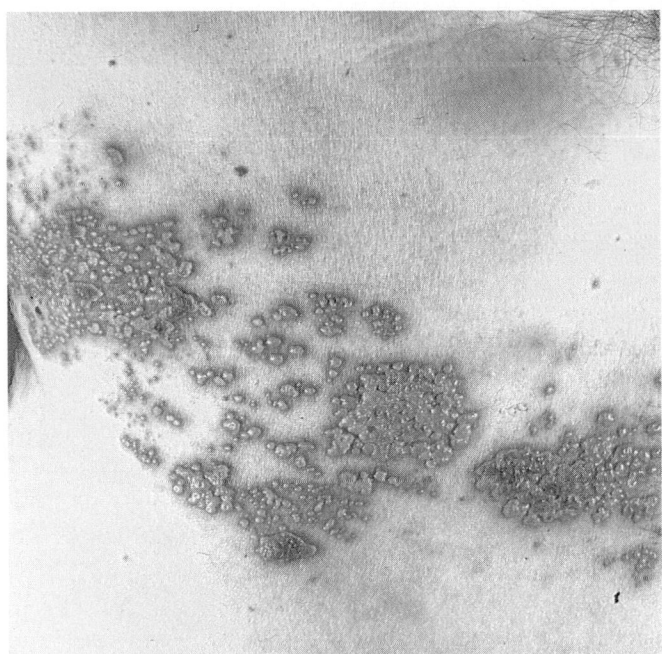

Figure 6–5. Herpes zoster.

Painful vesicles on an erythematous base in a dermatomal distribution is virtually pathognomonic for this condition caused by the varicella zoster virus. This infection may be a harbinger that the patient may later develop bona fide AIDS.

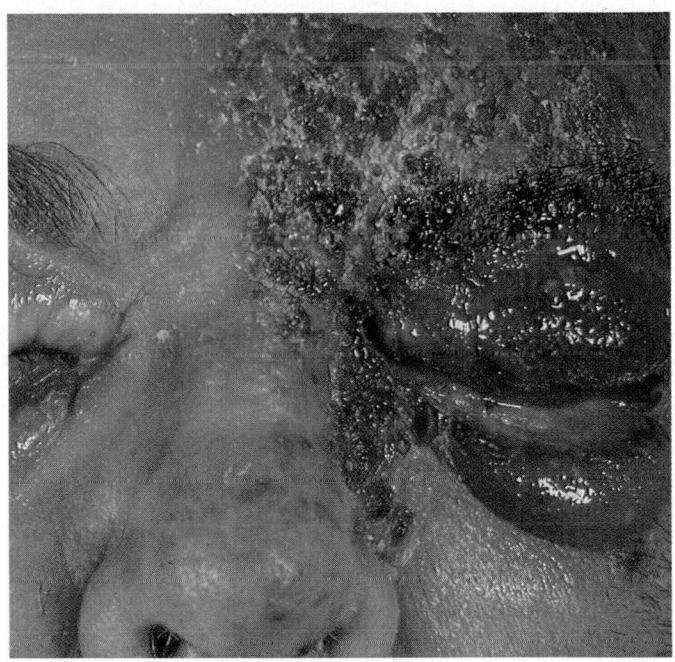

Figure 6–6. Herpes zoster.

Infections may be severe and fulminant in immunocompromised patients.

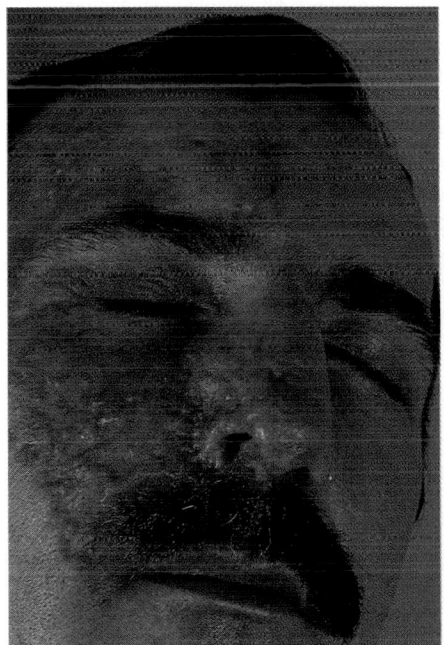

Figure 6–7. Herpes zoster.

Severe residual scarring of the face occurring as a sequela to herpes zoster. This complication is more frequent in patients with AIDS.

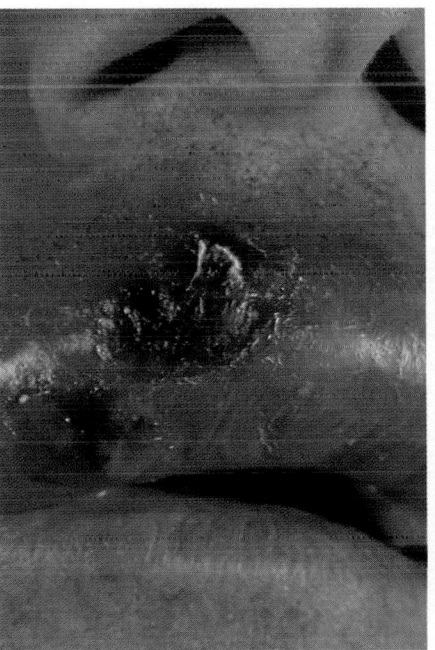

Figure 6–8. Herpes simplex ulcers.

Herpes simplex infections may be persistent and result in chronic necrotizing ulcers.

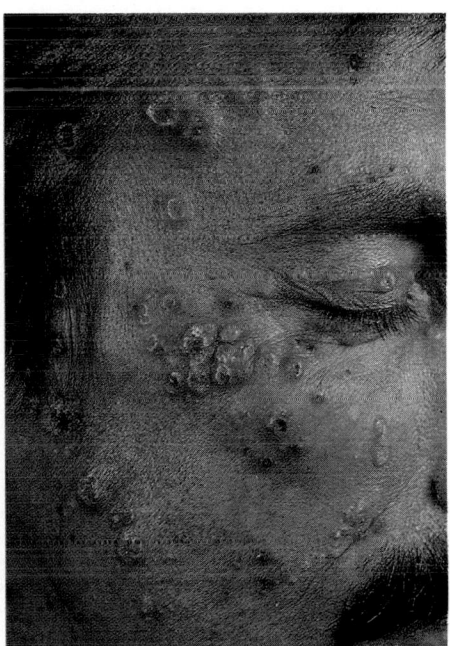

Figure 6–9. Molluscum contagiosum.

Numerous large umbilicated waxy papules of molluscum contagiosum are seen on the face of this patient with AIDS. They have coalesced to form crusted plaques. They may be seen on other body parts as well.

Verruca Vulgaris and Condylomata Acuminata (Figures 6–10 to 6–12)

Other viral skin infections, such as verruca vulgaris, are often seen in patients with AIDS. They tend to occur in the same areas as in healthy adults, but in greater numbers, and seem to be quite resistant to standard therapies. There are no data regarding the specific subtype of human papillomaviruses which are involved in these patients. However, the warts may be of several different clinical varieties: extensive flat and filiform warts, often found in the bearded area of the face, exuberant cauliflower-like plaques of confluent condylomata acuminata of the anogenital region; or multiple and large hyperkeratotic verruca vulgaris, commonly seen especially on or around the fingers. Multiple plantar warts have also been observed.

Hairy Leukoplakia (Figures 6–13 to 6–16)

A unique oral mucosal lesion known as "hairy leukoplakia" has recently been described exclusively to date only in patients at risk for AIDS and those afflicted with AIDS. Whitish, corrugated, verrucous plaques are seen on the lateral margins of the tongue and buccal mucosa.[8] Clinically, these lesions may resemble and be misdiagnosed as candidiasis. Unlike thrush, when plaques of hairy leukoplakia are scraped with a tongue depressor or other blunt instrument, the whitish surface cannot be rubbed away. Histochemical and electron microscopic evidence demonstrates the presence of human papillomavirus as well as Epstein-Barr virus particles in these lesions. It has been suggested that this unique mucosal lesion may be due to the Epstein-Barr virus.[9] Histologic examination of tissue is required for confirmation of the diagnosis. A recent clinical treatment trial showed that the hairy leukoplakia lesions resolved during treatment with acyclovir, an antiviral agent, in high doses of 800 mg qid for two weeks.[10] These findings support the hypothesis that the lesions are caused by a member of the herpes group of viruses.

Hairy leukoplakia has been seen almost exclusively in HIV-antibody–positive homosexual men, even those who are asymptomatic individuals, although it is more common among gay men with HIV-related diseases, including those with persistent generalized lymphadenopathy, AIDS-related complex (ARC), and with AIDS. A few cases of hairy leukoplakia have been reported in women with HIV infection and a hemophiliac with AIDS.[11]

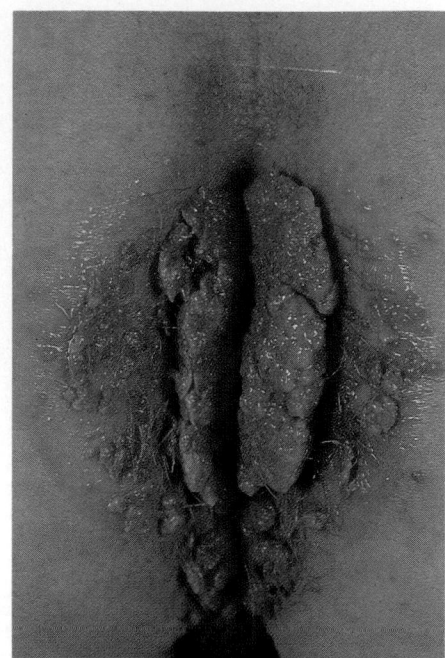

Figure 6–10. Condyloma acuminatum.

Multiple vegetating coalescing condyloma acuminatum in the perianal area of a patient with AIDS. When this is extensive, problems with anal blockage may occur.

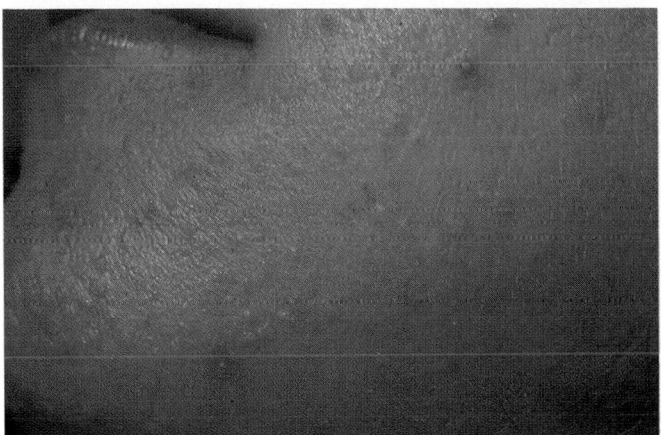

Figure 6–11. Warts.

Myriad skin-colored flat warts can occasionally be seen in patients with AIDS. Such lesions are virtually impossible to eradicate.

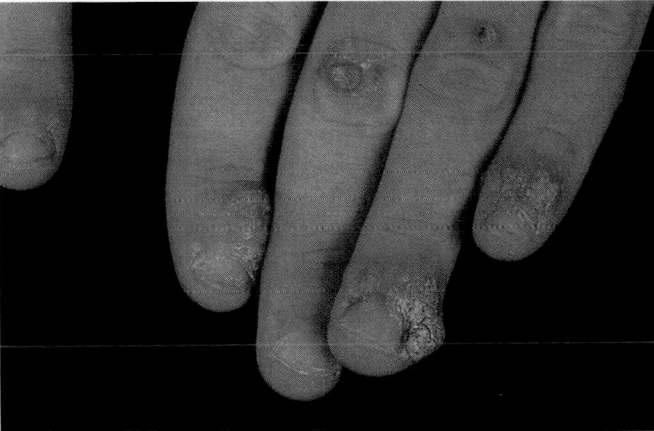

Figure 6–12. Verrucous papules.

Hyperkeratotic verrucous papules that coalesce, especially in the periungual area, may pose a therapeutic as well as a cosmetic problem in the AIDS patient.

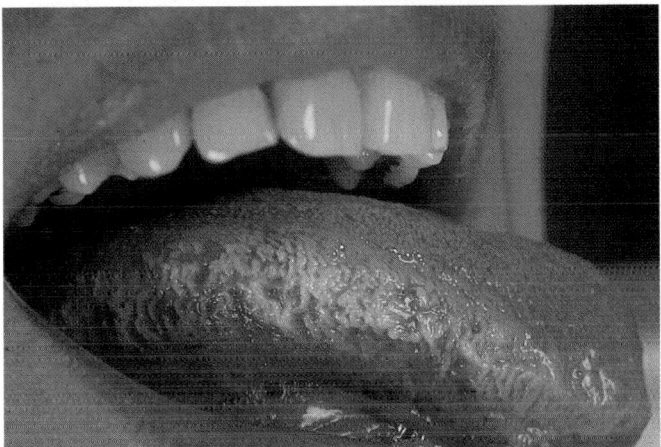

Figure 6–13. Hairy leukoplakia.

Λ whitish verrucous corrugated plaque commonly seen on the lateral surfaces of the tongue is characteristic of this condition; it may be caused by the Epstein-Barr virus. When scraped with a tongue blade or other instrument, the lesion does not wipe away.

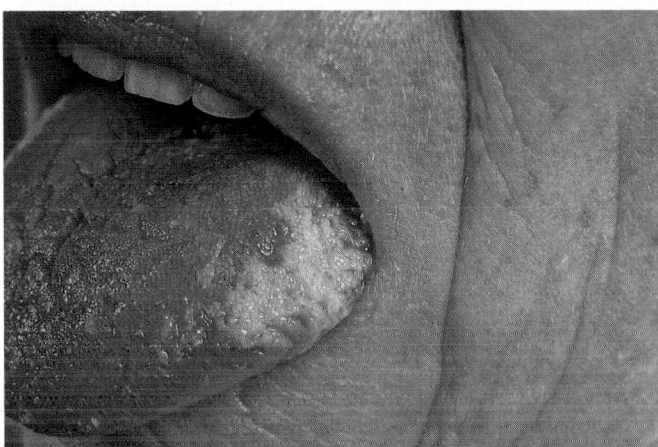

Figure 6–14. Another example of hairy leukoplakia.

In this case, the patient was a woman who had received blood transfusions.

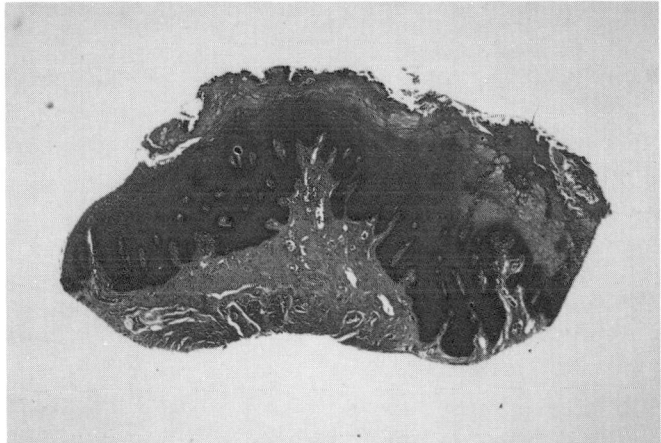

Figure 6–15. Punch biopsy of hairy leukoplakia.

Note the epidermal hyperplasia and pallor of the uppermost portion of the epithelium.

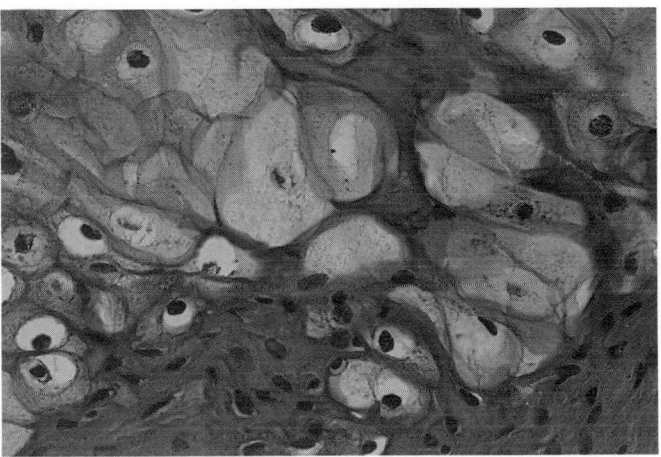

Figure 6–16. Hairy leukoplakia.

Marked ballooning of keratinocytes responsible for pallor seen at lower magnification. The extensive ballooning degeneration is characteristic of hairy leukoplakia.

Folliculitis, Abscesses, Furuncles, and Impetigo

Because the B-cell arm of the host's immune system is also defective in patients with AIDS, infections caused by common bacterial organisms as well as those caused by more virulent bacteria can cause serious but not necessarily life-threatening diseases in a given individual. Acneiform papules and pustules may be widely distributed over the trunk, extremities, and face. Bacterial cultures of such lesions have been found to grow not only "diphtheroids" but *Staphylococcus aureus* and *Streptococcus pneumoniae* as well. In some cases, gram-negative organisms such as *Proteus* species were found. Like many of the other infectious diseases encountered in the patient with AIDS, bacterial infections are often refractory to the usual antibiotic therapy. Of interest is that pustules examined histologically have, in some cases, been distinguished by having numerous eosinophils within the infundibula of hair follicles.[12] The significance of this finding is not yet understood.

Folliculitis may progress to form localized abscesses, furuncles, and even carbuncles (Figure 6–18). Occasionally, cellulitis may supervene. Whereas an immunocompetent individual might be managed as an outpatient, treated with oral antibiotics, the patient with AIDS may require hospitalization and treatment with intravenous antimicrobial agents because the risk of systemic spread of the infection is much greater.

When attempting to isolate the organism causing an abscess, the physician should alert the clinical laboratory to the fact that the patient is immunocompromised so that a search for unusual opportunistic infectious organisms will be undertaken. This may require special handling and culturing methods. Clinically, one may not be able to distinguish a pyogenic infection caused by *Staphylococcus aureus* from one caused by a mycobacterium. Delays in accurate diagnosis can be detrimental for the patient.

Another common skin infection of childhood that is seen quite frequently among patients with AIDS is impetigo, which is caused by coagulase-positive staphylococci and by beta-hemolytic streptococci (Figures 6–17 and 6–19). Although impetigo in children is seen most commonly on the face, in individuals at risk for AIDS and among patients with AIDS-related disease, impetigo is seen more often in the axillary, inguinal, and other intertriginous locations. The infection usually begins as painful red macules which may develop into bullous impetigo with superficial vesicles that rupture, oozing serous or purulent fluid. A characteristic honey-colored surface crust forms, and satellite lesions may develop. Usually, the infection responds readily to systemic and sometimes topical antibiotics. However, in the patient with AIDS, therapeutic response may be delayed.

Not infrequently, impetigo may be superimposed upon and may complicate a herpes infection of the skin.

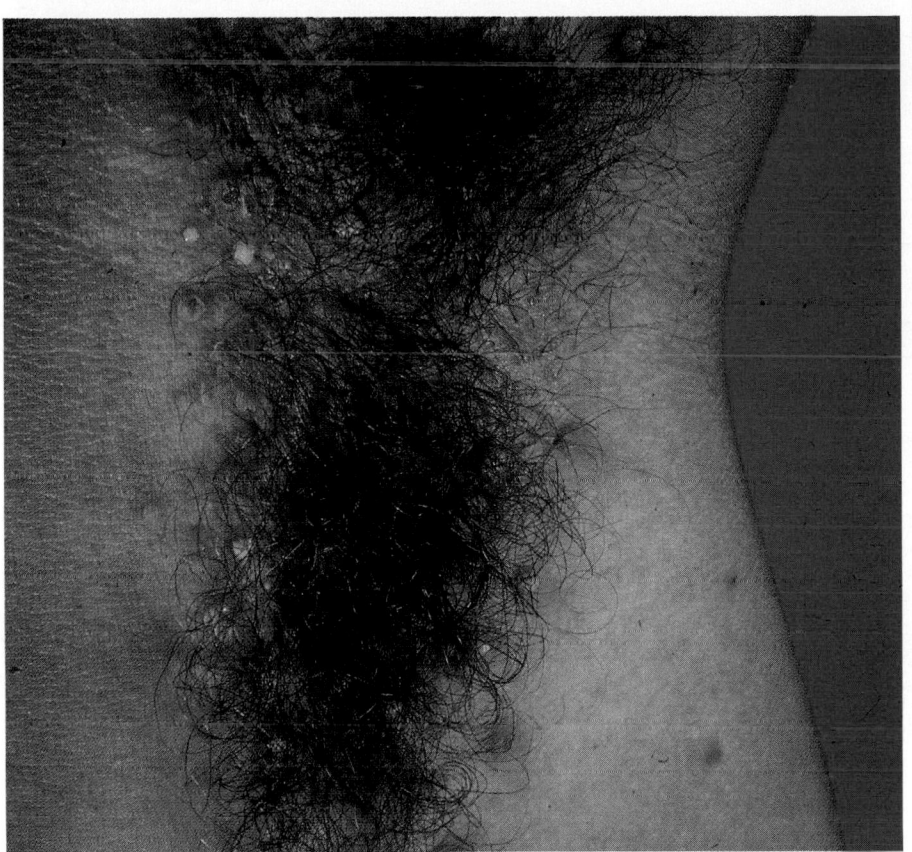

Figure 6–17. Impetigo.
This infection may be widespread and fulminant in patients with AIDS.

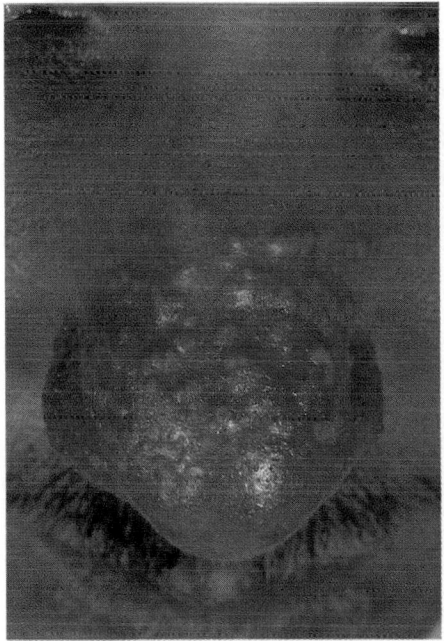

Figure 6–18. Pyoderma.
A severe pyoderma as pictured here may be seen in patients with AIDS. Many different bacterial organisms can cause this clinical syndrome.

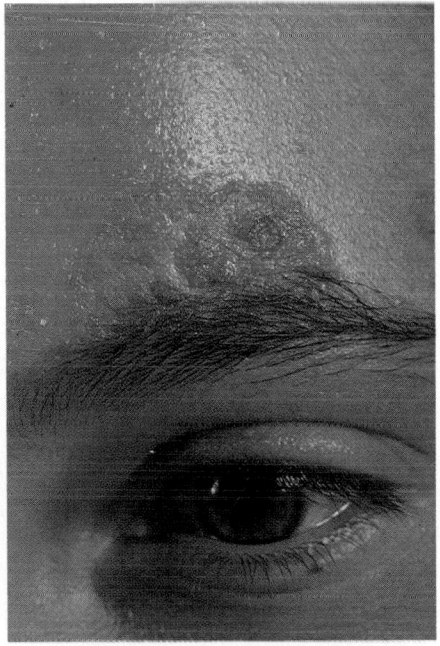

Figure 6–19. Impetigo.
The characteristic erosion covered by a honey-colored crust is pictured here. These infections may be widespread and fulminant in patients with AIDS.

Syphilis
(Figures 6–20 to 6–23)

Although syphilis is a quite common sexually transmitted disease in patients with AIDS, lately it has been observed that many patients have unusual manifestations of this condition and respond to treatment in an unusual fashion. Although the usual characteristic widespread eruption of papules with slight scale involving the trunk, extremities, palms, soles, and mucous membranes is characteristically seen, a number of more unusual manifestations have recently been described. Neal Gregory at New York University Medical Center has seen several patients with rapid progression of syphilis from a primary to a tertiary stage in a matter of months.[13] In one such case florid lesions of secondary syphilis were present on the trunk while a palatal gumma was present concomitantly. In addition, patients have been found to be seronegative for syphilis despite findings of spirochetes in biopsy specimens when silver stains or special immunoperoxidase studies for spirochetes were performed. On some occasions, when secondary lesions were present clinically, the seronegativity observed was found to be due to a prozone phenomenon as a consequence of an improperly diluted very high antibody titer. On the other hand, true seronegative titers have been found as well.

In addition to the unusual cutaneous manifestations of syphilis, increased severity of central nervous system involvement has been noted in patients with AIDS.[15] Severe lancinating pain and meningovascular syphilis have been seen in patients following presumed adequate treatment of secondary syphilis. Often patients require chronic penicillin therapy to keep the infection in check. Furthermore, on occasion, fully developed secondary syphilis, including cutaneous manifestations, has been seen to develop following the usual treatment regimens with intramuscular penicillin G benzathine (Bicillin). Finally, in one unusual case the patient developed a relapse of syphilis following the administration of vaccine, which implied that the alteration of the immune status was enough to trigger latent yet viable organisms of syphilis present within the patient even though he had been treated adequately.[13] Thus, the immune system seems to be unable to totally eradicate syphilis, even with the usual intramuscular regimens of penicillin in this patient population, and consequently careful evaluation for neurosyphilis must be carried out. Furthermore, the serologic testing usually considered quite reliable for patients with syphilis may be completely unreliable in patients with AIDS, and the best test remains a search for treponemes in tissue.

Norwegian Scabies
(Figures 6–24 and 6–25)

Like other patients with immunocompromised states, patients with AIDS may occasionally develop Norwegian scabies. Clinically, this may appear as obvious hyperkeratotic plaques present on the palms, soles, trunk, or extremities, but in some cases, there may be simply scattered pruritic papules, accompanied by slight scale present on the trunk or extremities and genitalia. What distinguishes this variant of Norwegian scabies from classical Norwegian scabies is that there may be only slight crusting but myriad mites are found. When scrapings are taken, several mites often may be seen with relative ease. The treatment of this condition consists of the usual antiscabetic medications, but because of the number of organisms and the relative immunocompromised state of the patient, the condition may be relatively difficult to eradicate. Often severe pruritus develops following destruction of the mites.

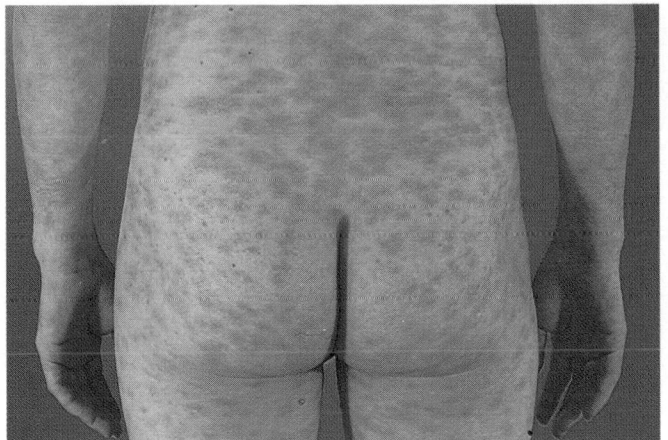

Figure 6–20. Secondary syphilis.

Widespread eruption of reddish-brown papules with scales is characteristic of this condition. In patients with AIDS, it may be more florid and may be associated concomitantly with a lesion of tertiary syphilis.

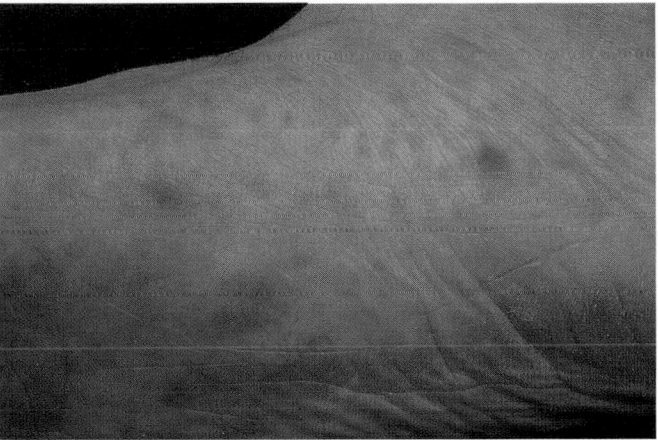

Figure 6–21. Secondary syphilis.

Characteristic reddish-brown papules on the soles. Such lesions on occasion have been mistaken for Kaposi's sarcoma.

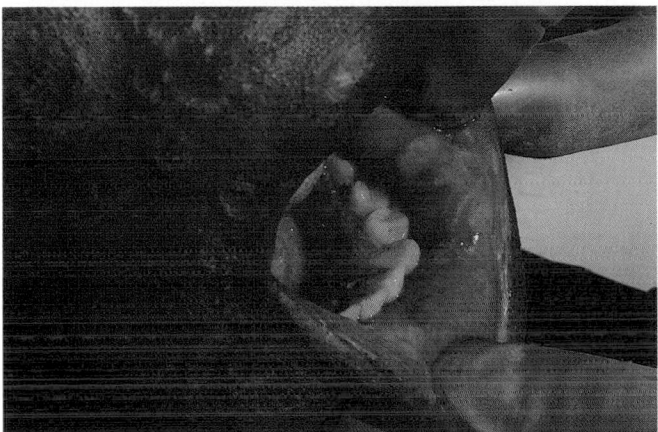

Figure 6–22. Mucous patches of secondary syphilis.

Notice the annular configuration of the lesions on the skin and the whitish, erosive plaques present on the labial mucosa. Such lesions are teeming with spirochetes.

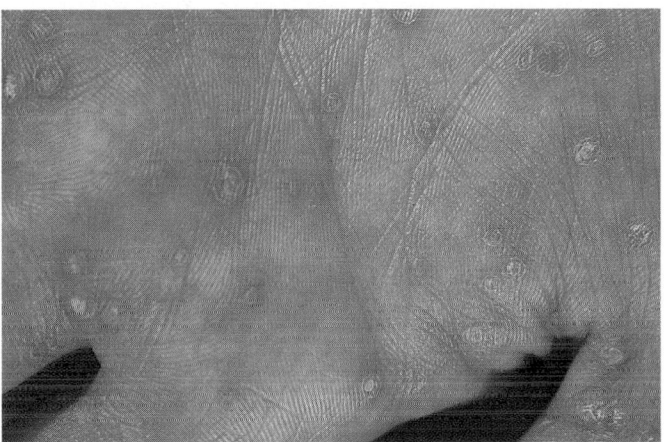

Figure 6–23. Secondary syphilis.

Close-up view of papules of secondary syphilis to demonstrate the scaling and slight crusting present on the surface.

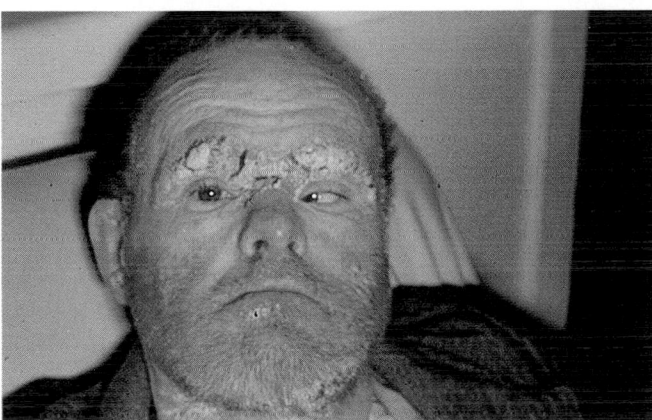

Figure 6–24. Norwegian scabies.

These markedly hyperkeratotic and crusted plaques were found to have innumerable mites of *Sarcoptes scabei*. This is a florid example of Norwegian scabies.

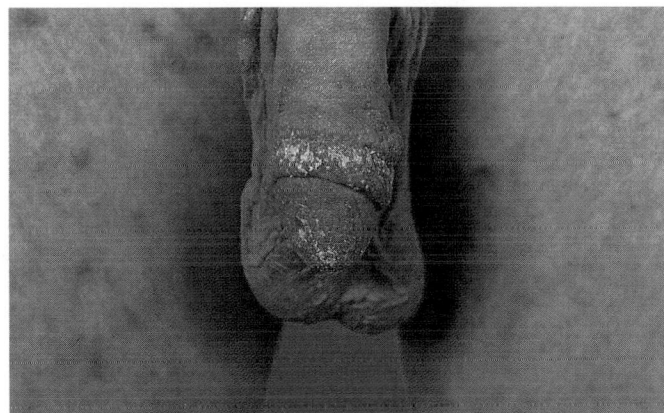

Figure 6–25. Norwegian scabies.

Papules and slight scaling and crusting were the manifestations of Norwegian scabies in this patient. Notice the marked lack of hyperkeratosis and crusting, as seen in Figure 6–24.

Mycobacterial Infection
(Figures 6–26 to 6–29)

Although uncommon, AIDS patients with systemic mycobacterial infections may develop cutaneous lesions. Clinically, the mycobacterial skin lesions appear as small papules and pustules that resemble folliculitis;[16] however, cultures and specially stained biopsy specimens demonstrate mycobacteria histologically. In four AIDS patients, who were intravenous drug users, seen at New York University Medical Center with cutaneous mycobacterial disease, three eventually were found to have *Mycobacterium tuberculosis* and one had *Mycobacterium avium.* In the patients with *M. tuberculosis,* pustular lesions of the skin were secondary to reactivated pulmonary foci.

Other cutaneous manifestations of tuberculosis, such as lupus vulgaris, occasionally, albeit rarely, are seen in patients with AIDS.

It should be re-emphasized that the individual lesions appear virtually identical to those of simple folliculitis. Because this diagnosis can be confirmed with certainty only by culture or examination of tissue stained for acid-fast bacilli, such studies should be performed on any patient with AIDS who has such lesions.

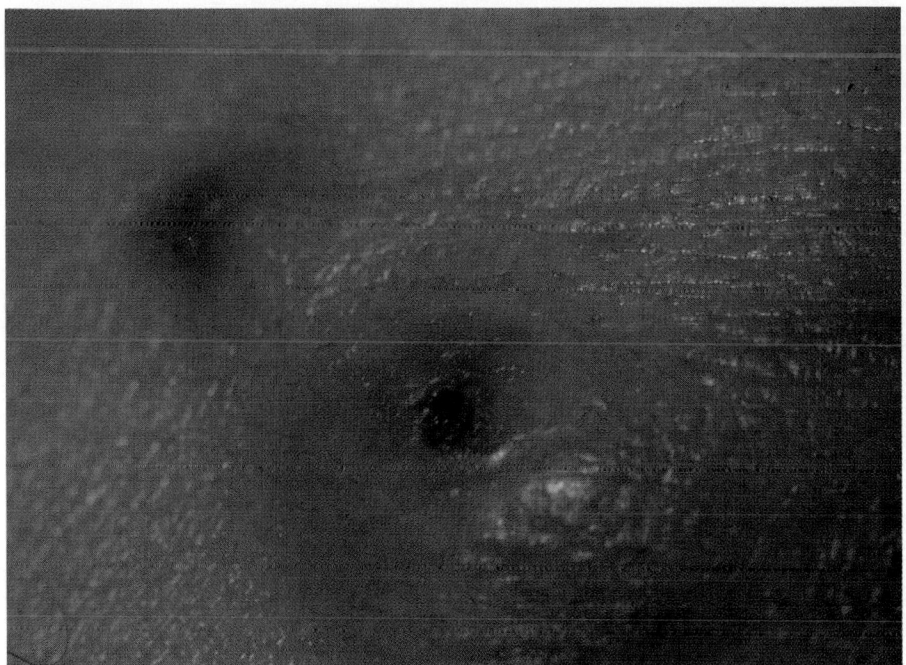

Figure 6–26. Cutaneous tuberculosis.

Individual acneiform crusted papules present on the trunk and extremities clinically had a very nondescript appearance but histologically revealed myriad acid-fast bacilli. In this case, the organism was *Mycobacterium tuberculosis.*

Figure 6–27. Cutaneous tuberculosis.

Another example of the relatively nondescript nature of these lesions. This is distinct from the usual clinical appearance of cutaneous tuberculosis.

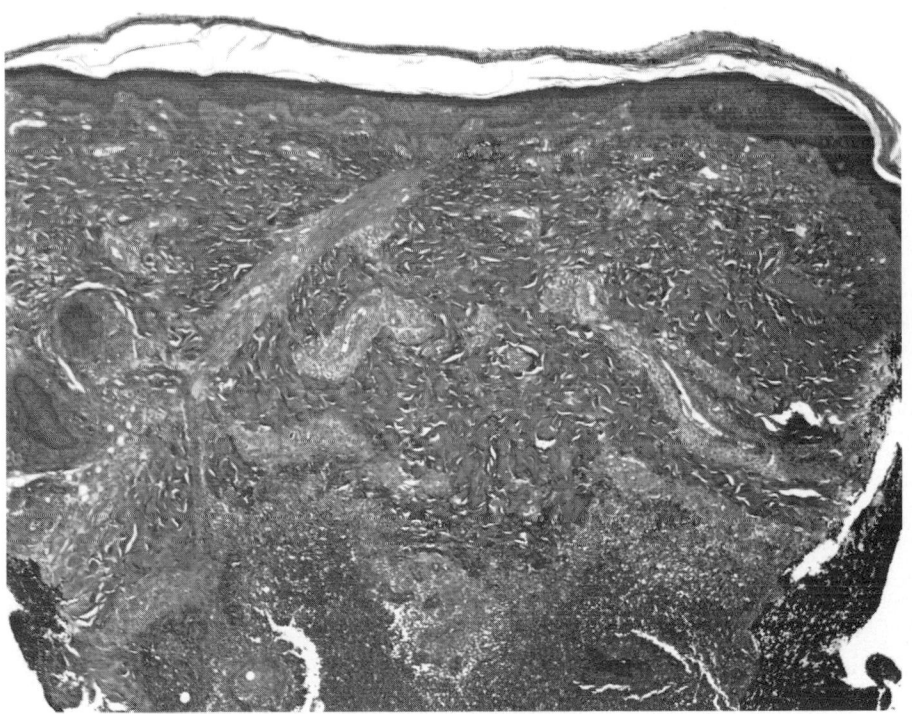

Figure 6–28. Abscess.

There is a diffuse dermatitis present in the depths of the specimen consisting of numerous neutrophils and some histiocytes. These are the features of an abscess.

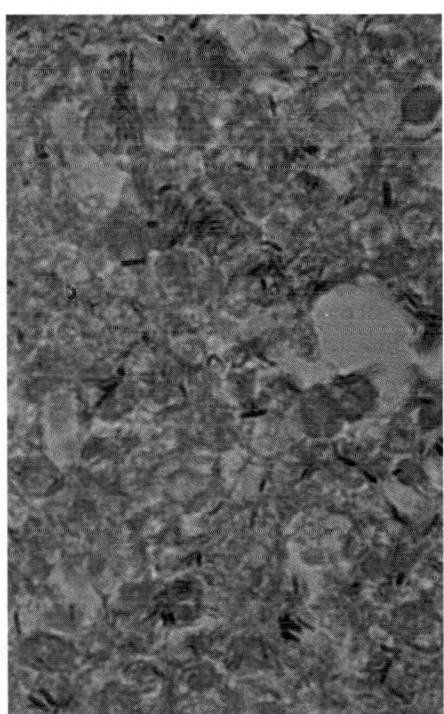

Figure 6–29. *Mycobacterium tuberculosis* infection.

Stains for mycobacteria revealed innumerable acid-fast bacilli. These proved to be *Mycobacterium tuberculosis,* but *Mycobacterium avium-intracellulare* may produce identical clinical and histologic features.

Superficial Fungal Infections
(Figures 6–30 to 6–33)

White patches of the buccal mucosa or tongue in a patient at high risk for HIV-infection and AIDS should cause one to suspect the diagnosis of candidiasis (moniliasis, thrush). It has been shown that such individuals who have oral infections with *Candida albicans* have a very high likelihood of being infected with HIV and of later developing symptomatic diseases such as AIDS-related complex or AIDS.[17] Clinically, one usually sees whitish, curd-like exudates on the dorsal or lateral tongue, oropharynx, or buccal mucosa that can be easily scraped away with a cotton swab or tongue depressor. A reddish friable surface that may be associated with a burning sensation is often found underneath the candidial exudate. Sometimes, only a beefy red, eroded surface of the tongue is seen. Microscopic examination of exudate scraped from the tongue surface treated with 10 per cent potassium hydroxide solution will be shown to contain numerous pseudohyphae and budding yeasts. It is also important to evaluate these patients

for esophageal candidiasis. This complication may be associated with dysphagia, which can lead to anorexia and consequent malnutrition. Cutaneous and perianal candidal infections occasionally occur as well.

Treatment may be difficult because the condition often recurs following discontinuation of therapy. Oral administration of clotrimazole or nystatin may help to suppress candidal overgrowth. Ultimately, ketoconazole may be required.

In addition to *Candida albicans,* other fungi may cause severe cutaneous or systemic infections that fail to respond to available topical and systemic antifungal therapy. Widespread dermatophytosis, especially that caused by *Trichophyton rubrum,* involving palms, soles, nails, and intertriginous areas have been observed in individuals with or at high risk for AIDS. Neither systemic griseofulvin, ketoconazole, nor topical antifungal medications have been found to be completely effective in eradicating such infection.

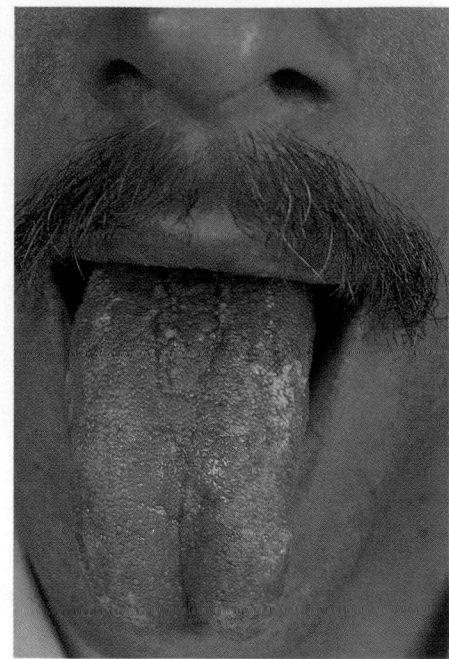

Figure 6–30. Candidiasis.
A whitish, curd-like exudate present on the tongue or buccal mucosa that can easily be scraped away is characteristic of this condition. This may be an indication that a patient will later develop AIDS.

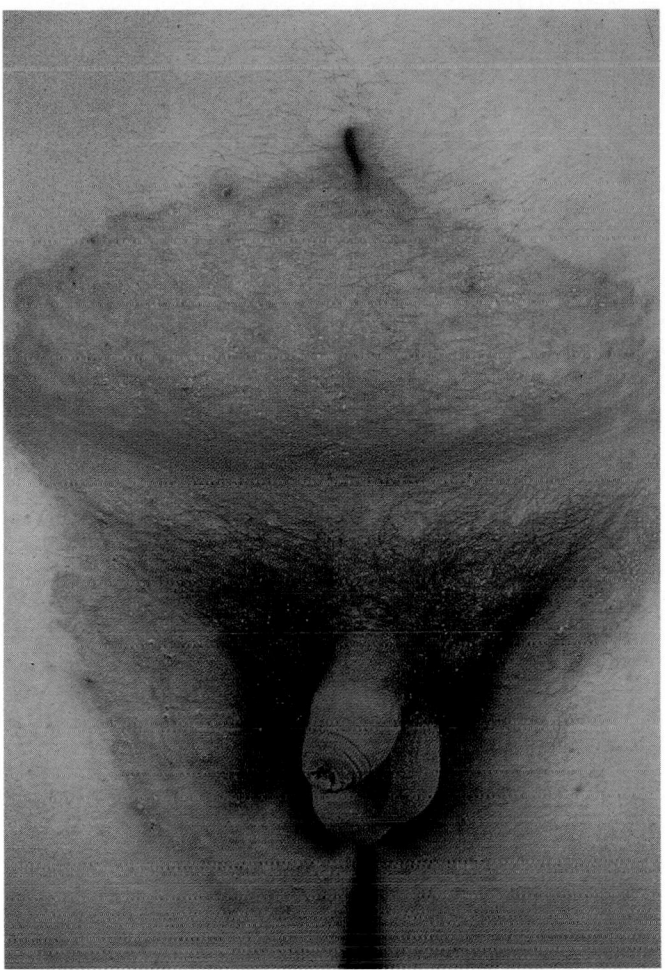

Figure 6–31. Mucocutaneous candidiasis.

Chronic mucocutaneous candidiasis seen in patients with AIDS. Note the extensive crusting and scaling as well as the subungual hyperkeratosis.

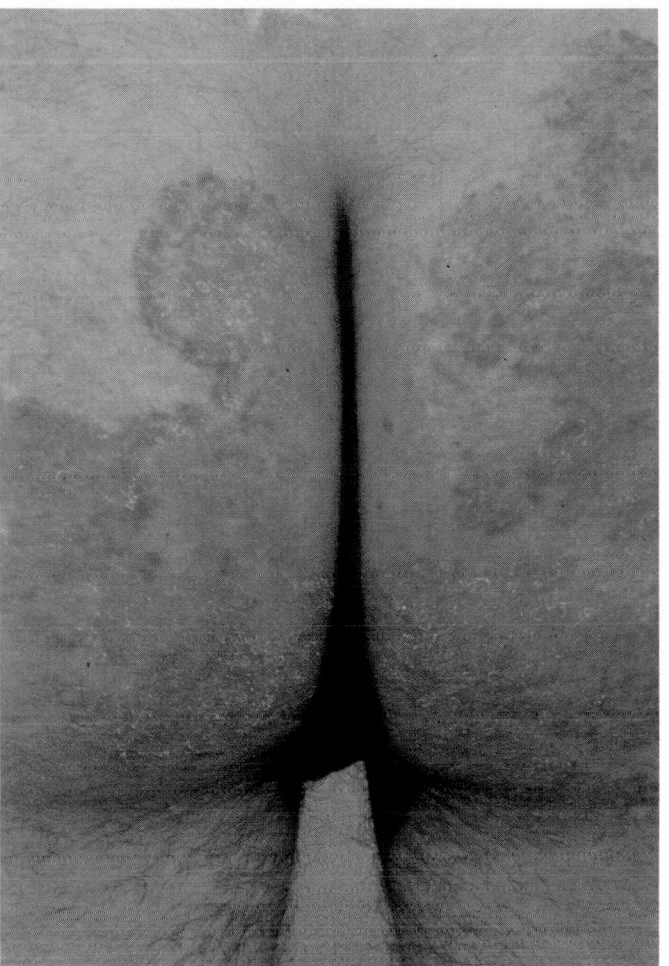

Figure 6–32. Dermatophyte infections.

Common dermatophyte infections in patients with AIDS on occasion may become rampant because of the immunosuppression. Scrapings for microscopic examination and culture should be obtained when such lesions are encountered.

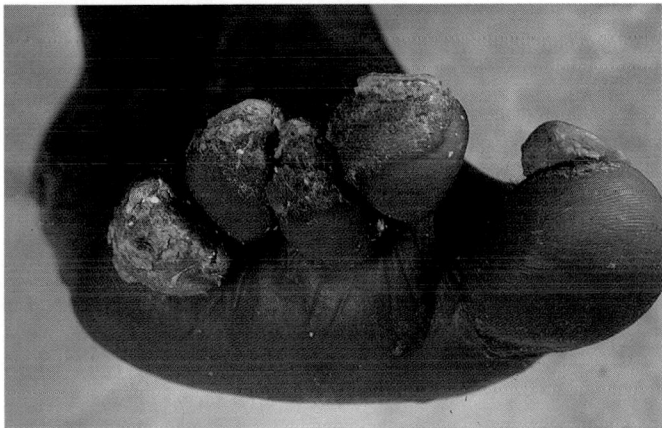

Figure 6–33. Onychomycosis.

Severe onychomycosis with marked subungual hyperkeratosis and nail dystrophy may also be seen in patients with AIDS. This is usually a chronic condition seen in elderly patients; however, it may have an early onset in the patient with AIDS.

Systemic Fungal Infections

When highly pathogenic fungi which often cause systemic disease in immunocompetent individuals infect AIDS patients, the outcome may be fatal. The systemic fungal infections most commonly found among patients with AIDS are due to *Cryptococcus neoformans* and *Histoplasma capsulatum*.

***Cryptococcus neoformans* (Figures 6–34 to 6–38).** Cryptococcosis most often causes a meningitis, although the skin is rarely involved. This fungus may cause single or multiple red to purple 5-mm to 1-cm papules, nodules, and indurated plaques of the integument that resemble the cutaneous lesions of bacterial cellulitis. Superficial erosion and crusting of the cryptococcal skin lesions may be found. One of the most common presenting signs of cutaneous cryptococcosis that has been observed has been the presence of widespread, skin-colored, dome-shaped, and sometimes slightly umbilicated papules that bear a striking resemblance to the papules of molluscum contagiosum, a benign cutaneous viral infection frequently seen in patients with AIDS or at high risk for the disease.[18] Occasionally, an AIDS patient may have both infections simultaneously, and individual lesions of each may be clinically indistinguishable. It is often necessary to biopsy and to culture papular lesions thought to be molluscum contagiosum to exclude the more serious diagnosis of cryptococcosis. Patients with cryptococcosis may be asymptomatic; on occasion, however, a careful history and neurologic examination will reveal subtle changes in personality, memory loss, thought disorders, or a poorly defined psychiatric illness. In such cases, a spinal fluid examination including fungal culture is indicated. Treatment of this condition is difficult and is best conducted in concert with a specialist in infectious diseases.

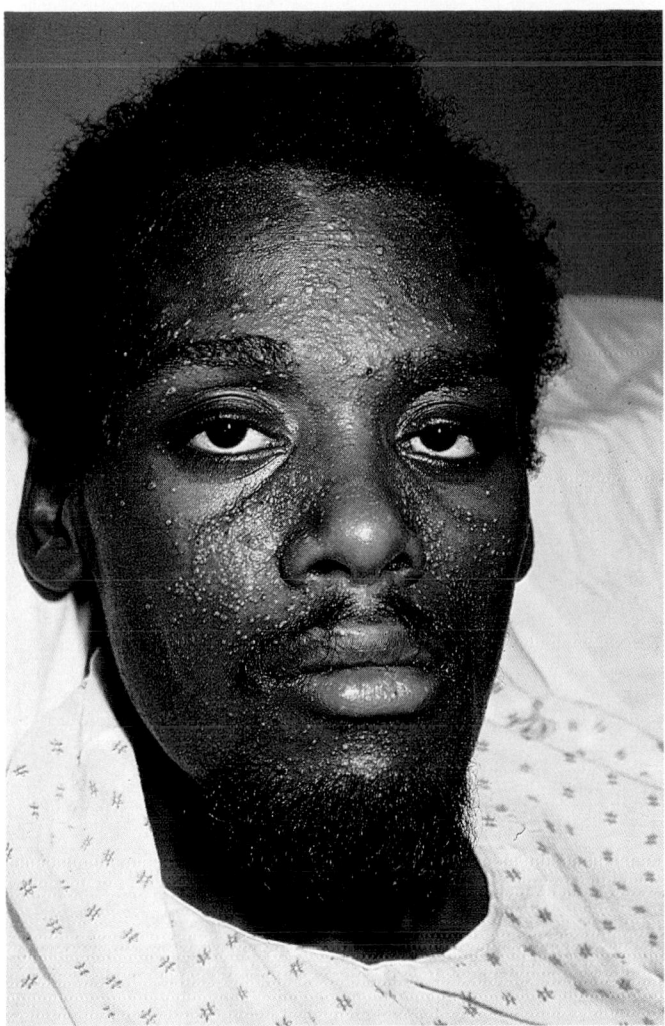

Figure 6–34. Cryptococcosis.
Crusted umbilicated follicular and perifollicular papules may mimic lesions of molluscum contagiosum infection. They are often multiple and may tend to confluence in both conditions.

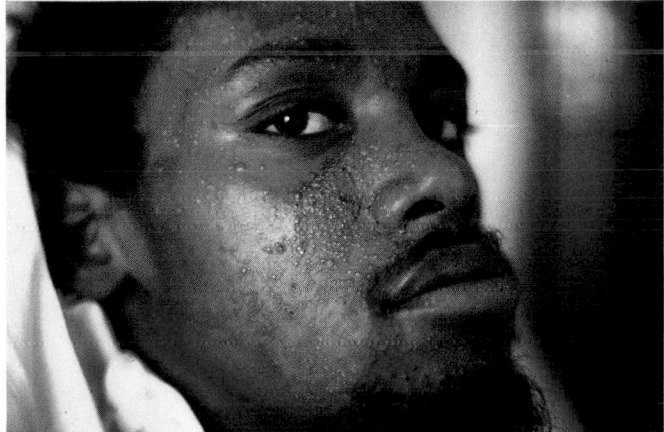

Figure 6–35. Cryptococcosis.
Close-up view revealing the umbilicated nature of the papules. A biopsy is essential to distinguish this condition from molluscum contagiosum infection.

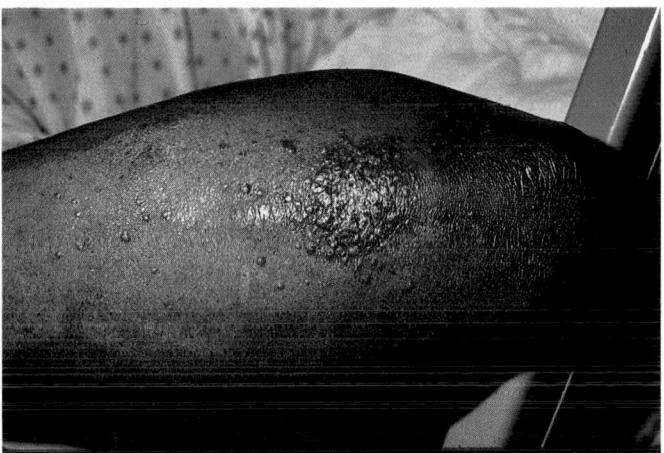

Figure 6–36. Cryptococcosis.
The lesions have coalesced to form a plaque on the arm.

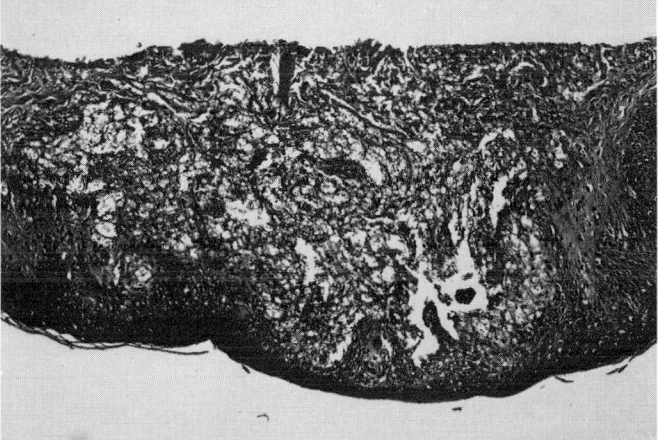

Figure 6–37. Cryptococcosis.
Shave biopsy of a lesion of cryptococcosis. Note the clear-staining cells present in the dermis.

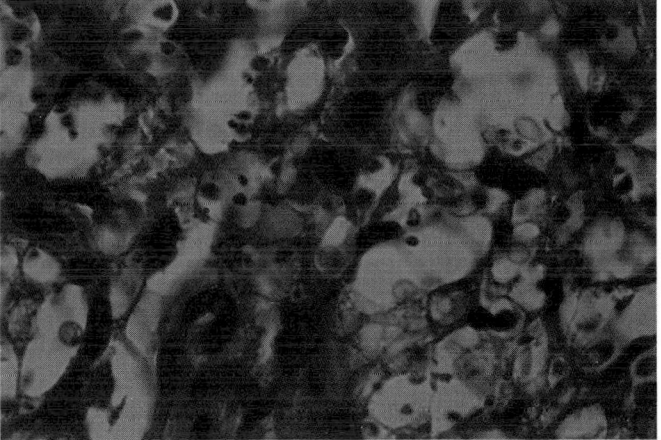

Figure 6–38. Cryptococcosis.
Higher magnification of the same specimen as in Figure 6–39 reveals numerous organisms of *Cryptococcus neoformans*. The whitish areas represent the abundant mucinous capsular material.

***Histoplasma capsulatum* (Figures 6–39 to 6–41).** The incidence of cutaneous histoplasmosis is even rarer than cryptococcosis in patients with AIDS. Examination of the skin may reveal scattered acneiform papules, a widespread eruption of reddish macules and papules, or one to a few indurated, pinkish red crusted plaques.[19, 20] A specific diagnosis can be made with certainty only by fungal culture and histopathologic evaluation of biopsy specimens. It is important to alert the pathologist that the patient has or is suspected of having AIDS, for the diagnosis of histoplasmosis can be subtle even with microscopic examination. As in the case with cryptococcosis, patients with cutaneous histoplasmosis may not be acutely ill or have any evidence of systemic or central nervous system involvement. AIDS patients with cutaneous histoplasmosis are often not aware of prior pulmonary disease.

Any infectious disease in patients with AIDS may have an unusual appearance. The physician should maintain a high index of suspicion and should perform biopsies and viral, bacterial, or fungal cultures of any atypical skin lesion in order not to miss a potentially fatal infectious disease.

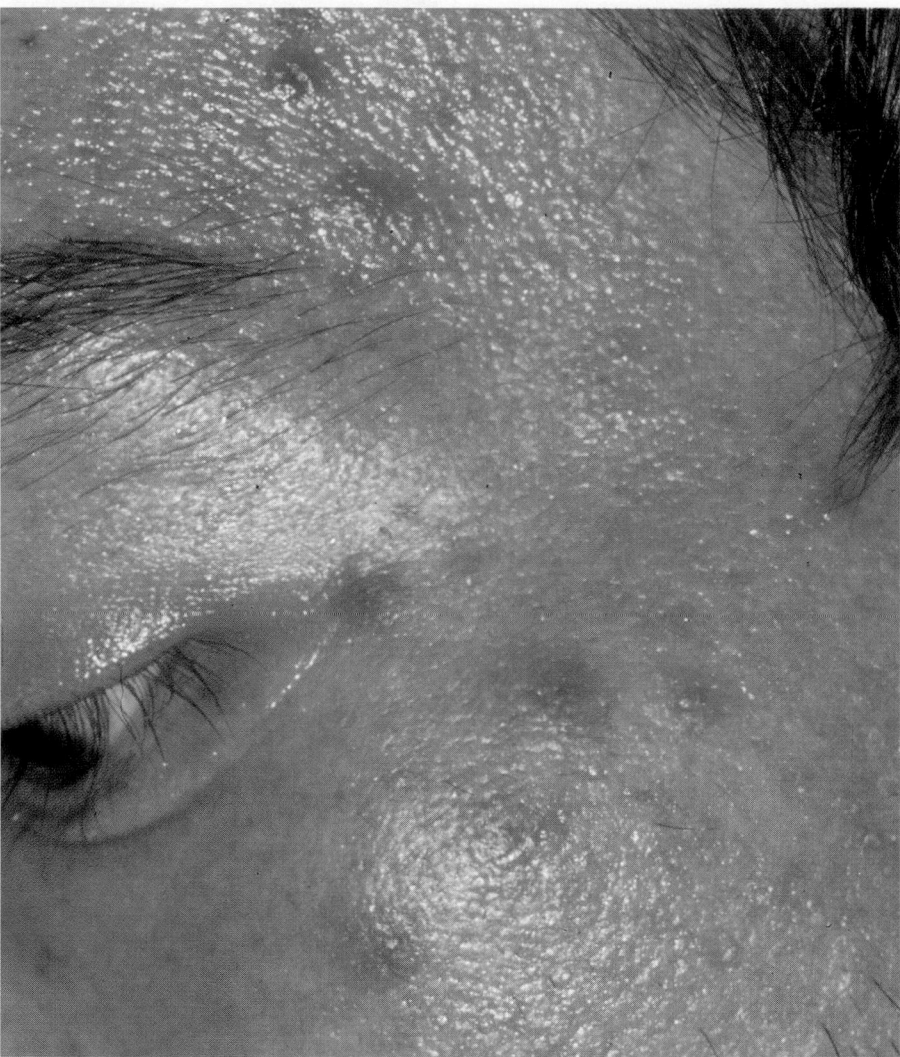

Figure 6–39. *Histoplasma capsulatum* infection.
Scattered and sometimes widespread acneiform papules or nodules may be caused by a number of different systemic infectious organisms. In this case the cause was *Histoplasma capsulatum;* however, cutaneous cryptococcosis and cutaneous *Mycobacterium avium-intracellulare* infection may appear identical.

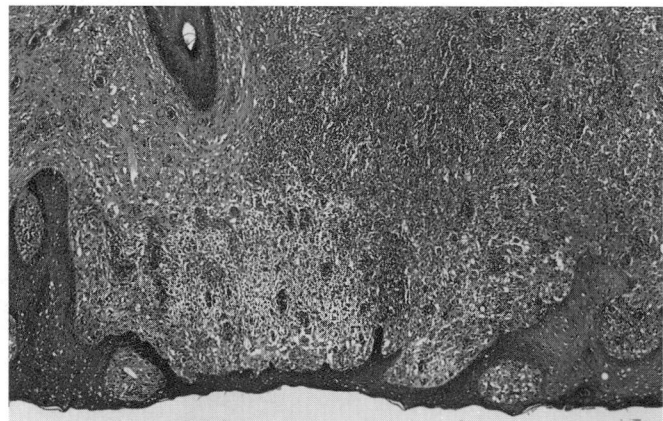

Figure 6–40. Histoplasmosis.
Note the epidermal hyperplasia and the infiltrate of pale-staining cells in the dermis.

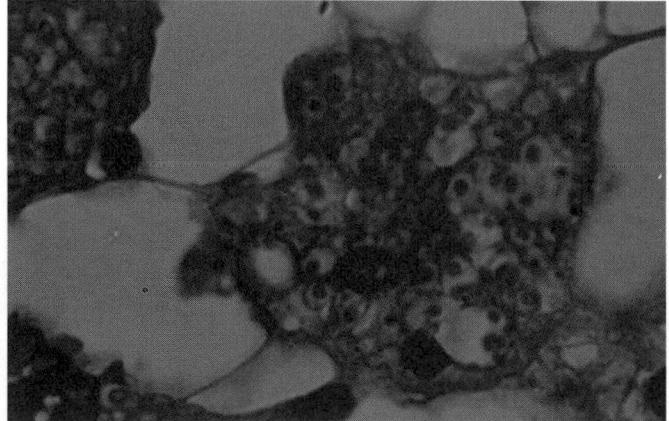

Figure 6–41. Histoplasmosis.
This histiocyte is virtually filled with *Histoplasma capsulatum* organisms.

Noninfectious Skin Conditions

In addition to infectious diseases, a number of secondary noninfectious cutaneous signs and symptoms have been described in patients with AIDS or the AIDS-related complex (ARC), such as nonspecific severe pruritus or hives. It should be emphasized that the occurrence of these should alert one to consider AIDS in the differential diagnosis.

Seborrheic Dermatitis–like Eruption
(Figures 6–42 to 6–46)

One of the most commonly observed skin conditions associated with HIV-infection or AIDS is an eruption that resembles seborrheic dermatitis, usually involving the scalp and face. This eruption appears as slightly indurated, often diffuse or confluent, pinkish red, scaly plaques. Occasionally these may be large, thickened, and heavily crusted.[21] This seborrheic dermatitis–like condition may occur on the upper anterior chest, back, groin, and extremities. The eruption tends to be somewhat refractory to the usual treatment modalities used for seborrheic dermatitis, such as topi-

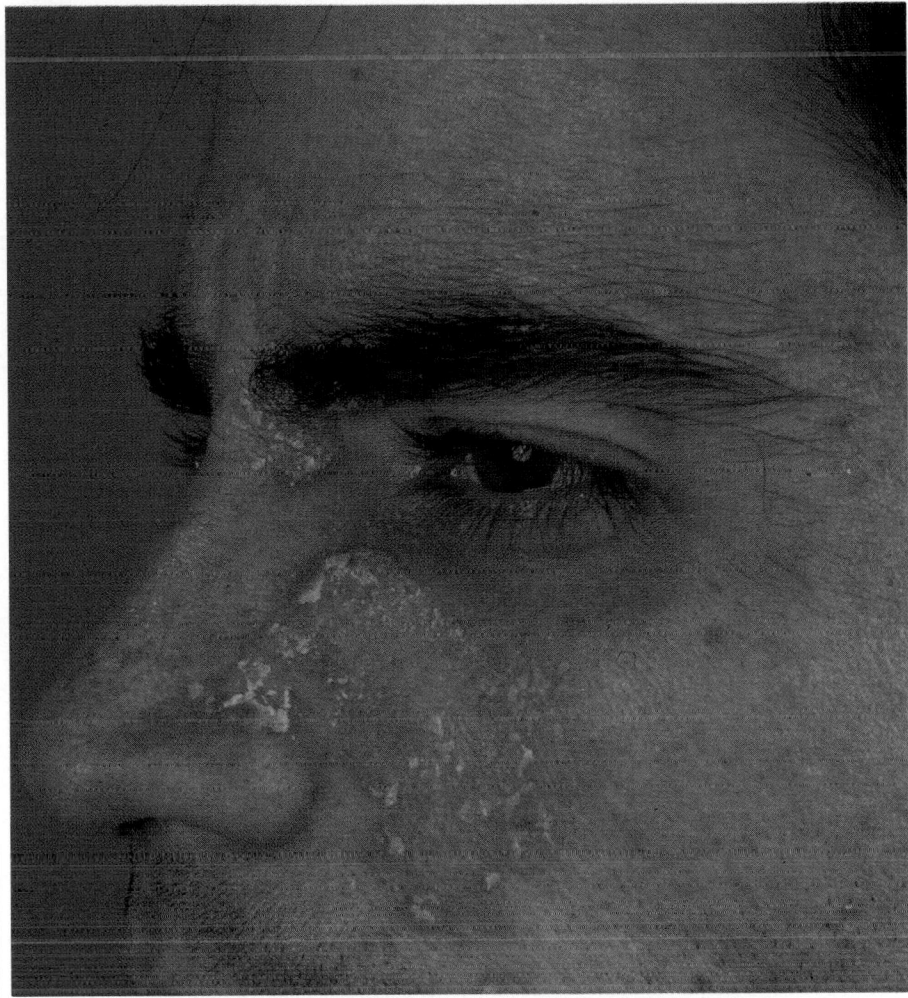

Figure 6–42. Seborrheic dermatitis-like eruption.
This eruption is seen in a patient with AIDS. Pinkish red scaly and crusted plaques seen in the malar areas but also in other locations are characteristic of this condition. It is refractory to treatment in most cases.

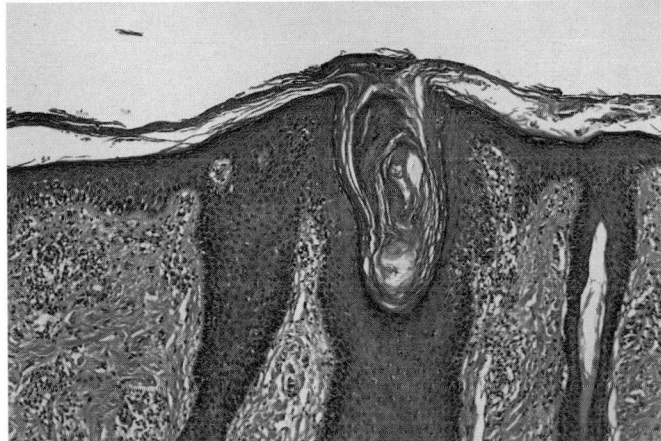

Figure 6–43. Seborrheic dermatitis-like eruption.
Photomicrograph. The parakeratosis is present over most of the epidermis as opposed to being located in the lips of the follicular ostia.

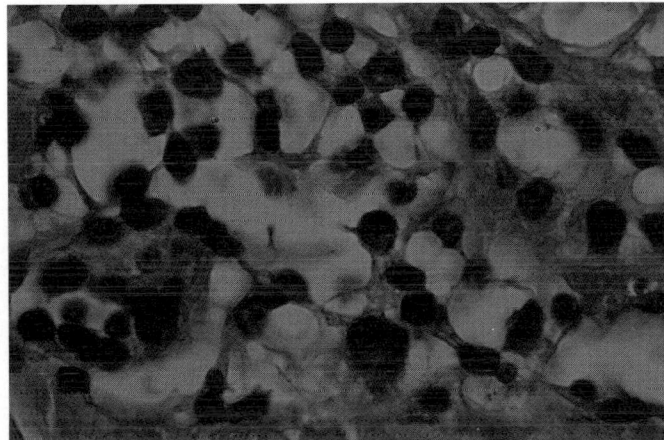

Figure 6–44. Seborrheic dermatitis-like eruption.
The inflammatory cell infiltrate in the eruption often consists of many plasma cells.

cal corticosteroids. In some patients, this eruption may be the presenting complaint in an otherwise asymptomatic HIV seropositive individual, who may later develop AIDS. Most cases were initially diagnosed simply as seborrheic dermatitis.

When the eruption is especially florid, it may resemble psoriasis, but it can be distinguished from that condition because it does not involve extensor surfaces of the extremities such as the elbows and knees and has a superficial surface scale or crust rather than the thickened "micaceous" scale of typical psoriasis. Patients with AIDS, however, may develop psoriasis that is often of a severe and diffuse nature. In some individuals with prior history of psoriasis, this condition may be exacerbated and can become widespread.

The concurrence of Reiter's syndrome and AIDS has recently been noted.[22] Reiter's syndrome was noted to be unusually severe and had its onset either concomitant with, preceding, or succeeding the diagnosis of AIDS (Figures 6–47 to 6–49). The development of this condition was thought to be precipitated by infections with enteric bacteria, either *Shigella flexneri* or *Campylobacter fetus*. Of importance was the fact that immunosuppressive therapy, especially methotrexate, administered for Reiter's syndrome, resulted in a profound immunodepression. Thus, it is important to be alert to the possible presence of AIDS in patients with Reiter's disease.

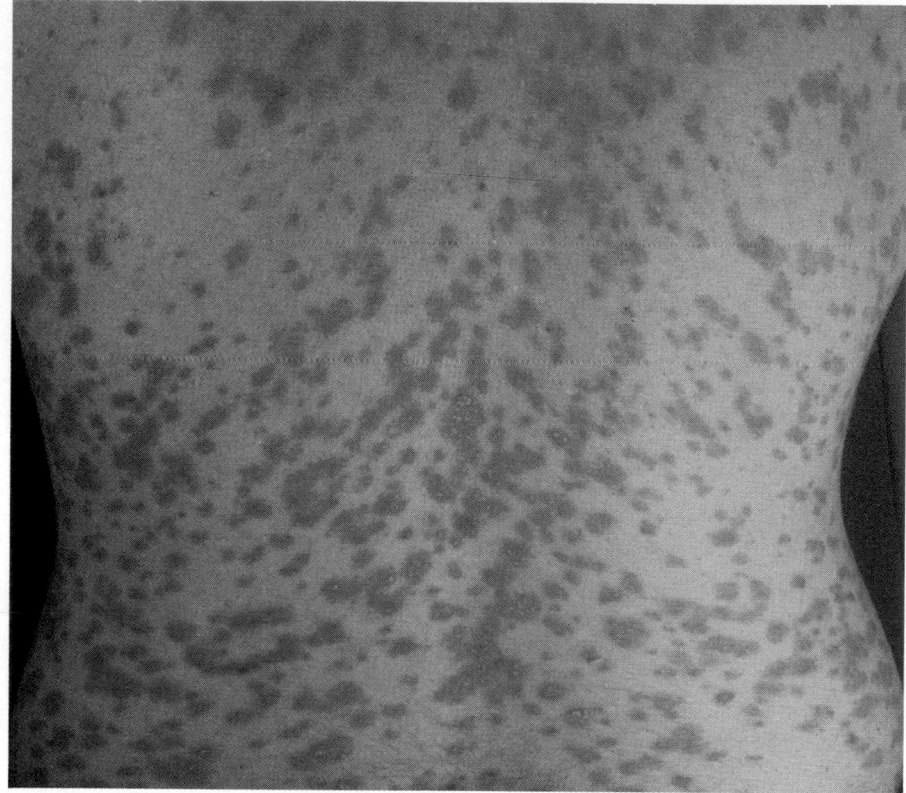

Figure 6–45. Psoriasis.

Psoriasis in a patient with AIDS. Common psoriasis may be markedly exacerbated in this patient population, and erythroderma may result.

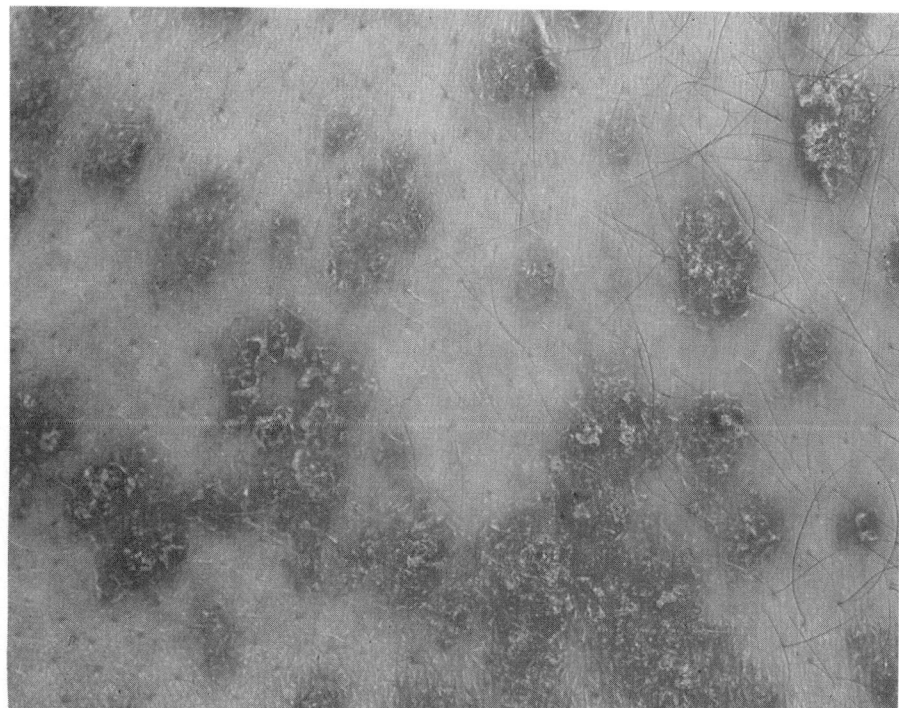

Figure 6–46. Eruptive psoriasis.

Close-up view of eruptive psoriasis in a patient with AIDS.

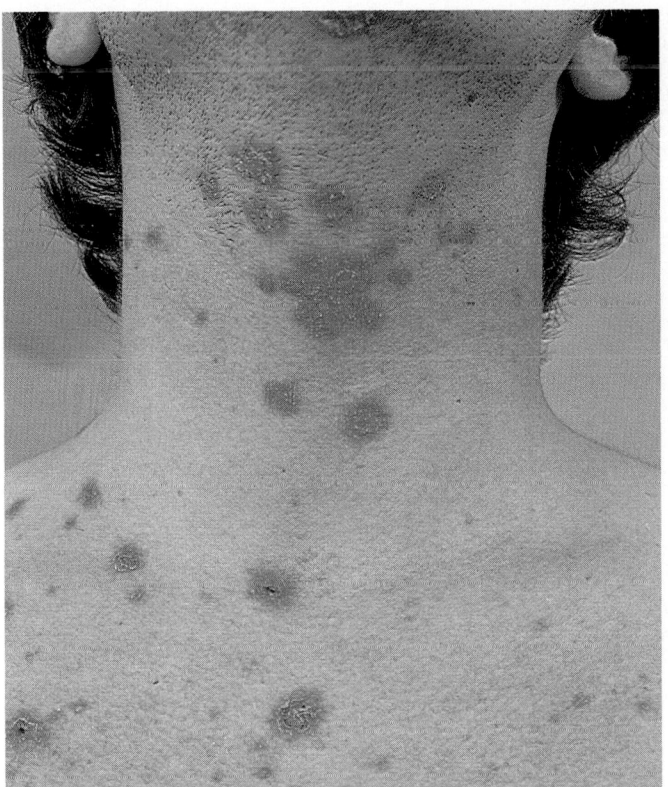

Figure 6–47. Reiter's disease.

A thick, scaly, and crusted plaque present on the trunk and extremities and the acral surfaces is characteristic of Reiter's syndrome.

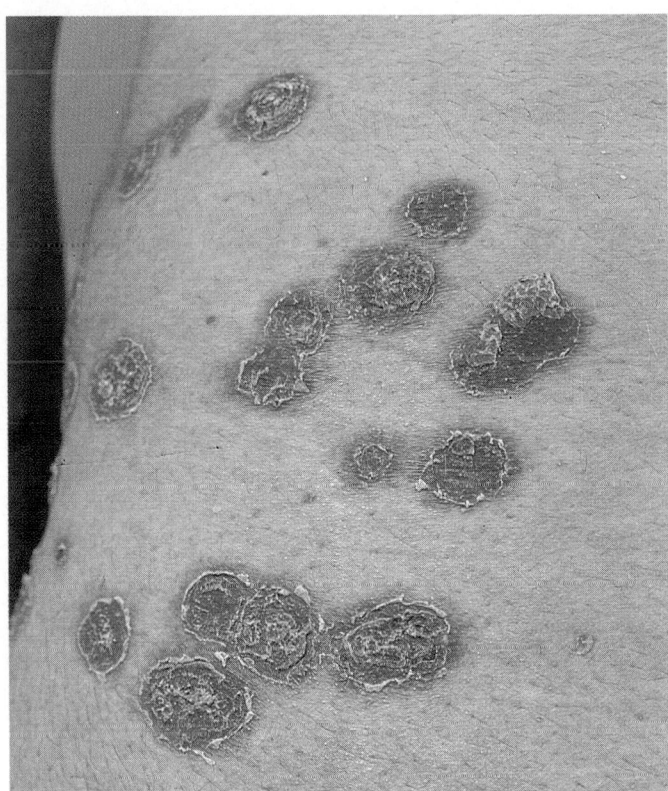

Figure 6–48. Reiter's syndrome.

Close-up view of individual crusted plaques of Reiter's syndrome. This may simply represent an unusual, florid manifestation of psoriasis.

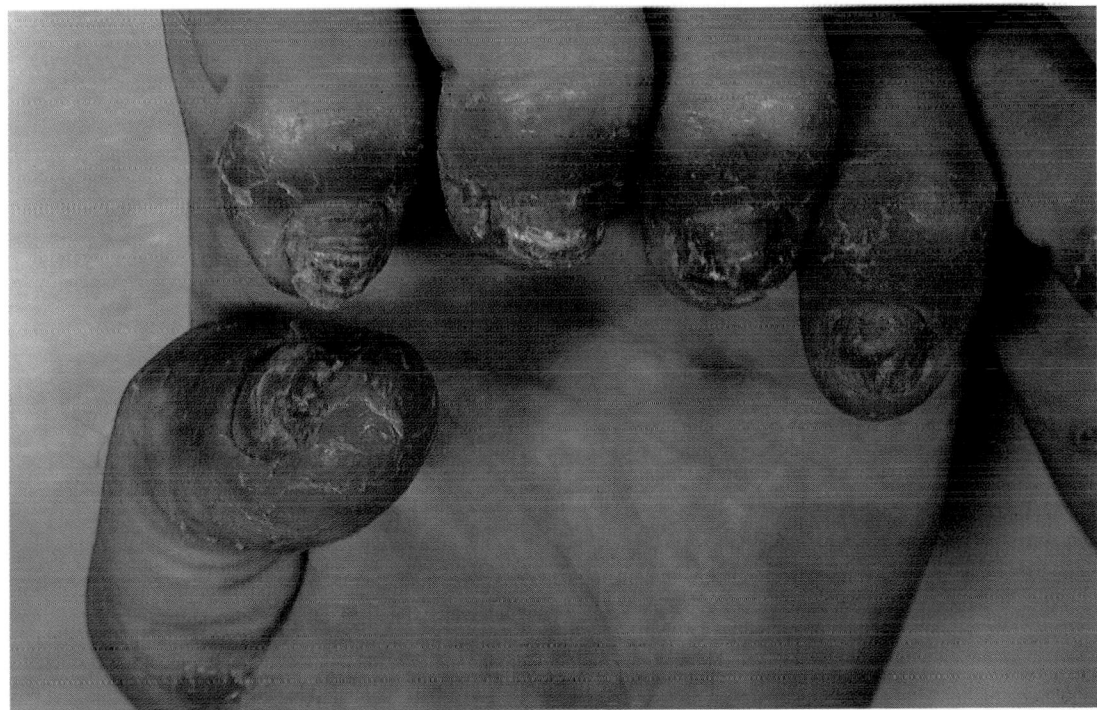

Figure 6–49. Reiter's disease.

Acral erythema, crusting, and subungual hyperkeratosis are characteristic of the acral lesions of Reiter's disease.

Morbilliform Drug Eruption
(Figures 6–50 and 6–51)

A widespread eruption consisting of pruritic, pinkish red macules and papules, many often urticarial, frequently develops following the administration of certain drugs in patients with AIDS. One agent which is especially likely to result in this complication is trimetho-prim-sulfamethoxazole (Bactrim), the primary drug used in the treatment of *Pneumocystis carinii* pneumonia. Up to 60 per cent of AIDS patients may develop a morbilli-form drug eruption following administration of this medication.[23] Although this drug eruption is similar to the allergic drug eruption that is seen frequently in patients with infectious mononucleosis who have received ampicillin, no definite correlation with a viral infection has been established. In some instances, the eruption may persist for several weeks, even months, after the administration of the drug has been discontinued. The particular incidence of this eruption is much higher in the population of those afflicted with AIDS; it is also more persistent, and for these reasons, it differs from similar allergic eruptions which are less commonly seen in non-AIDS patients to whom this drug is given. Treatment consists of the combined use of antihistamines, cool compresses, emollients, and topical steroids.

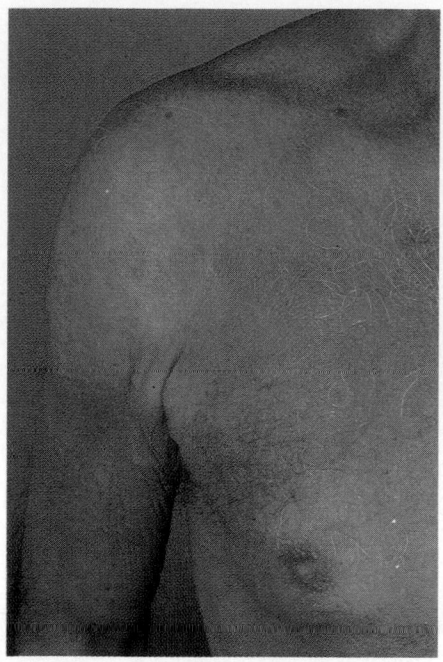

Figure 6–50. Morbilliform drug eruption.

A widespread eruption consisting of pruritic, pinkish red macules and papules is commonly seen following administration of trimetho-prim-sulfamethoxazole for *Pneumocystis carinii* pneumonia. The morphologic appearance of this eruption is quite similar to that seen in patients with infectious mononucleosis who have received ampicillin.

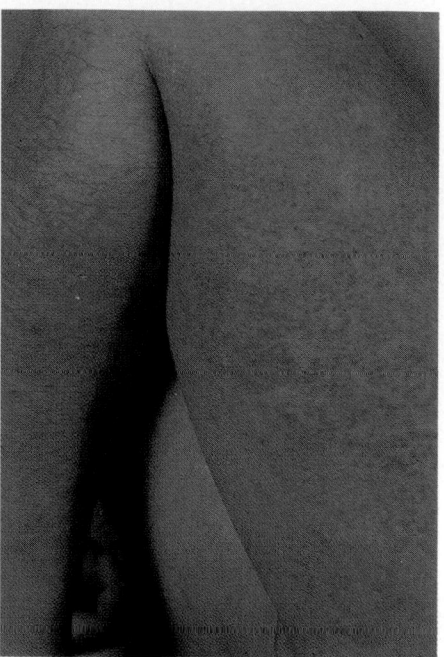

Figure 6–51. Morbilliform drug eruption.

Close-up view shows fine, morbilliform macules and papules.

Papular Urticaria
(Figures 6–52 to 6–54)

One of the most peculiar and unusual nonspecific cutaneous signs of AIDS is "papular urticaria," characterized by the onset of itchy red to pink, urticarial, dome-shaped papules with a widespread distribution over the trunk and extremities. Individual lesions may resemble insect bites. The patients complain of severe pruritus, and like certain other conditions seen in AIDS patients, the symptoms as well as the eruption are not readily responsive to conventional treatment modalities. The eruption may persist for several months, although the lesions may subside and recur intermittently. This cycle may continue relentlessly.

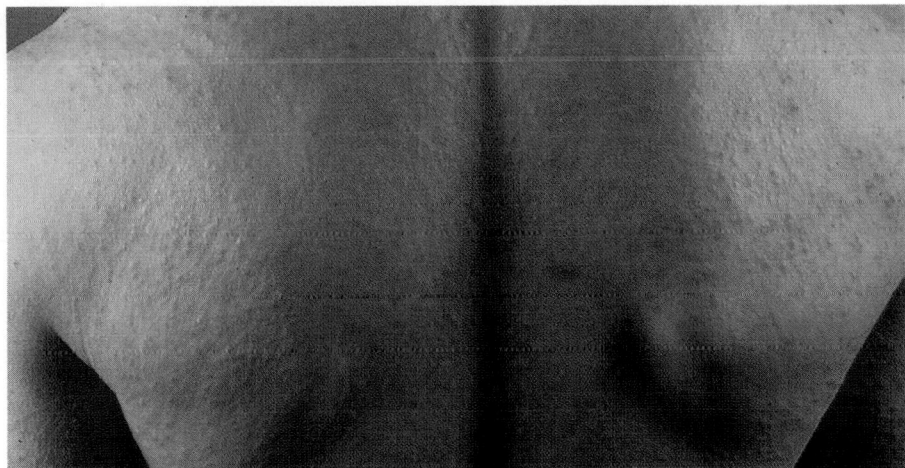

Figure 6–52. Papular urticaria.
This widespread eruption consists of pinkish red, dome-shaped urticarial papules that are often excoriated. Individual lesions have morphologic appearances similar to those of insect bites.

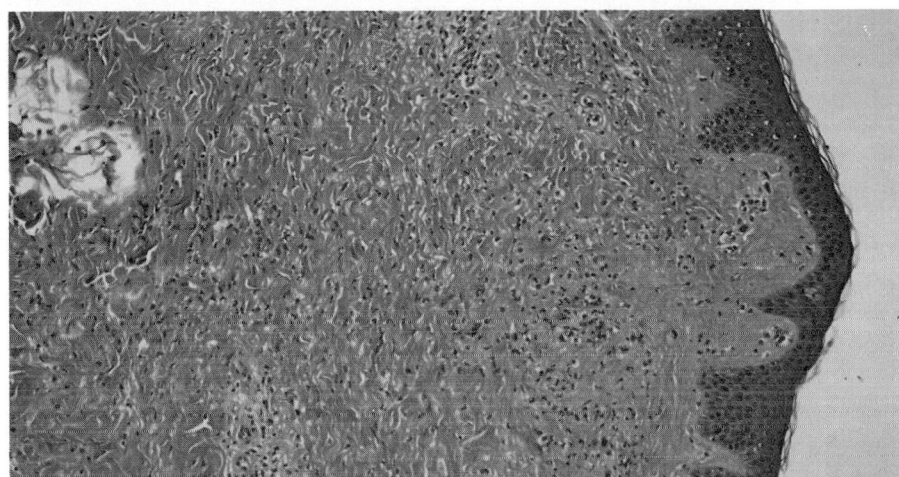

Figure 6–53. Papular urticaria.
Punch biopsy demonstrates a superficial and deep perivascular and interstitial infiltrate in the dermis.

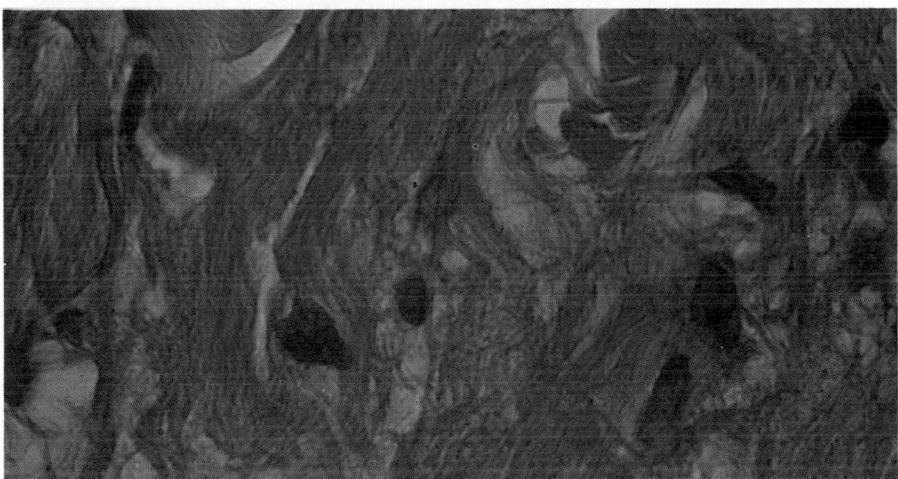

Figure 6–54. Papular urticaria.
The infiltrate consists of lymphocytes, histiocytes, and numerous eosinophils. The histologic differential diagnosis includes a response to an arthropod assault.

Eosinophilic Pustular Folliculitis
(Figures 6–55 to 6–59)

A peculiar generalized acneiform, follicular, and papular eruption often associated with severe pruritus that clinically resembles urticarial papules surrounding a central pustule has been seen with increasing frequency among HIV-infected individuals. It is of interest that biopsy specimens of these pustular lesions are histologically distinguished by the presence of numerous eosinophils within the infundibula of hair follicles.[24] The nature and significance of this unique eruption in the HIV-infected immunostressed patient are not yet understood. The symptoms of this condition often respond to topical acne medications; antihistamines are used to control the pruritus, and more recently, therapy with ultraviolet B has been shown to relieve pruritus and result in partial resolution of the process.[25]

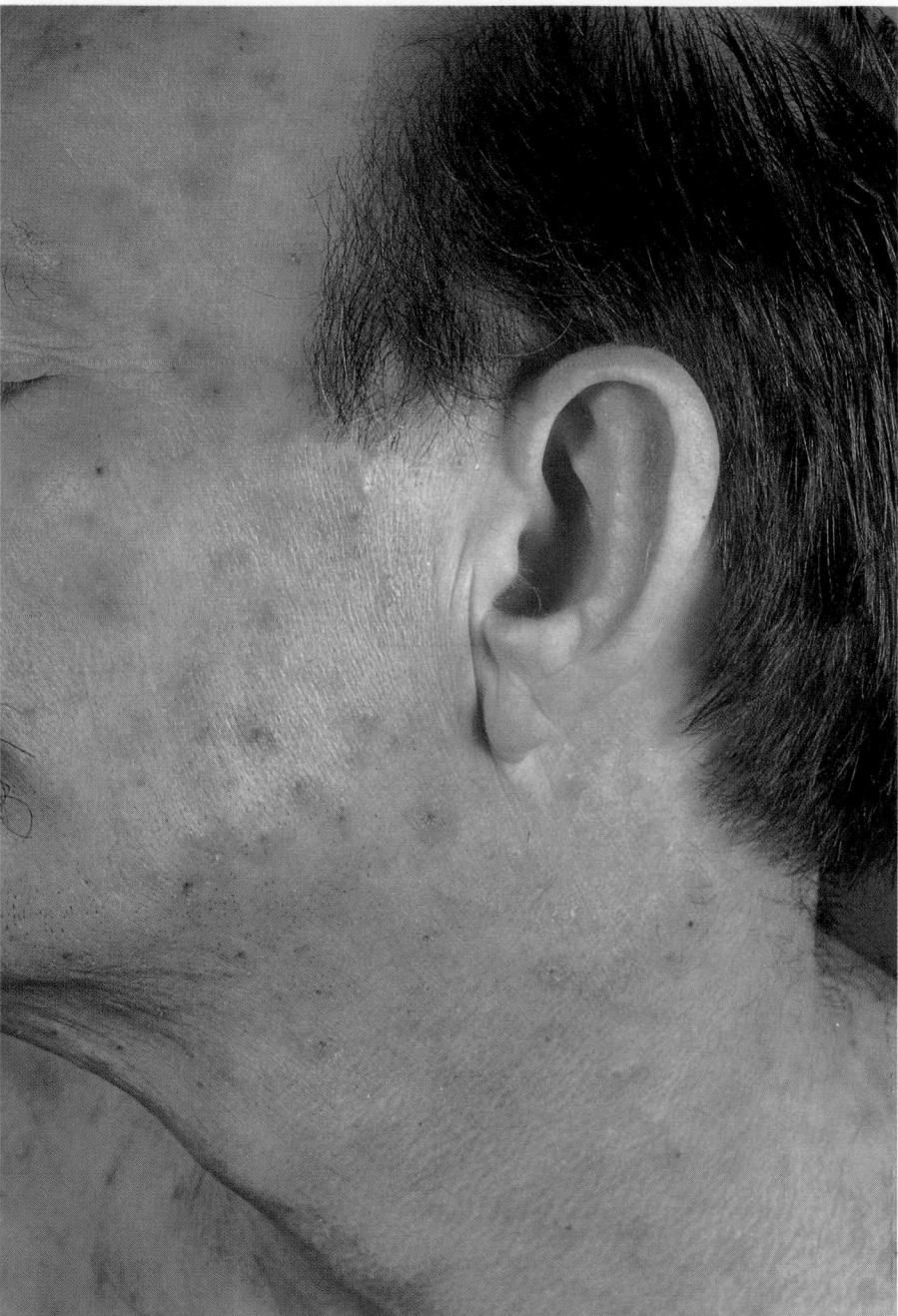

Figure 6–55. Eosinophilic pustular folliculitis.

This severely pruritic eruption is characterized by generalized perifollicular pustules often involving the head, neck, chest, and back and is often one of the earliest symptoms of HIV infection.

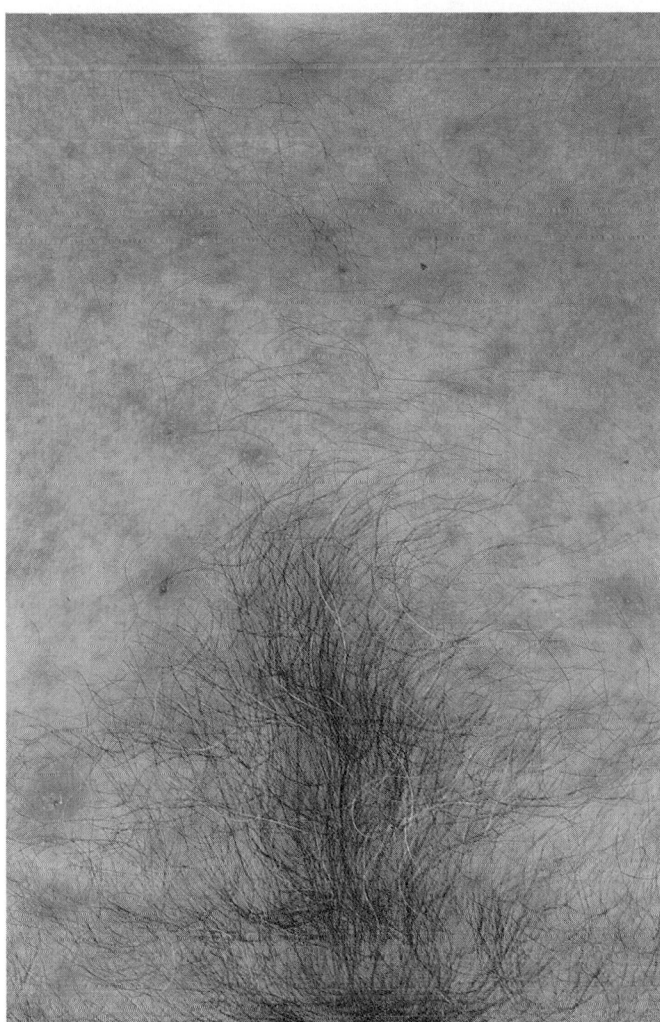

Figure 6–56. Eosinophilic pustular folliculitis.
Widespread follicular papules, often crusted and excoriated, are seen in this unusual manifestation of AIDS. It is clinically indistinguishable from the appearance of banal folliculitis.

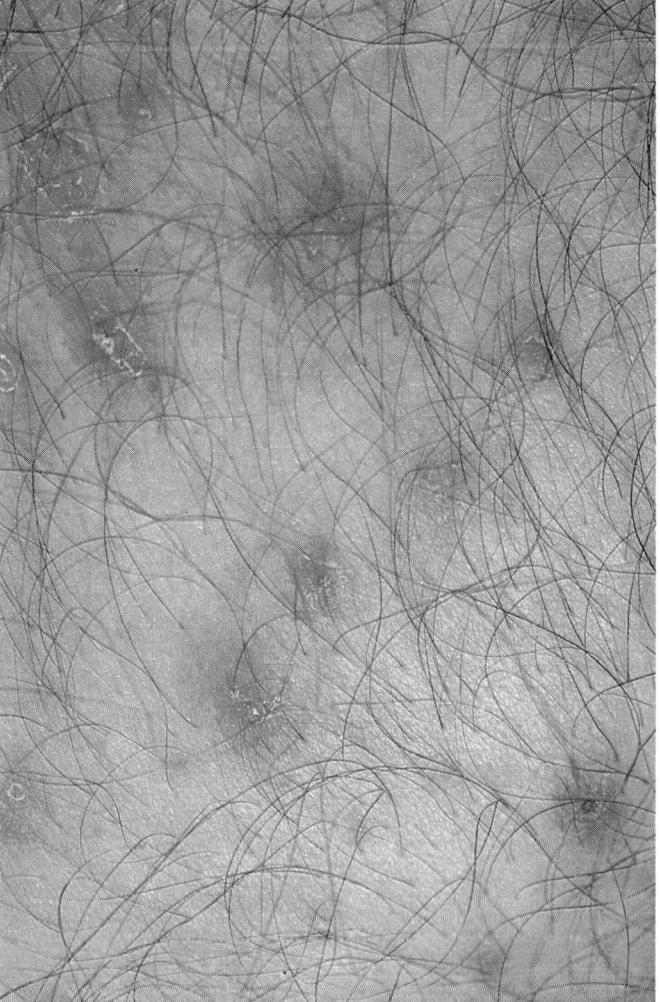

Figure 6–57. Eosinophilic pustular folliculitis.
Close-up view.

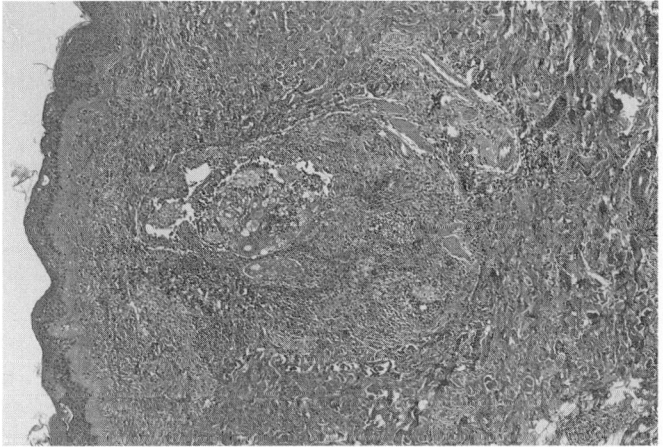

Figure 6–58. Eosinophilic pustular folliculitis.
Photomicrograph. The inflammatory cell infiltrate is centered within the lumen of the hair follicle, and some is present around it.

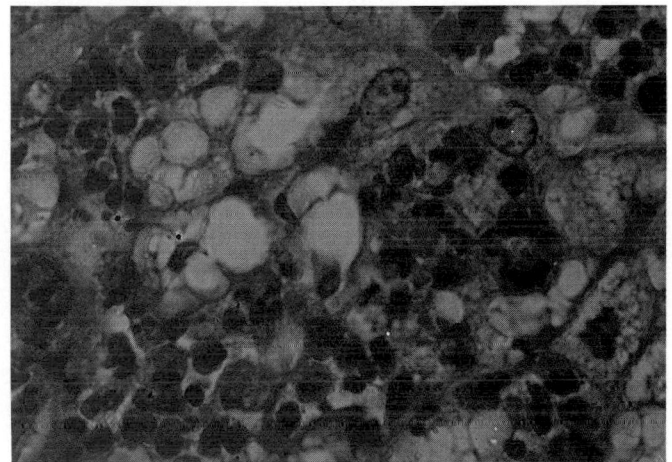

Figure 6–59. Eosinophilic pustular folliculitis.
Myriad eosinophils in a collection within the affected follicle.

Other Unusual Manifestations (Figures 6–60 to 6–68)

A unique form of pseudothrombophlebitis called "hyperalgesic pseudothrombophlebitis" has been described in several patients with AIDS. This syndrome is characterized by induration, erythema, and edema of the calf and is accompanied by severe pain and exquisite tenderness of the overlying skin.[26] Venography yields consistently negative results for the presence of deep vein thrombosis. The majority of patients with this type of pseudothrombophlebitis also have cutaneous systemic Kaposi's sarcoma. Whether this entity is an unusual manifestation of Kaposi's sarcoma itself or whether it results from unknown systemic medications is yet to be determined.

A curious side effect of recombinant leukocyte A interferon has been reported in two patients with B-cell lymphomas.[27] These patients experienced pronounced growth of their eyelashes over the two years of therapy necessitating periodic trimming of the lashes (Figure 6–60). We have seen this in one other patient with *Pneumocystis carinii* pneumonia who was receiving treatment with intramuscular injections of pentamidine. The mechanism of this phenomenon is unclear; it may be that these drugs modify the three stages of the hair cycle, resulting in a prolonged anagen, the growth phase.

We recently described an unusual vascular proliferative process in patients with AIDS, which we have termed epithelioid angiomatosis[28] (Figures 6–61 to 6–65). This vascular process is distinct from Kaposi's sarcoma and different from common hemangiomas in that it is composed of peculiar large, cuboidal, endothelial cells with the histologic and histochemical features of histiocytes. In addition, there are no bizarre, jagged blood vessels, and the inflammatory cell infiltrate seen in the lesion consists of lymphocytes, histiocytes, and often numerous neutrophils, as opposed to plasma cells. These lesions are virtually indistinguishable from pyogenic granulomas and from the *verruca peruviana* lesions of bartonellosis. The term "histiocytoid hemangioma" has also been used to describe similar lesions.[29] Nine patients with these lesions have recently been seen in New York City; the lesions have been seen in multiple, widely disseminated disease or as a solitary subcutaneous lesion. It has recently been observed that these lesions are probably infectious and may be caused by an organism similar to the cat-scratch disease bacillus.[30] Lesions stained with Warthin-Starry stains revealed numerous small clumps of interstitial bacteria, which were also demonstrated by electron microscopy. Studies with specific monoclonal antibodies to the cat-scratch disease bacillus suggest that these organisms are closely related. We have recently cultured the putative organism isolated from the lesions of two of these patients. At this time, the organism is being further characterized and appears to be distinct from the cat-scratch disease bacillus.[31]

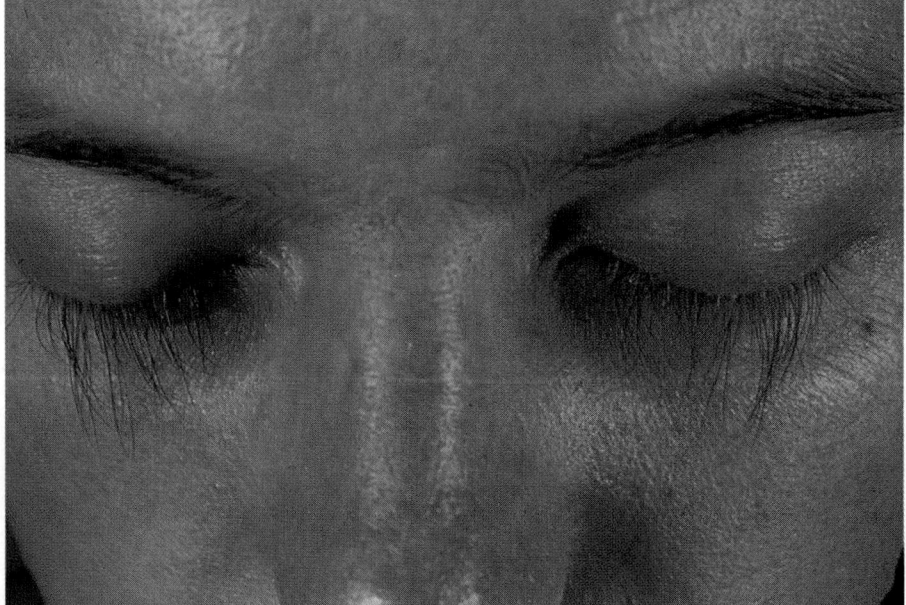

Figure 6–60. Long eyelashes.

This unusual phenomenon has been observed in patients who received recombinant leukocyte A interferon. It has also been seen in one patient with AIDS who received intramuscular pentamidine.

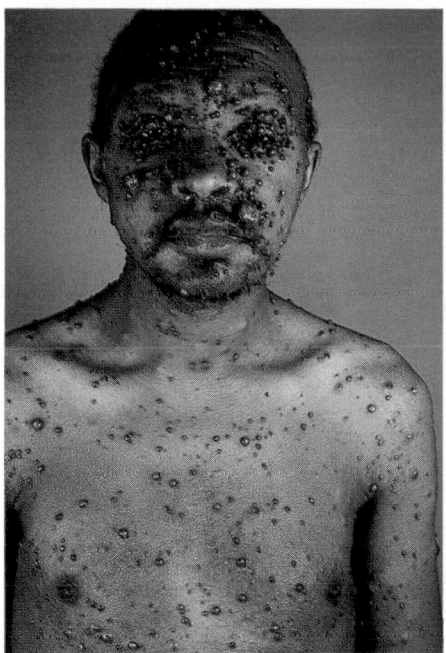

Figure 6–61. Epithelioid angiomatosis.

This rare and unusual vascular proliferation is sometimes seen in patients with AIDS. It is distinct from Kaposi's sarcoma.

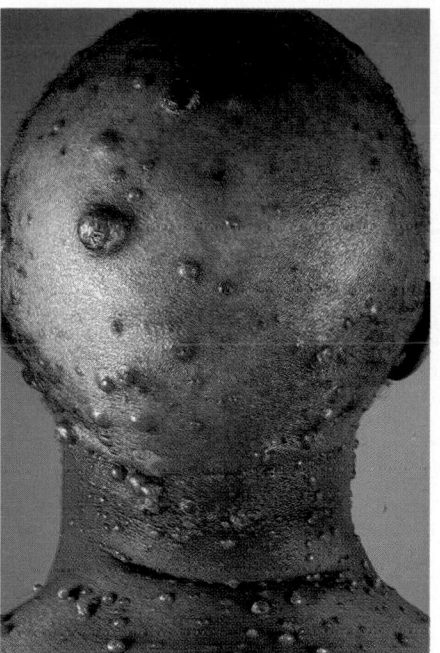

Figure 6–62. Epithelioid angiomatosis.

In contradistinction to Kaposi's sarcoma, these lesions are friable and pedunculated. The histopathologic findings are distinct from those of Kaposi's sarcoma.

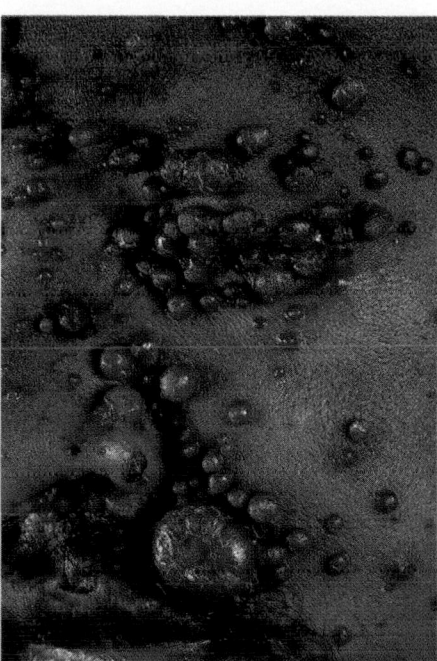

Figure 6–63. Epithelioid angiomatosis.

Close-up view demonstrating the dome-shaped sessile and pedunculated papules and nodules of epithelioid angiomatosis.

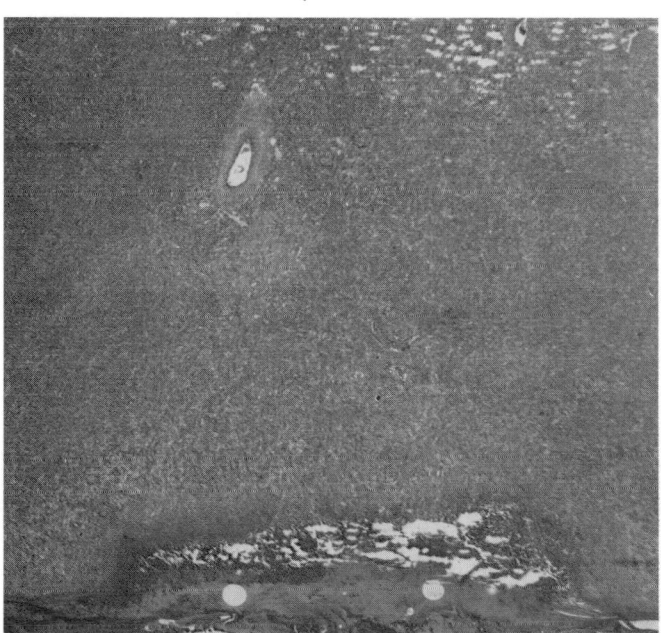

Figure 6–64. Epithelioid angioma.

Histologic photomicrograph of epithelioid angioma. There is a vascular proliferation characterized by pale-staining cells with scattered vascular spaces.

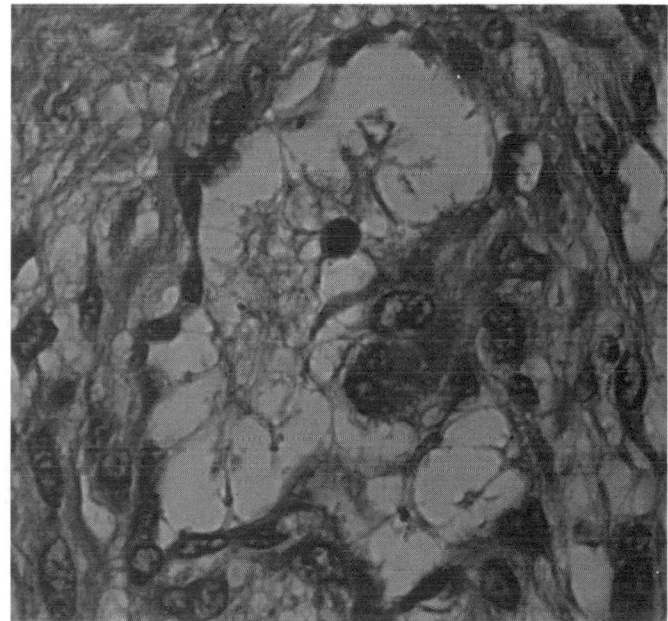

Figure 6–65. Epithelioid angioma.

High magnification reveals the cells to have cuboidal shapes with abundant pale-staining cytoplasm and plump endothelial cells that protrude into the lumen of the vessel. This appearance is distinct from that of Kaposi's sarcoma.

It has been noted that patients with AIDS often have a diffuse, fine, downy alopecia (Figures 6–66 and 6–67). This may or may not be associated with slight scaling of the scalp. It may be seen in individuals with relatively early manifestations of AIDS, but in some cases it is seen as a late sequela. Although not many cases have been studied histologically, when the material is biopsied, there is a perifollicular inflammatory cell infiltrate consisting of lymphocytes, plasma cells, and histiocytes, and some of the histiocytes are multinucleated. There is a decreased number of follicles in anagen and an increased number of follicles in telogen. Special stains for microorganisms have been negative. In all probability, the granulomatous inflammation is a consequence of rupture of follicles. Thus, the precise etiology of this alopecia is not clear. It may be progressive, and patients may eventually lose their entire pelage.

Multiple basal cell carcinomas as well as metastatic basal cell carcinoma have recently been described in patients with AIDS[32] (Figures 6–68 and 6–69). The multiple basal cell carcinomas may be either superficial or nodular. The number has ranged anywhere from a few to many. Therefore, patients with AIDS should be examined carefully for the presence of such lesions, especially if there is a history of prolonged sun exposure. In addition, any basal cell carcinoma or other cutaneous neoplasm should be treated as soon as possible after a diagnosis is made to prevent possible metastatic spread.

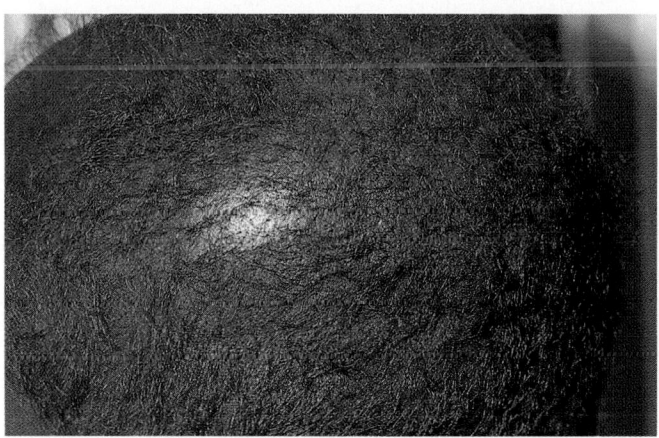

Figure 6–66. Alopecia of AIDS.

There is a fine, downy quality to the hair, which is increased in density. Notice the relative lack of inflammation seen clinically.

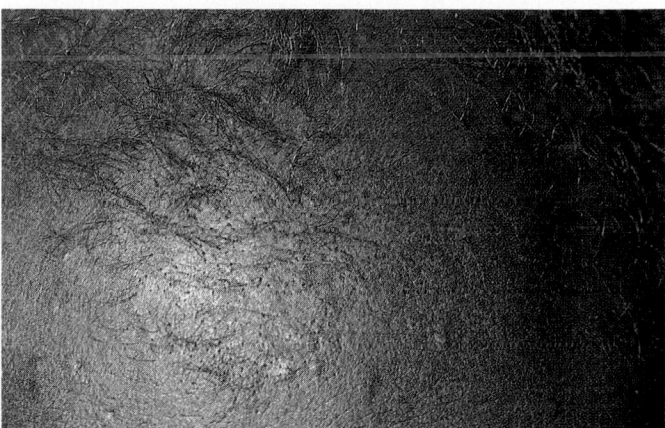

Figure 6–67. AIDS alopecia.

Close-up view. Occasionally scattered follicular papules may be seen that probably represent slight folliculitis.

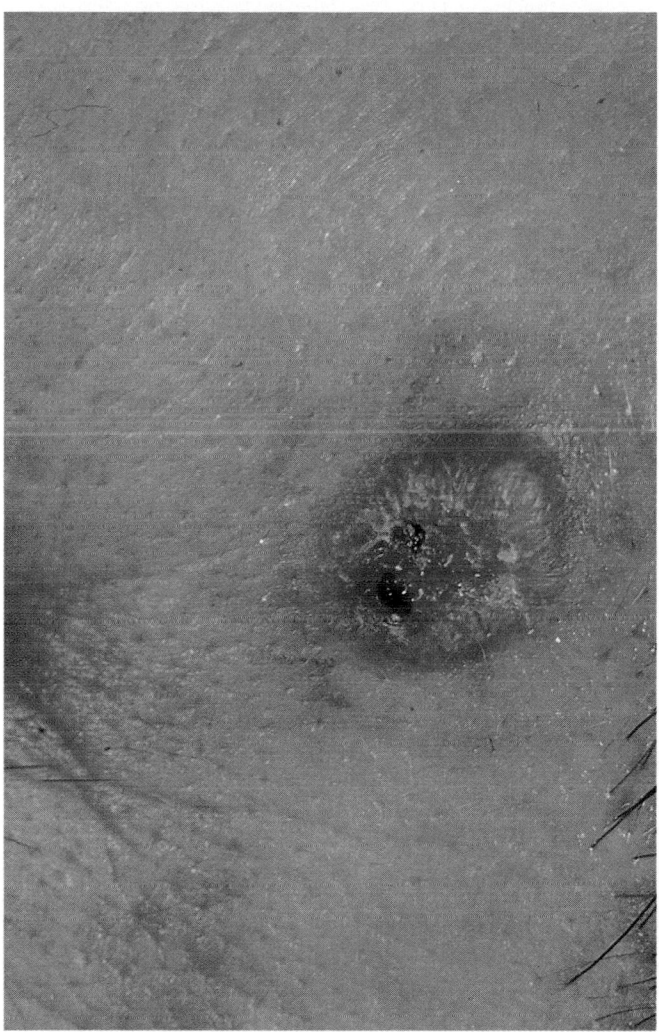

Figure 6–68. Basal cell carcinoma.

A characteristic reddish, ulcerated, pearly nodule seen on the side of the face of a patient with AIDS. Basal cell carcinomas often develop more aggressively in this patient population.

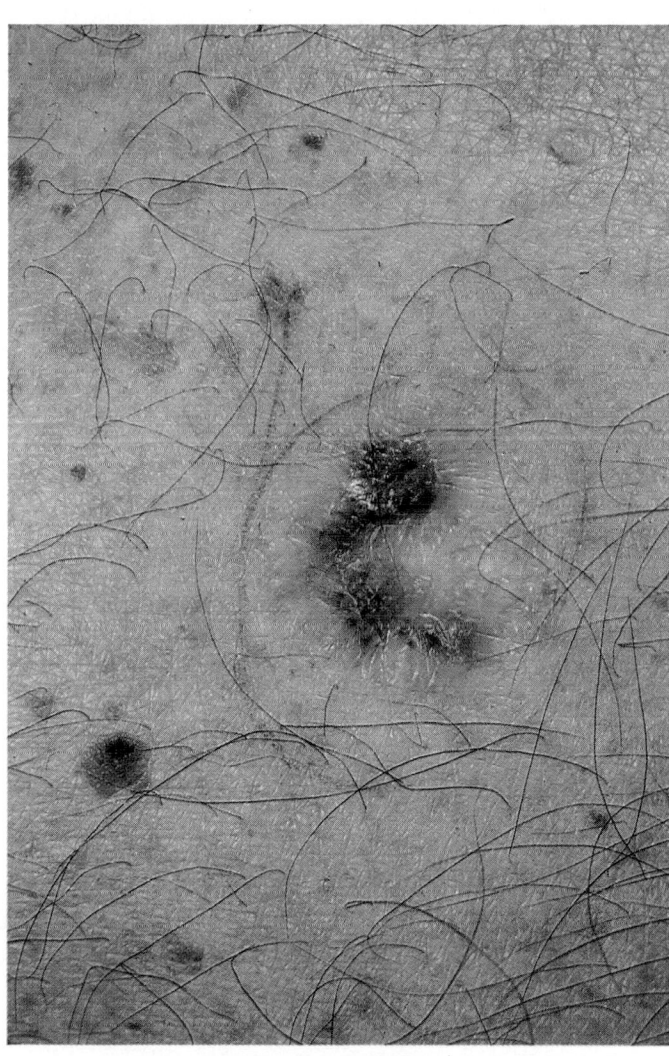

Figure 6–69. Basal cell carcinoma.

This multifocal pigmented basal cell carcinoma is another example of the types of lesions that may be seen in patients with AIDS. It should be remembered that these may be multiple and have been reported to metastasize.

Acknowledgments

Thanks to Alvin E. Friedman-Kien, M.D., for reviewing the manuscript. Ellen C. Gendler, M.D., Clinical Instructor of Dermatology, New York University Medical Center, assisted in the preparation of parts of this manuscript. Many of the clinical photographs are from the Clinical Photography Section of New York University Department of Dermatology and were taken by William Slue.

My thanks also to Dr. Sheri Lagin, Clinical Instructor at New York University Medical Center, for providing photographs of cryptococcosis, shown in Figures 6–34 and 6–35.

References

1. Linn CS, Pinha PD, Krishnan MN, et al: Cytomegalic inclusion disease of the skin. Arch Dermatol *117*:282, 1981.
2. Feldman PS, Walker AN, Baker R: Cutaneous lesions heralding disseminated cytomegalovirus infection. J Am Acad Dermatol *7*:545, 1982.
3. Muehler-Stamou A, Sen HJ, Emodi G: Epidermolysis in a case of severe cytomegalovirus infection. Br Med J *3*:609, 1974.
4. Medearis DN Jr: Cytomegalic inclusion disease: An analysis of the clinical features based on the literature in six additional cases. Pediatrics *19*:467–480, 1957.
5. Minars N, Silverman JF, Escobar NR, et al: Fatal cytomegalic inclusion disease: Associated skin manifestations in a renal transplant patient. Arch Dermatol *113*:1569, 1977.
6. Kwan TH, Kaufman HW: Acid fast bacilli with cytomegalovirus and herpes virus inclusions in the skin of an AIDS patient. Am J Clin Pathol *85*:236, 1986.
7. Friedman-Kien AE, LaFleur FL, Gendler EC, Hennessey NP, et al: Herpes zoster: A possible early clinical sign for development of acquired immunodeficiency syndrome in high risk individuals. J Am Acad Dermatol *14*:1023, 1986.
8. Hollander H, Schiodt M, Greenspan D, et al: Hairy leukoplakia and the acquired immunodeficiency syndrome. Ann Intern Med *104*:892, 1986.
9. Greenspan JS, Greenspan D, Lenette ET, Abrams DI, et al: Replication of Epstein-Barr virus within the epithelial cells of oral "hairy" leukoplakia, an AIDS associated lesion. N Engl J Med *313*:1564, 1985.
10. Friedman-Kien AE: Viral origin of hairy leukoplakia. Letter to Editor. Lancet *ii*:694, 1986.
11. Greenspan D, Hollander H, Friedman-Kien AE, et al: Oral hairy leukoplakia in two women, a hemophiliac, and a transfusion recipient. Letter to Editor. Lancet *ii*:978, 1986.
12. Soeprono FF, Schinella RA: Eosinophilic pustular folliculitis in patients with acquired immunodeficiency syndrome. J Am Acad Dermatol *14*:1020, 1986.
13. Gregory AN: Unusual observations of syphilis in patients with human immunodeficiency virus infection. Paper in preparation.
14. Hicks CB, et al: Sero-negative secondary syphilis in a patient infected with the auto-immuno-deficiency virus (HIV) with Kaposi's sarcoma. Ann Intern Med *107*:492, 1987.
15. Johns DR, et al: Alteration of the natural history of neuro-syphilis by concurrent infection with the human immunodeficiency virus. N Engl J Med *316*:1569, 1987.
16. Brown FS, Anderson RH, Burnett JW: Cutaneous tuberculosis. J Am Acad Dermatol *6*:101, 1982.
17. Klein RS, Harris CA, Small CB, et al: Oral candidiasis in high risk patients as the initial manifestation of the acquired immunodeficiency syndrome. N Engl J Med *311*:354, 1984.
18. Rico NJ, Penneys NS: Cutaneous cryptococcosis resembling molluscum contagiosum in a patient with AIDS. Arch Dermatol *121*:901, 1985.
19. Hazelhurst JA, Vismer HF: Histoplasmosis presenting with unusual skin lesions in acquired immunodeficiency syndrome (AIDS). Br J Dermatol *113*:345, 1985.
20. Kalter DC, Tschen JA, Klima M: Maculopapular rash in a patient with acquired immunodeficiency syndrome. Arch Dermatol *121*:1455, 1985.
21. Soeprono FF, Schinella RA, Cockerell CJ, Comite SL: Seborrheic-like dermatitis of acquired immunodeficiency syndrome. J Am Acad Dermatol *14*:242, 1986.
22. Winchester R, Bernstein DH, Fischer HD, et al: The co-occurrence of Reiter's syndrome and acquired immunodeficiency. Ann Intern Med *106*:19–26, 1987.
23. Gordin FM, Simon GL, Wofsy CD, Mills J: Adverse reactions to trimethoprim-sulfamethoxazole in patients with the acquired immunodeficiency syndrome. Ann Intern Med *100*:495, 1984.
24. Seoprano FF, Schienella RA: Eosinophilic pustular folliculitis in patients with acquired immuno-deficiency syndrome. J Am Acad Dermatol *14*:1020, 1986.
25. Buschness MR, Lim HW, Hatcher VA, Sanchez M, Soter MA: Ultra-violet B phototherapy of eosinophilic pustular folliculitis in patients with the acquired immuno-deficient syndrome. Submitted for publication, 1988.
26. Abramson SB, Odajnyk CM, Grieco AJ, et al: Hyperalgesic pseudothrombophlebitis: New syndrome in male homosexuals. Am J Med *78*:317, 1985.
27. Foon KA, Dougher G: Increased growth of eyelashes in a patient given leukocyte A interferon. N Engl J Med *311*:1259, 1984.
28. Cockerell CJ, Whitlow MA, Webster GF, Friedman-Kien AE: Epithelioid angiomatosis: A distinct vascular disorder in patients with the acquired immuno-deficiency syndrome or AIDS-related complex. Lancet *ii*:654, 1987.
29. Rosai J, Gold J, Tandy R: The histiocytoid hemangioma: A unifying concept embracing several previously described entities of skin, soft tissue, large vessels, bone and heart. Hum Pathol *10*:707, 1979.
30. Le Boit PE, Egbert BM, Stoler MH, et al.: Epithelioid hemangioma-like vascular proliferation in AIDS: manifestation of cat-scratch disease bacillus infection? Lancet i:960-963, 1988.
31. Cockerell CJ, Tierno P, Zucker-Franklin D, and Friedman-Kien AE. Recent observations. 1988.
32. Sitz KZ, Kepden M, Johnson DF: Metastatic basal cell carcinoma in acquired immuno-deficiency syndrome-related complex. JAMA *257*:340, 1987.

7

Opportunistic Infections in Patients with Human Immunodeficiency Virus Infection

Kenneth H. Mayer
Steven M. Opal

Infection with the human immuno-deficiency virus* (HIV, formerly HTLV-III/LAV) may result in clinically inapparent immunologic abnormalities or culminate in life-threatening illnesses due to a multiplicity of viral, bacterial, fungal, or protozoal pathogens, as well as opportunistic malignancies[1,2] (Table 7-1). A unifying feature of these disparate processes, which may involve many organ systems, resulting in varied clinical presentations, is the underlying immunologic derangement that occurs after retro-

---

*The term human immunodeficiency virus (HIV) in this chapter refers to HIV-I unless HIV-II is specified. Please see Chapter One for further differentiation between HIV-I and HIV-II.

viral exposure.[3] The primary insult has been thought to be due to a diminution of both the absolute number and function of T-helper/inducer lymphocytes; however, recent work suggests that HIV may affect other cells of the immune system, particularly monocyte macrophages.[4]

The relation of the immune dysfunction with the development of opportunistic infections in AIDS is further complicated by the fact that some of the infections result from the exposure of immunoincompetent individuals to ubiquitous agents, such as *Pneumocystis carinii* or *Candida albicans*, whereas other illnesses represent the reacti-

vation of latent infections, e.g., *Toxoplasma gondii*. The prevalence of different AIDS-associated illnesses may vary among risk groups, e.g., people from Africa and the Caribbean tend to have more toxoplasmosis and *Mycobacterium tuberculosis* infections and relatively less *P. carinii* infections than persons from the United States and Western Europe.[5] Putative cofactors, such as drug use (e.g., inhalation of volatile nitrites) and exposure to other immunosuppressive viruses (e.g., CMV and Epstein-Barr virus), have been thought to modify disease expression among individuals; however, the data in this regard are not conclusive.

Table 7-1. Opportunistic Infections Indicative of a Defect in Cellular Immune Function Associated with AIDS

A. *Helminthic infection*
   1. Strongyloidiasis (disseminated beyond the gastrointestinal tract)*

B. *Protozoan infection*
   1. *Pneumocystis carinii* pneumonia
   2. Disseminated toxoplasmosis, or *Toxoplasma* encephalitis, excluding congenital infection
   3. Chronic *Cryptosporidium* enteritis (>1 month)
   4. Chronic *Isospora belli* enteritis (>1 month)

C. *Fungal infection*
   1. *Candida* esophagitis, bronchopulmonary candidiasis*
   2. Cryptococcal meningitis, or disseminated infection
   3. Disseminated histoplasmosis*

D. *Bacterial infection*
   1. Disseminated (not just pulmonary or lymphatic) *M. avium-intracellulare* or *M. kansasii*

E. *Noncongenital viral infection*
   1. Chronic (>1 month) mucocutaneous herpes simplex
   2. Histologically evident cytomegalovirus infection including liver or lymph node
   3. Progressive multifocal leukencephalopathy

*Not listed in original CDC definition of AIDS, but subsequently added.

Etiology

The origin of HIV is still uncertain. A similar retrovirus has been isolated from wild African green monkeys.[6] Another retrovirus, in Western Africa, has been identified which is remarkably similar to the simian T-lymphotropic virus (STLV-III) or SIV, simian immunodeficiency virus, and has been called HTLV-IV and more recently, HIV-II.[7] The evolutionary relationships between SIV, HIV-II, and HIV-I require further clarification. It is possible that mutations in simian retroviruses in close contact between primates and humans in Africa may explain the fairly recent appearance of HIV-I and HIV-II as fairly recent causes of human immunodeficiency. Although SIV-III does not result in clinical disease in infected African green monkeys, and humans infected with HIV-II have thus far remained asymptomatic, another primate, the macaque monkey, develops lethal immunodeficiency after receiving SIV-III via an intravenous injection.[8] HIV-I and HIV-II have biologic and structural similarities to other human T-lymphotropic viruses (HTLV-I and HTLV-II) but are more closely related to visna (a slow virus that causes neurologic destruction in sheep) and other lentiviruses.[9] HIV-I and HIV-II are more complex than most of the other known animal retroviruses, some of which have only three essential genes—env, pol, and gag—coding for envelope proteins, the reverse transcriptase enzyme, and core proteins, respectively[10] (Figure 7–1).

The HIV genome is 9000 base pairs in size, with a divergence of up to 10 per cent in its genetic material between isolates found in San Francisco and in Central Africa.[11–14] The ENV gene contains the most divergent regions; some areas are hypervariable and appear to be unique for each isolate, whereas other regions are constant between multiple strains.[15] The GAG gene codes for several structural proteins, of which the p24 protein appears to be the most highly antigenic, and may be one of the first antibodies to be detected after infection with HIV.[16] Two other genes are unique for this retrovirus and are termed tat-III (which codes for the trans-activating transcriber that controls the level of expression of other genes)[17] and art, which is also known as trs (which codes for the differential expression of regulatory and structural functions, i.e., acceleration of the regulation of transcription).[18] These gene products trigger the activation of other HIV genes, resulting in rapid transcription and translation which leads to an acceleration of viral replication up to 1000 times the basal rate. The tat and art gene products appear to exert their greatest effect at the posttranscriptional level. The products produced by the short open reading frame (sor) and the 3' open reading frame (3' orf) have not yet been characterized.[19–21] Thus, viral replication and pathogenesis are not yet fully understood despite many recent important discoveries.

Pathogenesis

Although the transmission of HIV infection has been associated with intimate sexual contact as well as parenteral exposure to infected blood and blood products, the initial events in the pathogenesis of HIV infection are not certain. HIV has been shown to be able to infect T-helper lymphocytes,[22] monocyte macrophages,[23] and neurologic cells of macrophage lineage,[24] as well as other cell lines in tissue culture. HIV is able to enter target T-helper lymphocytes via binding of the envelope glycoprotein (gp120) to the CD4 antigenic determinant of the lymphocyte[25] (Figure 7–2). Following attachment and entry into the lymphocyte, the viral RNA is transcribed, as a result of the action of reverse transcriptase, into single-stranded DNA. Some of the DNA remains free in the cytoplasm and may partially account for a cytopathic effect on target cells.[26] However, most of the DNA is integrated into the host chromosome as proviral DNA, which may remain latent as part of the host genome indefinitely. This observation indicates that after initial infection with HIV, a host will remain infected indefinitely. Although the virus may remain dormant for months to years, proviral DNA may become activated in response to antigenic signals. Under in vitro conditions, effective antigenic stimuli have included mitogens, exposure to other viruses, and certain immunosuppressive agents.[27, 28] Activated proviral DNA can produce gene products at extraordinarily rapid rates under the influence of the tat and art genes, with a production of multiple copies of free virus and the associated destruction of the host cell[17, 18] (Figure 7–1). The precise mechanisms of cellular destruction are not certain at present. Giant cell formation, including the recruitment of uninfected lymphocytes, has been demonstrated in vitro.[29] HIV-infected lymphocytes appear to undergo accelerated maturation and are functionally impaired, responding inadequately to new stimuli. Likewise, the function of monocyte-macrophages, also directly infected by HIV, is severely impaired.[23]

HIV-infected mononuclear cells do not respond appropriately to new antigenic stimuli, resulting in impaired production of lymphokines and monokines.[30] Whether, in addition, there is the production of soluble mediators which have a deleterious effect on the immune system is not certain at the present time. The immune dysregulation due to the T lymphocyte and monocyte infection, results in alterations of humoral immunity as well. Many individuals with HIV infection have polyclonal hypergammaglobulinemia but are unable to respond appropriately to new antigenic stimuli with the production of new antibodies.[31] Infants and children with congenitally acquired HIV infection are often hypogammaglobulinemic because their B cells have not had the opportunity to become sensitized to ubiquitous antigens in the environment. This hypogammaglobulinemia is associated with recurrent infections with pyogenic bacteria in patients with pediatric AIDS.[32]

The loss of cell-mediated immunity results in patients becoming susceptible to a wide range of opportunistic infections and malignancies. It is not known whether the extreme cachexia seen in individuals with progressive HIV infection is due to multiple infections that recur in impaired hosts or to the elaboration of humoral factors which independently augment their constitutional symptoms. The extreme debilitation of individuals after recurrent opportunistic infections, plus the inability to eradicate many of these pathogens (such as cytomegalovirus, *Mycobacterium avium intracellulare,* cryptosporidia), results in the high fatality of HIV infection.

Human immunodeficiency virus itself may have direct effects on specific organs in addition to those described for the host immune system. The direct effects of HIV on the central nervous system appear to be second only to the effects on the immune system as a cause of morbidity and death.[33] The virus can multiply in central nervous system cells of macrophage lineage.[34] A number of cell lines derived from the central nervous system have been productively infected *in vitro* with HIV. At least a third of patients with advanced HIV infection show progressive neurologic deterioration, and up to 10 per cent of HIV-related deaths are related to central nervous system disease.[33] Recent studies indicate that the central nervous system may be an early target of HIV infection, resulting in subtle neurologic abnormalities in otherwise asymptomatic individuals.

The Diagnosis of AIDS and HIV Infection

Because the initial case definition of AIDS was developed prior to the elucidation of HIV as the etiologic agent, the diagnosis of AIDS then required that an individual, with no other reason for cellular immunodeficiency, have one of a specific list of opportunistic infections or malignancies (see Tables 7–1 and 7–2). Subsequently, the Centers for Disease Control (CDC) has developed a new classification schema that incorporates new insights that have been developed about the natural history of HIV infection in recent years (Table 7–3). The diagnosis of HIV infection requires the use of corroborative screening tests that have been developed since 1984. The indications for these tests, outside well-designed clinical or epidemiologic studies, is still open to controversy because of the lack of therapeutic interventions available for the asymptomatic seropositive patient at the present time. However, the use of HIV tests for screening the national blood supply, for assisting clinicians in interpreting new patterns of infection among members of high- and low-risk groups, and as an adjunct in counseling for interested patients to supplement risk reduction education are accepted uses of the test at the present time. Over the past year, HIV diagnostic tests have been utilized more than 20 million times.

The most commonly employed screening test is the ELISA (enzyme-linked immunosorbent assay), in which disrupted virus proteins

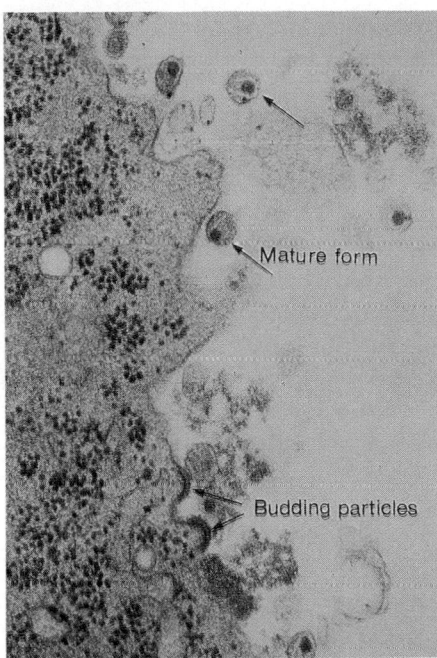

Figure 7–1. HIV.
Electron micrograph of HIV budding off a T lymphocyte.

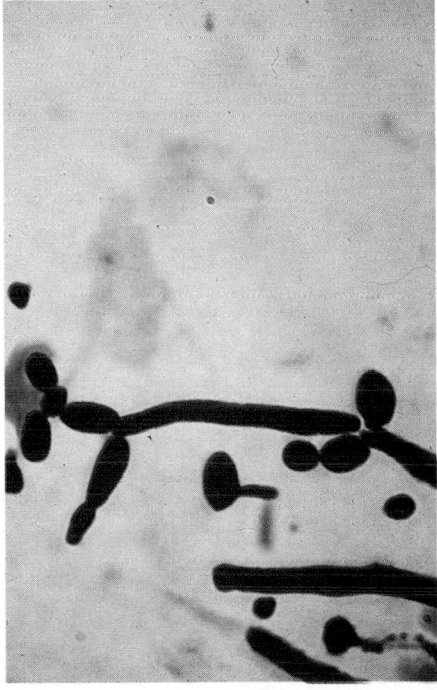

Figure 7–2. *Candida albicans.*
Potassium hydroxide stain of tongue scraping revealing budding yeast forms of *Candida albicans* causing thrush. (Courtesy of Jonathan W. M. Gold, MD, Associate Director, Special Microbiology Laboratory, Memorial Sloan-Kettering Cancer Center, New York.)

are applied to the surfaces of wells and microtiter plates or on polystyrene beads. Many companies have utilized these technologies in order to develop HIV screening tests which can be done rapidly with a high degree of reproducibility. Serum is added to these plates and if antibodies to HIV are present, they are sandwiched between the surfaces of the plate and an antiantibody which is conjugated to a chemical that can produce a color change when an additional specific reagent is added. Thus, a positive response is usually detected through a colorimetric reaction in a spectrophotometer with cut-offs being set on the basis of panels of known standards. The choice of the cut point has been set toward the more sensitive side so that the predictive value of the test is least accurate in low prevalence populations; this approach is clearly desirable for ensuring the safety of the blood supply but necessitates secondary corroborative tests in seropositive individuals, particularly from low-risk groups.[35]

Other tests for antibody detection include the Western Blot assay, the radioimmunoprecipitation assay as well as cytoplasmic or membrane immunofluorescence test.[36, 37] Second generation tests are being developed which include assays of antibodies to purified recombinant antigens[38] as well as tests to detect directly the presence of free serum antigen.[39] The clinical utility of these tests will require follow-up with larger cohorts over longer periods of time to assess whether the information provided sheds new light on the natural history of HIV infection, particularly in regard to the prognosis of infected individuals.

False positive ELISAs are more commonly found in multiparous women, drug users who are exposed to multiple human antigens, and individuals who have collagen-vascular diseases.[40, 41] Therefore, the Western Blot or another more specific test is necessary to corroborate the presence of HIV infection, particularly in low-risk individuals. Even the Western Blot test may occasionally yield a false-positive result,[42] especially in intravenous drug users.

In high-risk populations, the correlation of positive ELISA tests with positive Western Blot studies has been excellent; frequently, more than 93 per cent of ELISA positive individuals have corroborative Western Blot studies.[35] Although the "gold" standard for the diagnosis of HIV infection should be, in the theory, the ability to grow HIV from the patient's blood, growth of the virus in tissue culture has not been consistent, even in patients with clear-cut HIV infection.[43] A number of factors probably contribute to this, of which an important one is the very low titers of virus (usually no more than 1 in 10,000 peripheral blood lymphocytes are infected) in the blood of infected patients. Other problems in substantiating the antibody test with viral culture include technical difficulties of the culture techniques, and the possibility that humoral factors such as neutralizing antibodies may limit the ability to grow the virus from certain infected hosts at different stages of illness. Ongoing prospective epidemiologic cohort studies are addressing these questions. Certain individuals have had positive blood cultures for HIV without generating detectable antibodies.[44, 45] Some of these individuals, presumably recently infected, have subsequently seroconverted, but several have been followed for more than a year without the presence of detectable antibody by either ELISA or corroborative testing.

Clinical Manifestations of AIDS

Acute Retroviral Syndrome

After an initial intimate exposure in which HIV is transmitted, the newly infected person may remain asymptomatic for long periods of time or may develop an acute mononucleosis-like febrile illness within three to six weeks.[46] The symptoms may include fever, malaise, and generalized lymphadenopathy, which frequently lasts for about a week and then subsides completely. Other manifestations may include arthralgias, aseptic meningitis, and maculopapular or

Table 7–2. Prevalence of the Most Common Opportunistic Diseases in Among the First 12,000 Patients with AIDS*

Disease	Prevalence (%)
Opportunistic infections	
Pneumocystis carinii pneumonia	63
Candida esophagitis	14
Disseminated cytomegalovirus	7
Cryptococcosis	7
Atypical mycobacterial infection	5
Persistent herpes simplex	4
Cryptosporidiosis	4
Toxoplasmosis	4
Progressive multifocal leukencephalopathy	0.7
Opportunistic malignancies	
Kaposi's sarcoma	26
Brain lymphoma	0.7

*Data courtesy of the Centers for Disease Control: Note that many persons had >1 opportunistic illness.

urticarial rashes.[47] However, in one prospective study of a high-risk group in Amsterdam, the majority of newly infected individuals did not record any focal symptomatology other than fever around the time that they seroconverted.[38, 39] Thus, it is not known what proportion of patients develop such an "acute retroviral syndrome," and its clinical significance regarding subsequent progression of HIV infection is unknown at present. From the small number of individuals who have been studied intensively, antibodies to HIV are generally detectable within 4 to 12 weeks after a transmitting exposure.[48] The time between infection by HIV and seroconversion appears to be similar whether the exposure is via contaminated blood or via sexual contact.

Asymptomatic Infection

The majority of individuals currently infected with HIV worldwide are asymptomatic. The rates of development of AIDS and other clinical sequelae are uncertain at the present time because not enough large cohorts have been followed for sufficiently long periods of time. It is possible that the prevalence of cofactors such as other immunosuppressive viruses (e.g., cytomegalovirus and Epstein-Barr virus), malnutrition, or immunogenetic differences may play a role in the ultimate expression of illness after exposure to the HIV retrovirus. In the San Francisco hepatitis B cohort study, after a mean of five years follow-up of 51 homosexually active males, 18 per cent had developed CDC-defined AIDS, 5 per cent had constitutional symptoms, 30 per cent had generalized lymphadenopathy, 12 per cent had asymptomatic hematologic abnormalities, and 35 per cent were asymptomatic with normal laboratory test results.[49] After almost eight years of follow-up, a more recent update indicates

that almost 40 per cent of the men now have AIDs.[49a] These data suggest a tendency to progress from clinical conditions of less severity to more serious ones, without any evidence of improvement in immunologic function or clinical symptoms over time.[50]

Progressive Generalized Lymphadenopathy

Individuals at increased risk for HIV infection may have lymphadenopathy for multiple other reasons, including chronic infections with Epstein-Barr virus, cytomegalovirus, toxoplasmosis, and secondary syphilis, without the presence of HIV infection. However, early in the AIDS epidemic, it was recognized that a large number of high-risk individuals had developed generalized lymphadenopathy.[51] Over more than three years of follow-up, in San Francisco, 9 per cent of a cohort of 200 homosexually active males with generalized lymphadenopathy developed AIDS.[52] Other cohorts have found higher rates of progression of illness in individuals with generalized lymphadenopathy;[53] however, rates of development of clinical illness over time have been difficult to assess because the time of development of lymphadenopathy or HIV seroconver-

sion is frequently not known. A subgroup of individuals with generalized lymphadenopathy seem to do well for long periods of time as long as they are without systemic manifestations. The onset of constitutional symptoms, minor opportunistic infections such as thrush or zoster, and persistent hematologic abnormalities including leukopenia, lymphopenia, hypergammaglobulinemia, and an increase in the erythrocyte sedimentation rate may be harbingers of subsequent development of more serious opportunistic processes.

The AIDS-Related Complex

Various authors have described signs and symptoms which did not fit in the Centers for Disease Control classification for AIDS initially, but suggested that individuals had infections associated with HIV and might be at increased risk of developing the full-blown AIDS syndrome.[48, 49, 53] In addition to progressive generalized lymphadenopathy, symptoms that suggested the presence of progressive HIV infection included persistent fevers, diarrhea, anorexia, weight loss, and malaise that were not due to other underlying illnesses. The high prevalence of other infections which could independently produce these kinds of

Table 7–3. Summary of Centers for Disease Control Classification System for HIV Infections

Group I	Acute infection
Group II	Asymptomatic infection*
Group III	Persistent generalized lymphadenopathy*
Group IV	Other disease
Subgroup A	Constitutional disease
Subgroup B	Neurologic disease
Subgroup C	Secondary infectious diseases
Category C-1	Specified secondary infectious diseases listed in the CDC surveillance definition for AIDS†
Category C-2	Other specified secondary infectious diseases
Subgroup D	Secondary cancers†
Subgroup E	Other conditions

*Patients in groups II and III I may be subclassified on the basis of a laboratory evaluation.
†Includes those patients whose clinical presentation fulfills the definition of AIDS used by CDC for national reporting.

symptoms (e.g., cytomegalovirus, Epstein-Barr, and other virus infections) has made this a difficult group to characterize. The presence of oropharyngeal candidiasis has been suggested to be a particularly serious negative prognostic feature of individuals in this group[54] (Figure 7–2). Rates of development of AIDS among these individuals has ranged from 1.2 per cent[55] to more than 10 per cent[53] per year. Severe depression of the T lymphocyte subpopulation has been associated with the rapid onset of more severe manifestations of immunodeficiency.[76]

Protozoan Infections

Pneumocystis carinii

This organism is common in the environment so that the majority of immunocompetent children in the United States have detectable antibodies to *P. carinii*.[55] In addition to wide geographical dispersion, the organism has been found in multiple mammalian genera. Human cases of *P. carinii* pneumonitis have been noted in most countries, with the initial epidemics described among malnourished and premature infants found in displaced persons camps after World War II. Before the AIDS epidemic, the most frequent descriptions of *P. carinii* pneumonitis were of patients, particularly children, with hematologic malignancies.

The clinical disease usually only involves the lungs (Figure 7–3), although parasitemia, as well as liver, spleen, and lymph gland involvement, have been noted. One recent report suggested ocular involvement occurred in a patient with AIDS.[56] The organism may be found in either a cystic or trophozoite form. Cysts are spherical or cup-shaped and the wall stains brownish-black with Gomori methenamine-silver nitrate stain (Figure 7–4) and purple-violet with toluidine blue 0.[57] Neither method

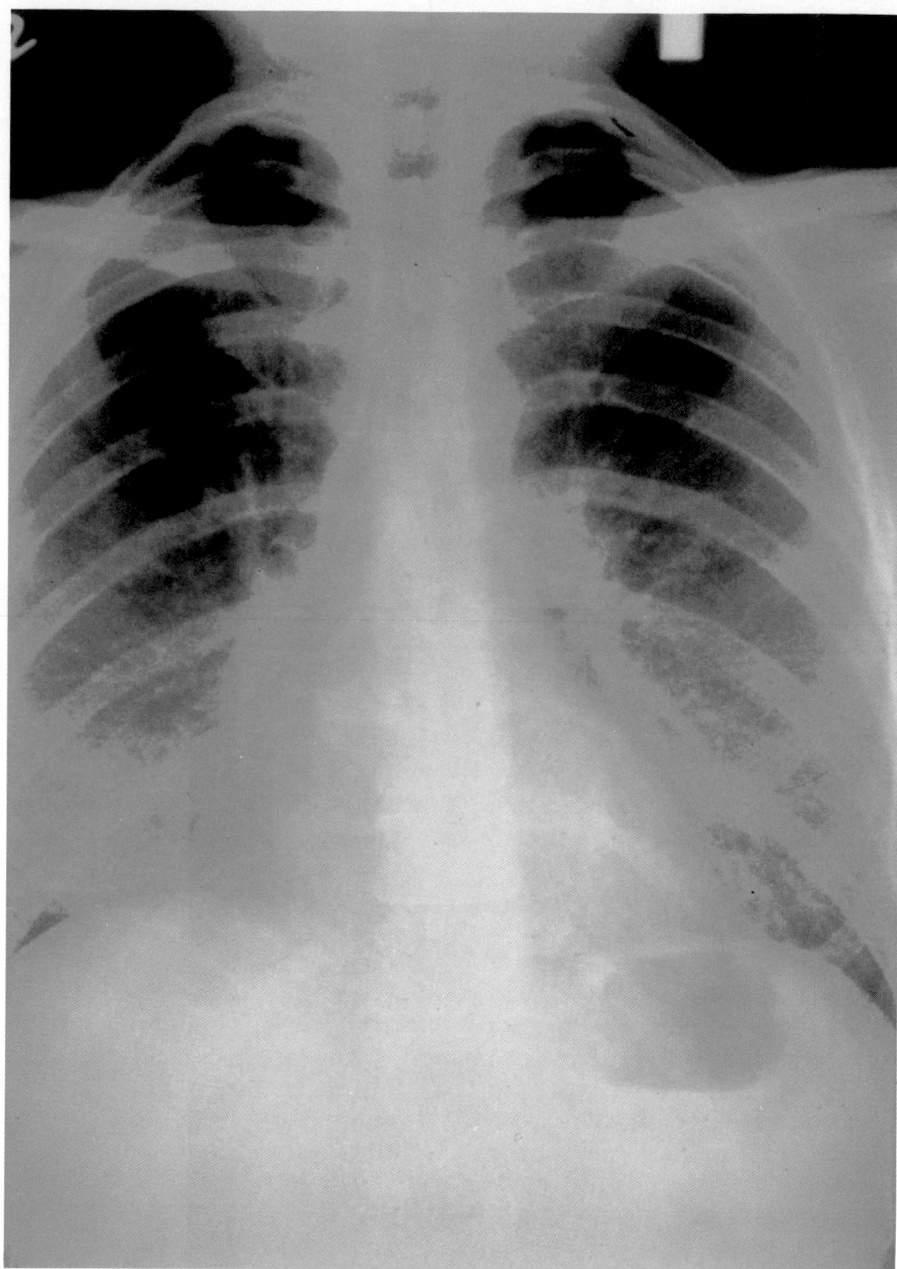

Figure 7–3. *Pneumocystis carinii*.
Chest x-ray showing bilateral lower lobar interstitial infiltrates.

will stain the trophozoite. Up to eight sporozoites may be found within a cyst, which may be demonstrated by Giemsa (Figure 7–5), Wright, Gram-Weigert, polychrome methylene blue or hematoxylin, and eosin stains (Figure 7–6), which also stain trophozoites but not the cyst wall.

Infection occurs after cyst forms are aerosolized and then multiply in pulmonary alveolar macrophages which may be associated with septal inflammation. If the organism proliferates extensively, a diffuse desquamative alveolitis may ensue. The alveolar lumen may fill with large numbers of organisms and macrophages, and the alveolar walls may thicken because of interstitial plasma cell infiltration resulting in a diffuse interstitial pneumonitis, tending to be more prominent in the lower lobes (see Figure 7–1). The chest x-ray, how-

ever, cannot be diagnostic in and of itself, as other interstitial pneumonitides may be seen with AIDS.[8, 9]

The clinical findings may appear subacutely or abruptly, most often including tachypnea and fever. A dry, nonproductive cough may be present, but more nonspecific symptoms such as anxiety, dyspnea on exertion, and malaise are more common. Evidence of pneumonitis on chest x-ray is generally only apparent after symptoms have been present for more than a week.[10] Pallor and cyanosis may be associated with more advanced illness. Rales are often absent, and the arterial oxygen tension may be in the normal range.

The diagnosis can be made effectively with bronchoalveolar lavage without a transbronchial biopsy;[58–62] recently, the use of sputum examination has been advocated.[63] The

majority of the patients respond to their first course of therapy with either trimethoprim-sulfamethoxazole or pentamidine isoethionate. However, more than a third of individuals manifest allergic reactions to these drugs (e.g., fever, rashes, granulocytopenia, hypoglycemia), necessitating changes in therapy.[64] Because relapses are frequent, it is suggested that individuals be treated for at least three weeks with systemic therapy.[65] Aerosolized pentamidine appears to be effective in the treatment of milder cases of *Pneumocystis carinii* pneumonia and may offer even greater promise as a prophylactic agent.[65a] Fansidar and trimethoprim have been used with some success.[66] Trials of *P. carinii* prophylaxis with oral trimethoprim-sulfamethoxazole, injections or inhalation of pentamidine, and trimetrexate (another dihydrofolate reductase inhibitor) are ongoing.

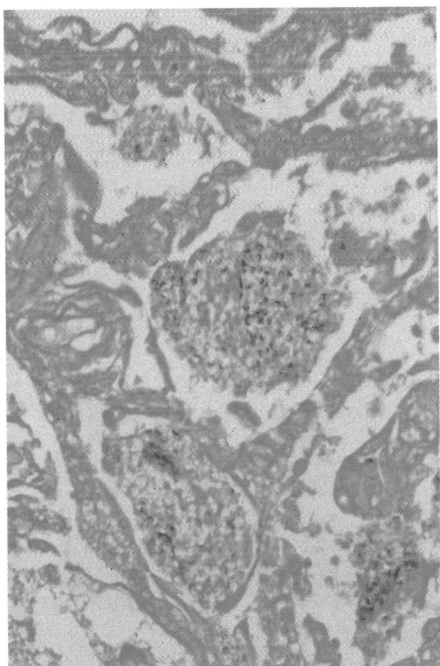

Figure 7–4. *Pneumocystis carinii* cysts.

These cysts are in alveolar spaces, stained black by Gomori methenamine silver stain. (From Still Picture Archives, Centers for Disease Control, Atlanta, Georgia.)

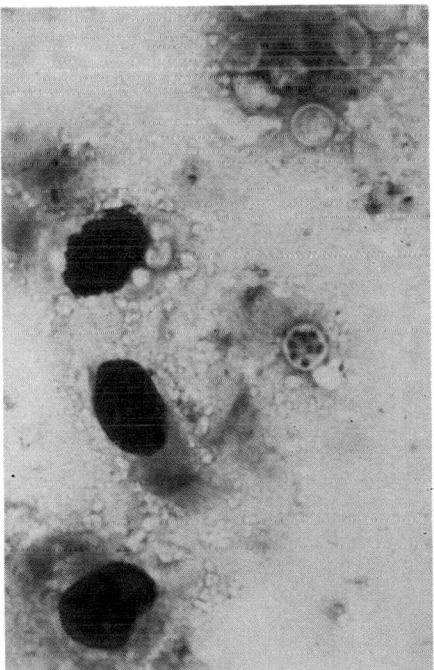

Figure 7–5. *Pneumocystis carinii.*

Pneumocystis carinii, lung impression smear; Giemsa stain. (×1125) (From Still Picture Archives, Centers for Disease Control, Atlanta, Georgia.)

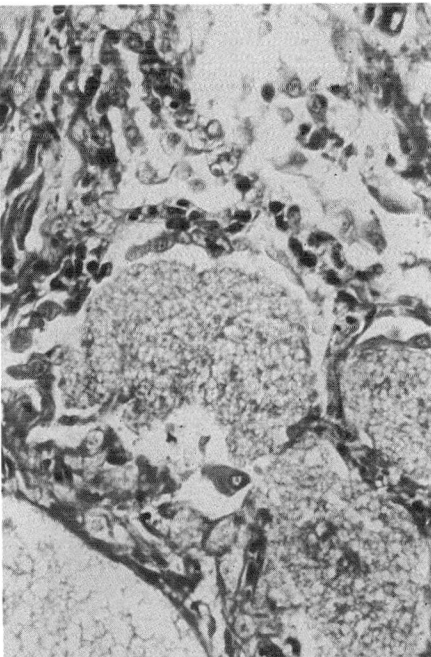

Figure 7–6. *Pneumocystis carinii.*

Pneumocystis carinii in alveolar spaces in human lung; hematoxylin and eosin stain. (From Still Picture Archives, Centers for Disease Control, Atlanta, Georgia.)

Toxoplasma gondii

T. gondii is an obligate intracellular protozoan that is ubiquitous in nature, resulting in varying degrees of infection and disease in animals and humans. Infection may be transmitted to many species of carnivores through the ingestion of cysts which release viable tachyzoites after the cyst wall is disrupted by gastric enzymes. These invade the mucosa of the gastrointestinal tract and, from there, disseminate widely through the body, most commonly encysting in the brain (Figures 7–7 and 7–8), heart, or skeletal muscle. Infection will persist for the life of the host, with reactivation occurring most frequently if the host becomes immunodeficient.

The majority of patients with toxoplasmosis in AIDS have findings referable to the central nervous system,[67, 68] which may present subacutely as personality changes (e.g., apathy, depression) or as acute meningoencephalitis, or commonly as a space-occupying lesion. Myocarditis, pneumonitis, and adult chorioretinitis have also been noted. *T. gondii* may be found rarely in the lymph nodes of persons with chronic generalized lymphadenopathy. The most common presentations include seizures, focal neurologic deficits, and encephalopathy.[69] CT scans frequently demonstrate the presence of one or multiple space-occupying lesions whose ring is enhanced by the use of contrast dye (Figure 7–9). Diagnosis involves clinical presentation and empiric therapy in many cases. However, use of brain biopsy is preferable to establish a definitive diagnosis, because individuals in some of the high-risk groups, such

as intravenous drug users, may have similar presentations with pyogenic brain abscesses.

Serologic studies, such as the Sabin-Feldman dye test, have been unreliable in the diagnosis of toxoplasmosis in patients with AIDS. The demonstration of tachyzoites in body fluids or tissue by Wright or Giemsa stains is diagnostic. Tissue cysts may be seen with the periodic acid–Schiff (PAS) stain, which will highly stain the tachyzoites within the cyst. They may reflect chronic infection, so that the clinical history is important in deciding the significance of only finding cysts without invasive tachyzoites. Increased numbers of tissue cysts in a specific location may be helpful in establishing a diagnosis of reactivated CNS toxoplasmosis, which can only be definitively diagnosed by brain biopsy.[69] Patients tend to respond to therapy with pyrimethamine and sulfadiazine, but frequently relapse because the cyst forms are resistant to these agents. Hence, patients must be treated for life.

Cryptosporidiosis

Cryptosporidia, and the associated species, *Isospora belli*, have been recognized as human pathogens only over the last 10 years. However, the spectrum of illness is now appreciated to include subclinical manifestations such as transient diarrhea in individuals whose immune systems are intact (Figure 7–10).[70] Many patients with AIDS have severe watery diarrhea, but only in a fraction of them can this be documented to be caused by cryptosporidia. The organism is a small bowel pathogen which proliferates widely on the surface of the GI mucosa resulting in a malab-

sorption-type syndrome (Figure 7–10).[71] Occasionally the organism may be isolated from other organs such as the gallbladder (associated with a sclerosing cholangitis-like syndrome)[72] as well as the lungs, but the primary disease is from the profuse, watery diarrhea that has been refractory to most antibiotic regimens in patients with AIDS. Symptoms may wax and wane, ranging from a few soft stools per day to a constant watery stream of diarrhea.

The organism cannot be identified by conventional stool staining techniques; however, it can be seen on iodine-stained wet mounts or in acid-fast stains of stool smears. However, the yield on identifying the organism is best if a sucrose flotation gradient technique is utilized (Figure 7–11).[73] The organism can be visualized on biopsy specimens of gastrointestinal mucosa by light or electron microscopy.

The therapy of cryptosporidiosis has been generally unsuccessful. Clinical studies have utilized a wide range of antiprotozoal drugs such as furazolidone, tetracycline, and antimalarials; however, the best success to date has been with spiramycin, a macrolide antibiotic.[74, 75] However, a good response has not been uniform, and relapses have occurred when the drug has been discontinued. DMFO, a potent *in vitro* antiprotozoal drug, has been suggested as a useful agent, given the generally poor response of AIDS patients with cryptosporidiosis to most regimens.[76] *Isospora belli*, a related coccidial protozoan which can cause a similar syndrome, has responded to therapy with trimethoprim-sulfamethoxazole.[77]

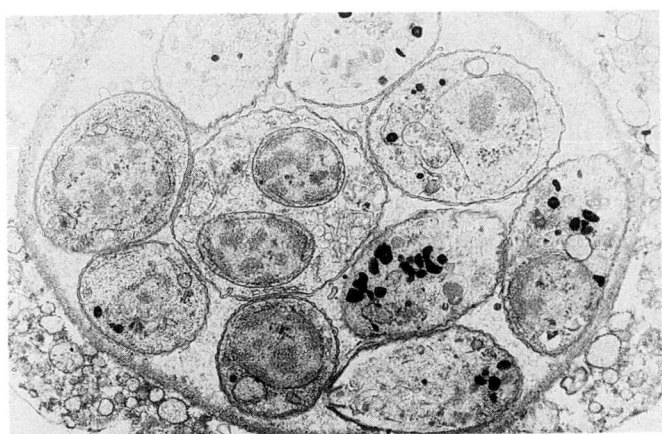

Figure 7–7. *Toxoplasma.*

Toxoplasma cyst, electron micrograph. (From Still Picture Archives, Centers for Disease Control, Atlanta, Georgia.)

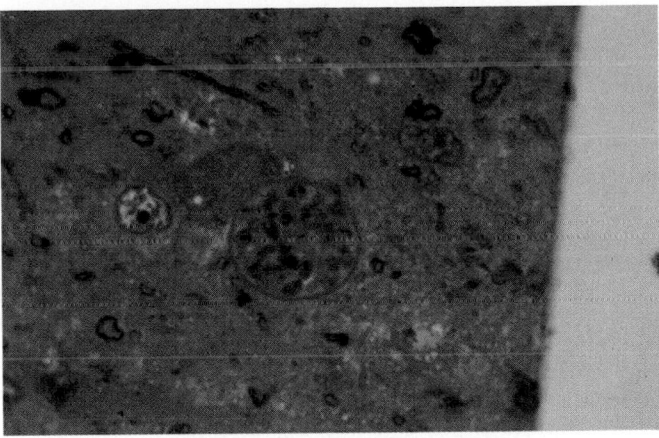

Figure 7–8. Toxoplasmosis.

Toxoplasmosis, section of brain. ($\times 1200$) (From Still Picture Archives, Centers for Disease Control, Atlanta, Georgia.)

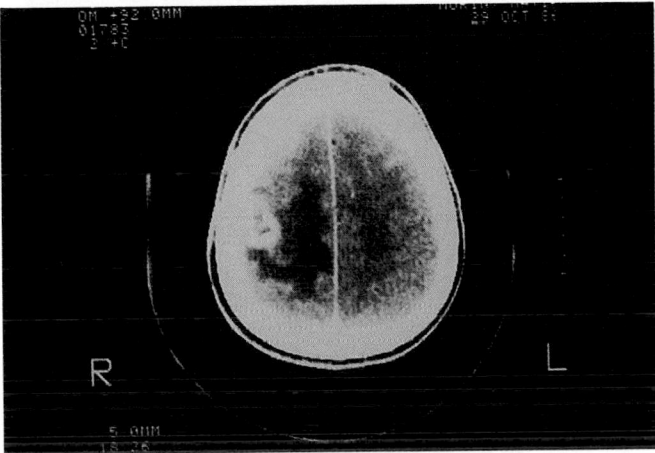

Figure 7–9. Toxoplasmosis.

Toxoplasmosis, space-occupying lesion on CT scan.

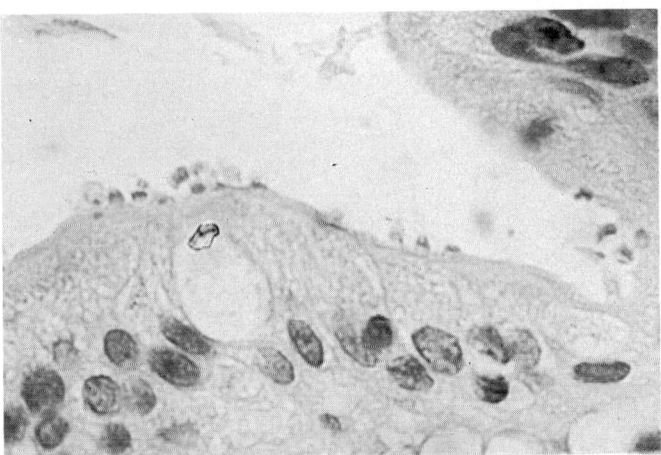

Figure 7–10. Cryptosporidiosis.

Cryptosporidiosis, small bowel biopsy; high-power magnification. (Courtesy of Jonathan W. M. Gold, MD, Associate Director, Special Microbiology Laboratory, Memorial Sloan-Kettering Cancer Center, New York.)

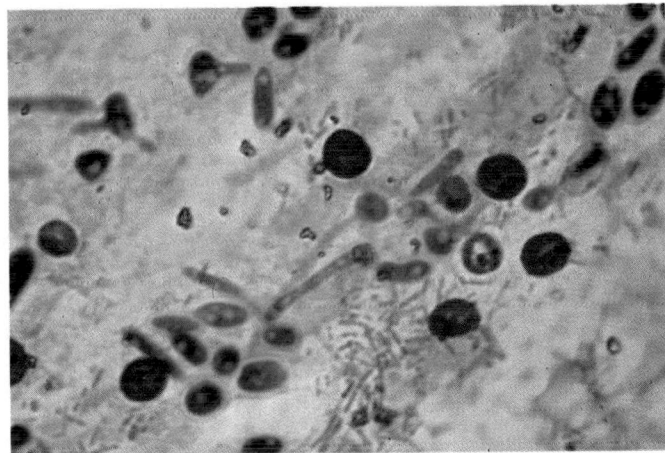

Figure 7–11. Cryptosporidiosis.

Cryptosporidiosis, modified cold Kinyoun acid-fast stain under oil immersion lens; oocysts (acid-fast) stain red; yeast cells (not acid-fast) stain green; direct fecal smear. (Courtesy of Dr. Pearl Ma, Director, Microbiology, St. Vincent's Hospital, New York.)

Other Protozoa

Although infection with *Giardia lamblia* (Figure 7–12) or *Entamoeba histolytica* (Figures 7–13 and 7–14) are not in and of themselves suggestive of immunodeficiency or HIV infection, these organisms may be found in high-risk patients more frequently than in the general population. Infected individuals may be asymptomatic carriers or may have persistent diarrhea and cramps as well as constitutional symptoms. Chronic infection may result in malabsorption and malnutrition, and possibly deleterious stimulation of the immune system of individuals who also carry HIV. Thus, prompt diagnosis by checking stools for cysts and trophozoites, with subsequent antiparasitic therapy, is desirable.

Fungal Infections

Candida albicans

Candidal infections of mucous membranes and the skin are common occurrences in patients with AIDS and related disorders. It is rare to see invasive disease, except in patients who have long-standing intravenous lines, or are extremely debilitated and cachectic. Case reports of candidal endocarditis or other systemic involvement have been noted (Figures 7–15 and 7–16).

Oropharyngeal candidiasis, or thrush, has been noted to be a common feature of AIDS-related symptoms in several of the risk groups.[78] Thrush is an uncommon finding in individuals who have not received broad-spectrum antibiotics or corticosteroids or who have other underlying immunologic or metabolic diseases. Candidal esophagitis is distinctly uncommon among any individuals except those who have AIDS so that individuals who are at risk for the syndrome who complain of dysphagia should undergo prompt endoscopy so that early treatment can be instituted (Figure 7–17). The differential diagnosis of dysphagia in these individuals also includes herpes esophagitis as well. Mucosal infections frequently respond rapidly to therapy with nystatin or clotrimazole troches or with mouthwash. However, some individuals, particularly those with esophagitis, will need treatment with ketoconazole and occasional refractory cases will need to be treated with systemic amphotericin B.

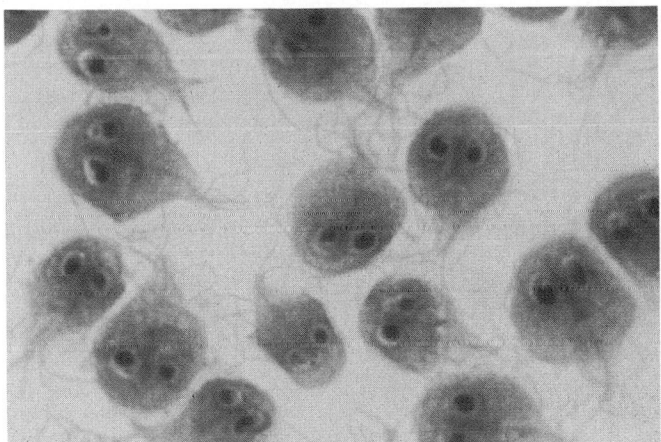

Figure 7–12. Giardia lamblia.

Giardia lamblia trophozooite from duodenal aspirate.

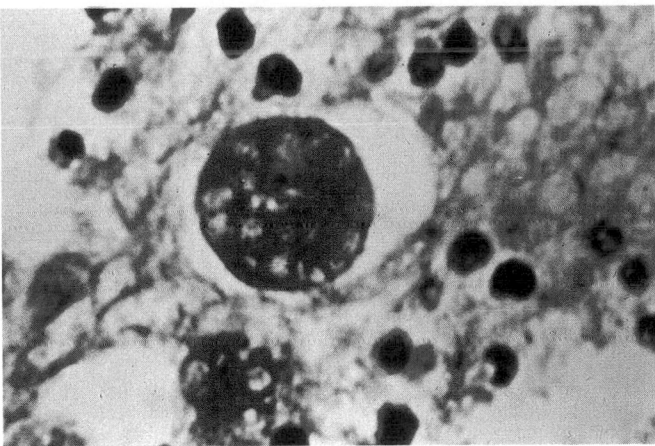

Figure 7–13. *E. histolytica*.

E. histolytica cyst in bowel preparation, surrounded by red blood cells.

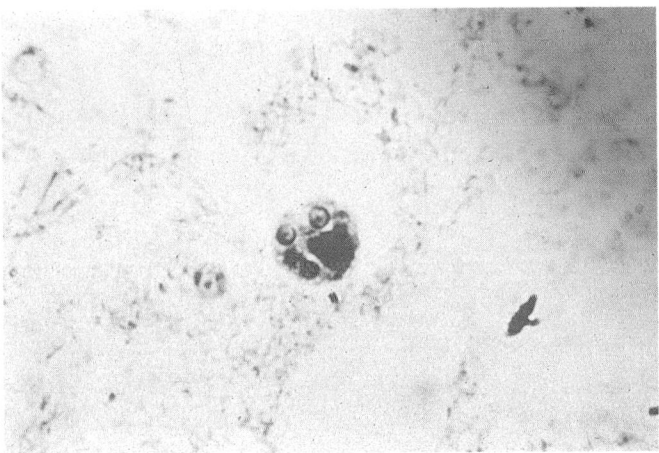

Figure 7–14. *E. histolytica*.

E. histolytica cyst with four nuclei and prominent chromatoidal body.

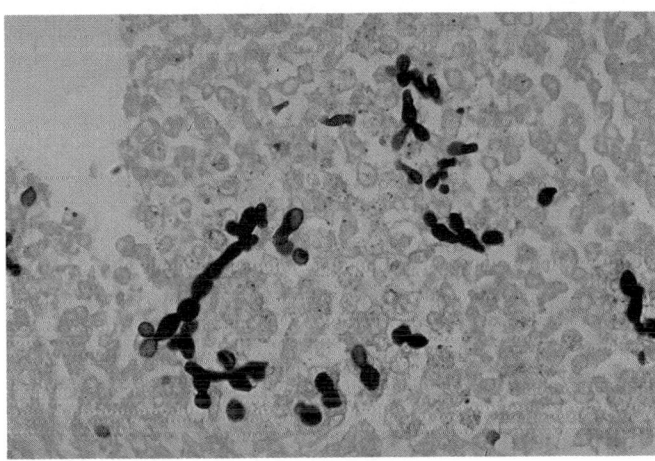

Figure 7–15. *Candida albicans*.

Candida albicans in human heart tissue; Gomori stain. (×500) (From Still Picture Archives, Centers for Disease Control, Atlanta, Georgia.)

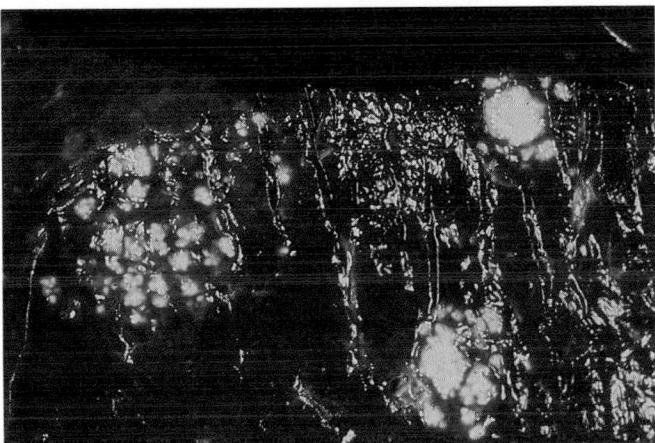

Figure 7–16. *Candida albicans*.

Human liver showing multiple granulomas caused by *Candida albicans*. (From Still Picture Archives, Centers for Disease Control, Atlanta, Georgia.)

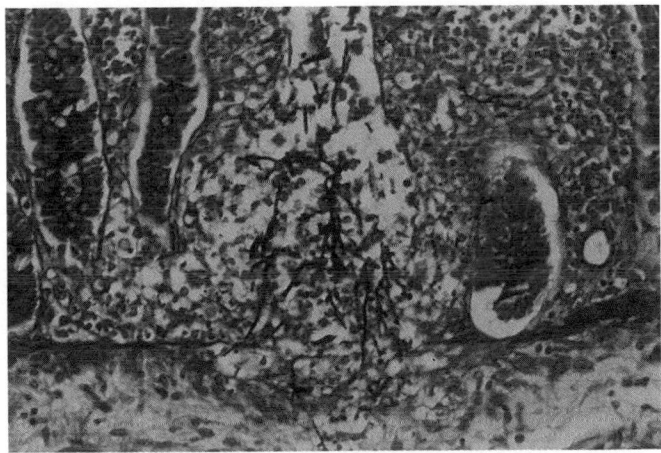

Figure 7–17. Candidal abscesses.

Esophageal biopsy reveals candidal abscesses, pseudohyphae extending through submucosa; periodic acid–Schiff stain. (From Still Picture Archives, Centers for Disease Control, Atlanta, Georgia.)

Cryptococcus neoformans

Cryptococcal infection in individuals with AIDS, as in other immunologic disorders, may present subacutely as a mild headache with a low-grade fever.[79, 80] More severe manifestations such as nausea, vomiting, and meningeal signs may develop subsequently. The cerebrospinal fluid usually reveals pleocytosis, low glucose and high protein. Definitive studies include the India ink test (Figure 7–18), latex agglutination testing for the cryptococcal antigen, as well as fungal cultures. In addition to cryptococcal meningitis, this organism may develop into mass lesions of the central nervous system (Figure 7–19). Patients with AIDS may also present with extra-meningeal manifestations of cryptococcal disease including hepatic (Figure 7–20), pulmonary (Figure 7–21), dermatologic (Figure 7–22), lymphadenopathic, and peritoneal involvement. Demonstration of this organism from any site in a patient with AIDS is a sufficient indication for the institution of prompt therapy.[80] Therapeutic regimens include low-dose amphotericin B (0.3 mg/kg per day) combined with flucytosine (150 mg/kg per day) for six weeks or high-dose amphotericin B alone (0.6 mg/kg per day) for at least 10 weeks.[81] Unfortunately, because the immunologic deficit in patients with AIDS does not remit during the course of therapy, relapses have been noted, and therefore, individuals with AIDS and cryptococcal disease may need longer courses of therapy, perhaps for an indefinite period of time.

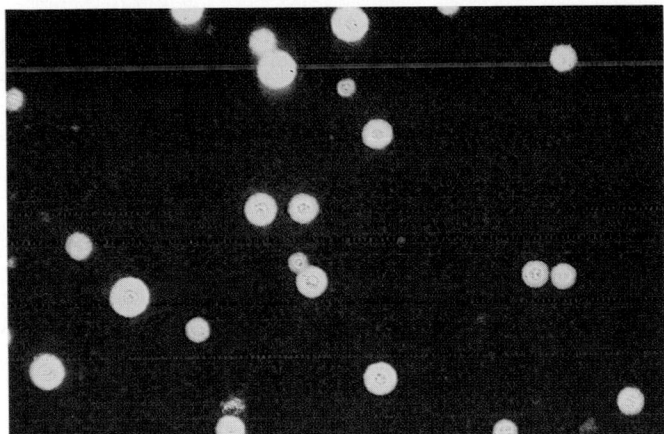

Figure 7–18. *Cryptococcus neoformans.*

Photomicrograph showing *Cryptococcus neoformans;* India ink mount. (×475) (From Still Picture Archives, Centers for Disease Control, Atlanta, Georgia.)

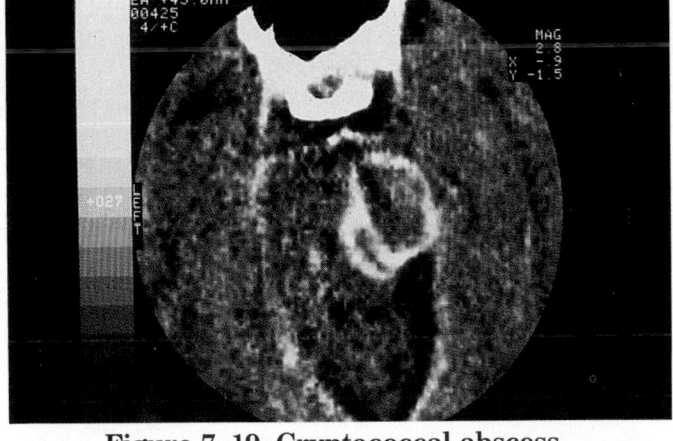

Figure 7–19. Cryptococcal abscess.

Cryptococcal abscess of the brainstem on CT scan. (From Still Picture Archives, Centers for Disease Control, Atlanta, Georgia.)

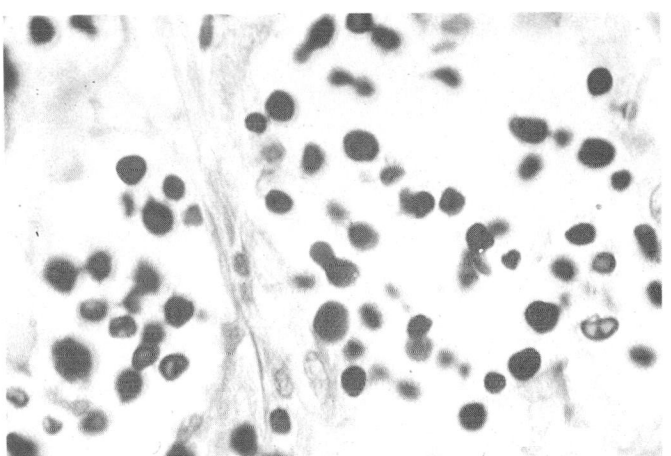

Figure 7–20. Cryptococcosis.

Cryptococcosis—tissue section of liver; periodic acid–Schiff stain. (×980) (From Still Picture Archives, Centers for Disease Control, Atlanta, Georgia.)

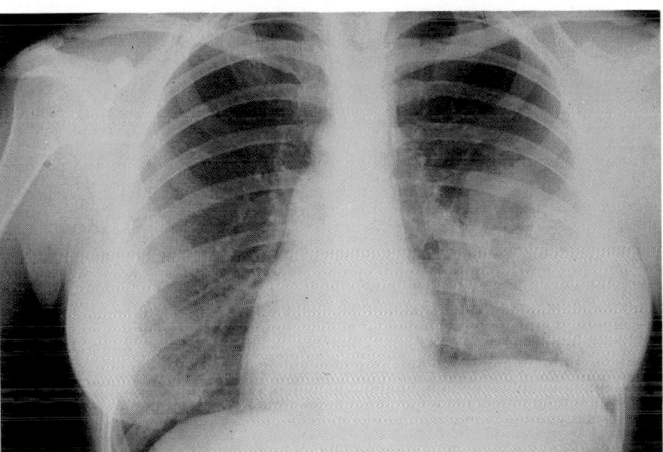

Figure 7–21. Cryptococcosis.

X-ray of patient showing nonencapsulated cryptococcosis. (From Still Picture Archives, Centers for Disease Control, Atlanta, Georgia.)

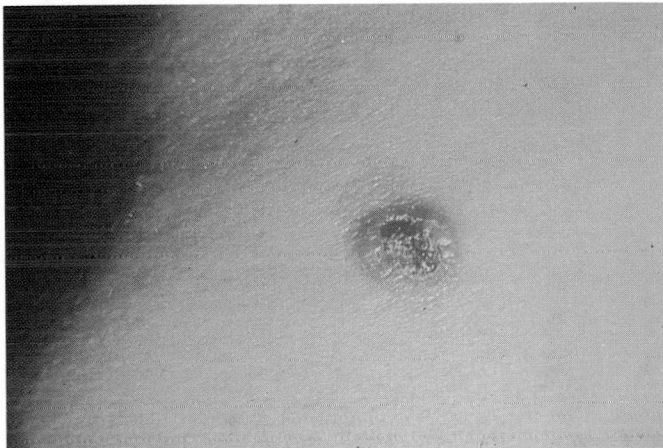

Figure 7–22. Cryptococcosis.

Cryptococcosis—skin lesion (close-up); disseminated case. (From Still Picture Archives, Centers for Disease Control, Atlanta, Georgia.)

Other Fungi

Immunocompromised patients, including those with AIDS, may develop disseminated fungal infections with a large number of pathogens. *Aspergillus* infection may result in a necrotizing pneumonitis (Figure 7–23) or spread widely and invade virtually any organ (Figure 7–24). In areas where histoplasmosis and coccidioidomycosis are endemic diseases, retrovirus-induced immunodeficiency may result in disseminated infection (Figures 7–25 and 7–26).

Bacterial Infections

Mycobacterium-avium intracellulare

Prior to the advent of the AIDS epidemic, *M. avium-intracellulare* was known to be a ubiquitous environmental contaminant that rarely caused disseminated disease in adults. In patients with AIDS, however, it has been found in up to one fifth of the number of cases that have been prospectively followed, presenting with fever, weight loss, and debilitation.[82, 83] The organism may be cultured from blood, lymph nodes, liver, spleen, lung, and bone marrow.[84] Granulomas may not be present and so the actual contribution of this organism to the morbidity of patients with AIDS is not always clear.[85] Several patients with *M. avium-intracellulare* have had chronic diarrhea and the organism has been found on small bowel biopsy (Figure 7–27).[86]

The organisms are acid-fast but are somewhat longer and thicker than *M. tuberculosis* upon staining. Cultures tend to grow more rapidly than tuberculosis and may often be recognized in two to three weeks (Figure 7–28). In addition to the acid-fast stain of blood cultures and other tissues, the organism may be demonstrated in macrophages utilizing the periodic acid–Schiff stain.

The treatment of this organism usually requires multiple antituberculous drugs because of high levels of resistance. In addition to conventional antituberculous medications such as isoniazid, ethambutal, and aminoglycosides, the organism is often sensitive to clofazimine and ansamycin, a rifampin derivative.[87] Treatment usually utilizes four of these drugs.[88] However, progressive cachexia, anemia, and fevers may be seen in individuals despite treatment with an optimal regimen. The clinical efficacy of these regimens has been questionable, and persistent inanition is very common despite treatment.

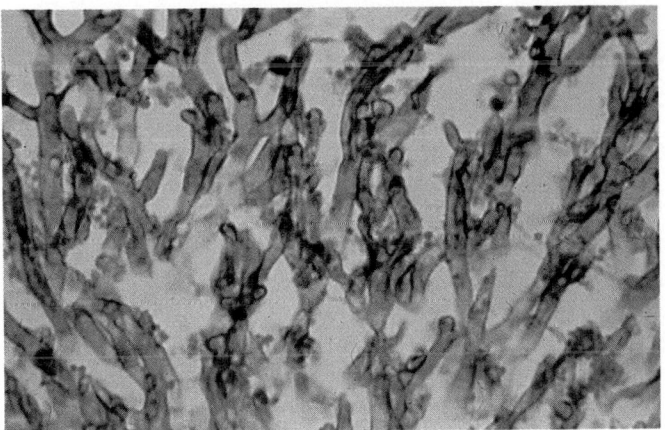

Figure 7–23. *Aspergillus fumigatus.*

Aspergillus fumigatus; hematoxylin and eosin stain of lung tissue with "forked stick" branching hyphae.

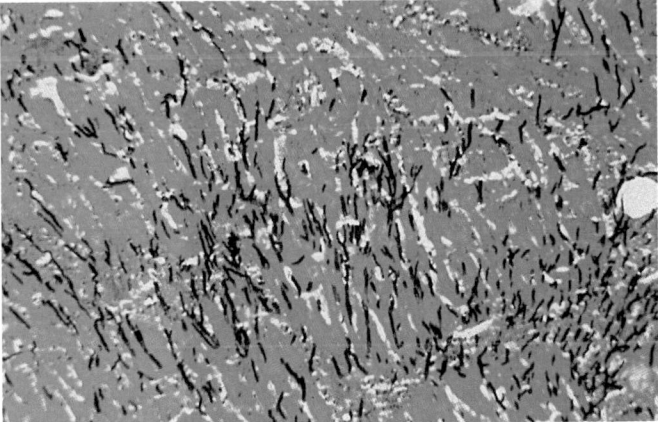

Figure 7–24. *Aspergillus fumigatus.*

Aspergillus fumigatus; Gomori methenamine silver stain of fungal invasion of myocardium.

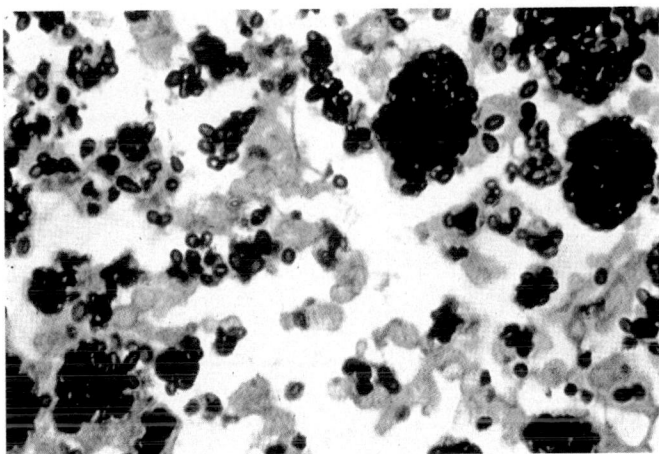

Figure 7–25. Histoplasmosis.

Histoplasmosis; Gomori methenamine silver stain of lung revealing narrow-based budding.

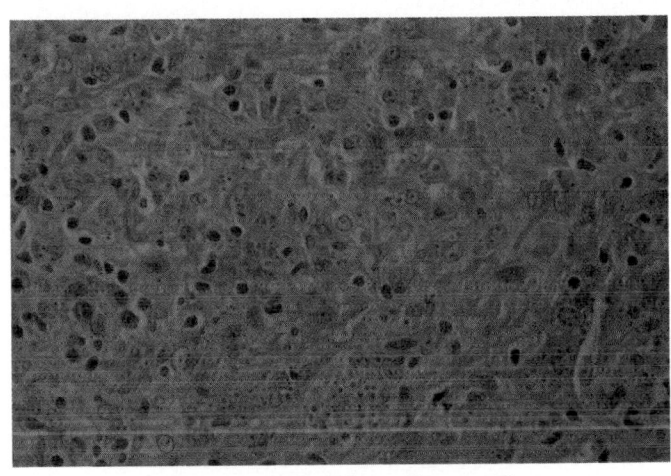

Figure 7–26. Histoplasmosis.

Histoplasmosis; periodic acid–Schiff stain.

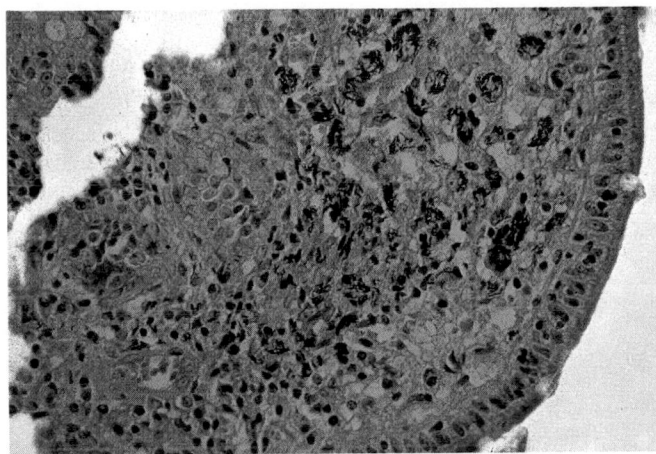

Figure 7–27. Mycobacterial infection.

Mycobacterial infection of small bowel; acid-fast stain. Biopsy specimen. (Courtesy of Jonathan W. M. Gold, MD, Associate Director, Special Microbiology Laboratory, Memorial Sloan-Kettering Cancer Center, New York.)

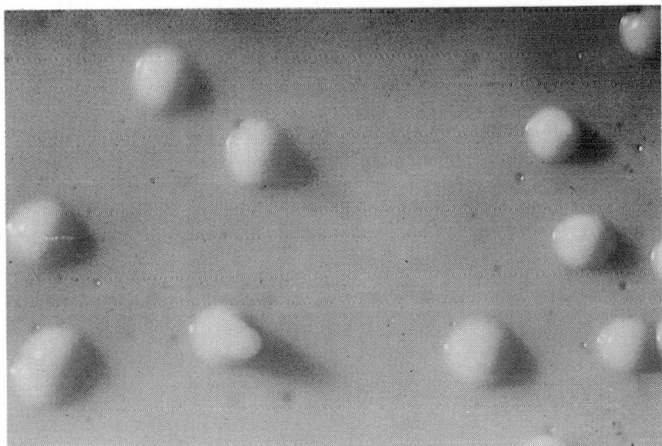

Figure 7–28. *Mycobacterium avium.*

Mycobacterium avium, colonial morphology. (From Still Picture Archives, Centers for Disease Control, Atlanta, Georgia.)

Mycobacterium Tuberculosis

Tuberculosis has been recognized with increasing frequency in individuals with AIDS who come from either the Caribbean, particularly Haiti, or Central Africa.[5, 89] Tuberculous infection has not been particularly common in individuals whose exposure to HIV occurred in the United States. This difference presumably reflects the high prevalence of endemic tuberculosis in underdeveloped countries which manifests itself as disseminated disease when individuals become immunosuppressed after infection with the retrovirus. Individuals may present with disseminated pulmonary tuberculosis (Figures 7–29 and 7–30), as well as extrapulmonary tuberculosis, including involvement of lymph nodes, liver (Figure 7–31), spleen, bone marrow, as well as the gastrointestinal tract.

Except in cases of meningeal or cavitary pulmonary tuberculosis, therapy may begin with two antituberculosis drugs, such as isoniazid and rifampin. The infection usually can be controlled with appropriate antibiotic therapy; however, because the immunodeficiency is generally not corrected in the course of antituberculosis chemotherapy, patients are at risk of relapse once the medications are stopped.

Salmonella Infection

Disseminated *Salmonella* infections have been associated with patients with other immuocompromised conditions such as hematologic malignancies. Individuals from Central Africa and Haiti as well as gay and bisexual men may have an increased prevalence of intestinal infections due to either environmental factors or specific behavioral practices. Individuals with AIDS who develop *Salmonella* infection of the gastrointestinal tract may have a higher incidence of persistent bacteremia.[90–92] These organisms may be routinely cultured using MacConkey, EMB, or SS media (Figure 7–32) and are frequently susceptible to conventional antibiotics. Given the ability for salmonellae to persist intracellularly in Peyer's patches in the gut, it is not surprising that the organism may be able to multiply and cause disseminated disease in immunocompromised patients with AIDS and related symptom complexes.

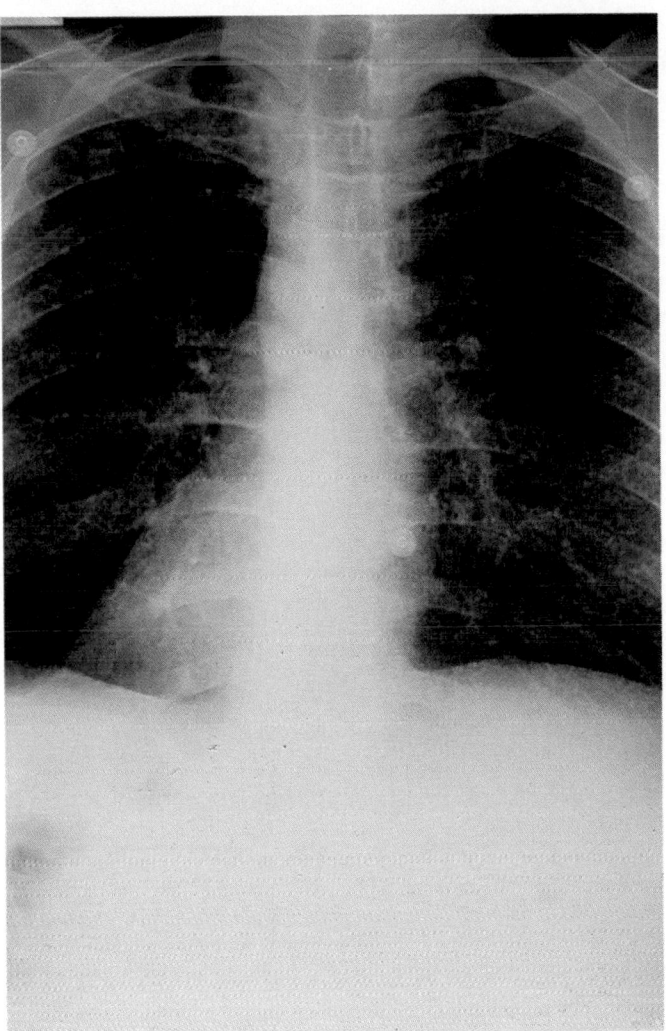

Figure 7–29. Miliary tuberculosis.
Chest x-ray in miliary tuberculosis.

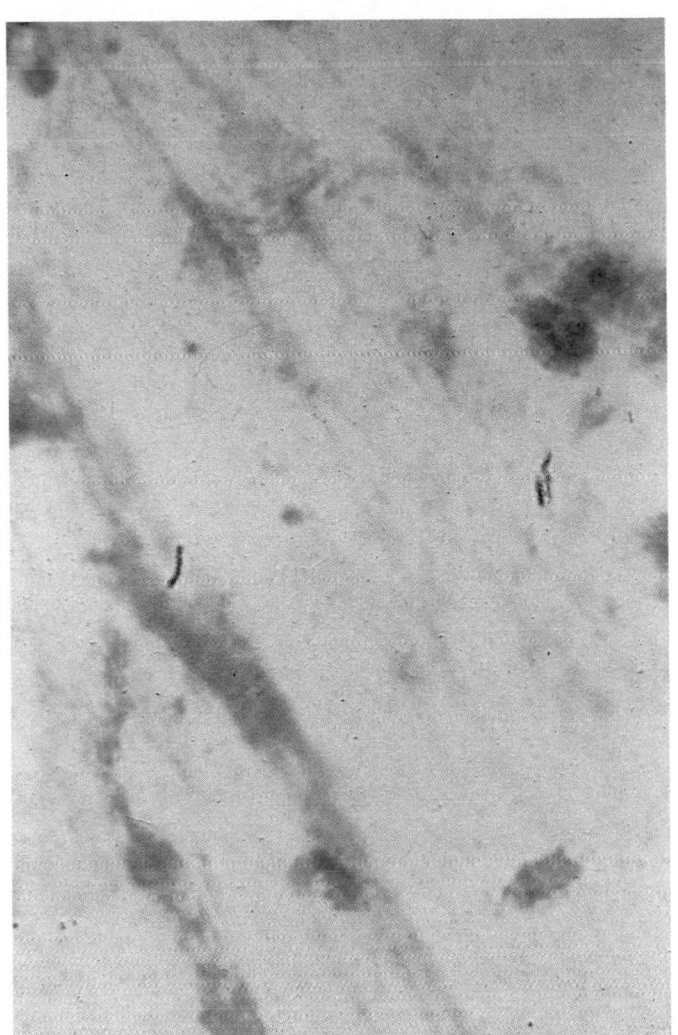

Figure 7–30. *M. tuberculosis*.
Ziehl-Neelsen stain of *M. tuberculosis*.

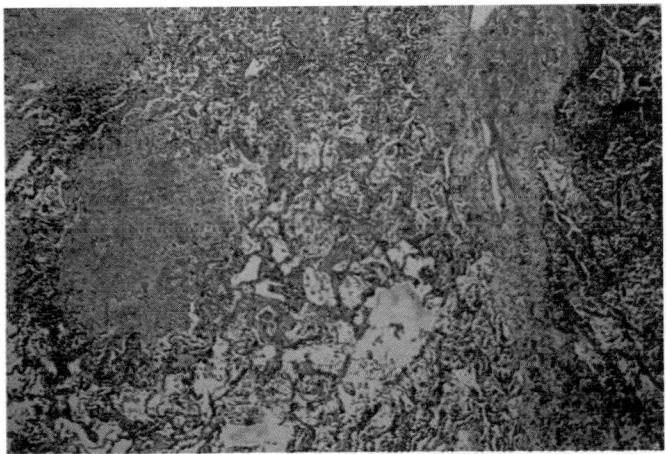

Figure 7–31. Hepatic granuloma.
Liver-hematoxylin and eosin stain of hepatic granuloma.

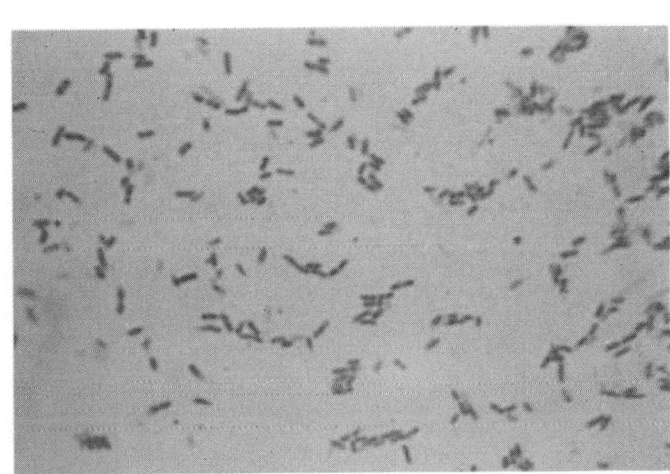

Figure 7–32. *Salmonella typhimurium*.
Gram stain of blood subculture revealing *Salmonella typhimurium*.

Other Bacteria

Immunocompromised patients with HIV infection may also be subject to disseminated infections with other bacteria that may be intracellular parasites. Thus, disseminated infection with *Nocardia* (Figures 7–33 and 7–34) and *Legionella* pneumonia (Figures 7–35 and 7–36) may be seen. Nocardiosis is preferably treated with intravenous sulfonamides, and legionellosis is treated with systemic erythromycin.

Viruses

Herpes Simplex and Zoster

In individuals who acquired AIDS because of increased sexual activity, frequently there is a history of exposure to herpes simplex earlier in life. Once individuals become immunodeficient because of HIV infection, herpes simplex may cause extensive mucosal and cutaneous ulcers in perioral or perirectal areas (Figure 7–37).[93, 94] Herpetic encephalitis or visceral involvement has not been commonly reported in individuals with AIDS. The major morbidity from these herpetic lesions is the failure to resolve, even with appropriate antiviral therapy with acyclovir. Clinical complaints may include rectal pain, bleeding, or a purulent discharge. The lesions may be up to 10 cm in diameter. Genital herpes may also occur in patients with AIDS; however, the progressive erosive disease noted with perioral and perianal involvement has not been reported. Part of the differential diagnosis of candidal esophagitis includes herpetic esophagitis and must be differentiated by endoscopy. Lesions that are suspected of being herpetic in origin may be swabbed, and Tzanck smear preparations using Wright stain can be performed for a rapid office or bedside diagnosis (Figure 7–38). In addition, herpetic ulcers can be cultured and virus can be retrieved within two weeks and generally in less than a week. Patients with AIDS-related symptoms who have recurrent herpetic disease may be best managed with long-term suppressive therapy with acyclovir, although on occasion immunocompetent hosts have developed resistant strains when treated for protracted periods with this drug.

The reactivation of the herpes zoster virus resulting in shingles frequently may be seen in individuals with HIV infection (Figures 7–26 and 7–39). Disseminated disease and encephalitis have been seen, but are uncommon. Particularly severe cases may benefit from high-dose intravenous acyclovir.[95]

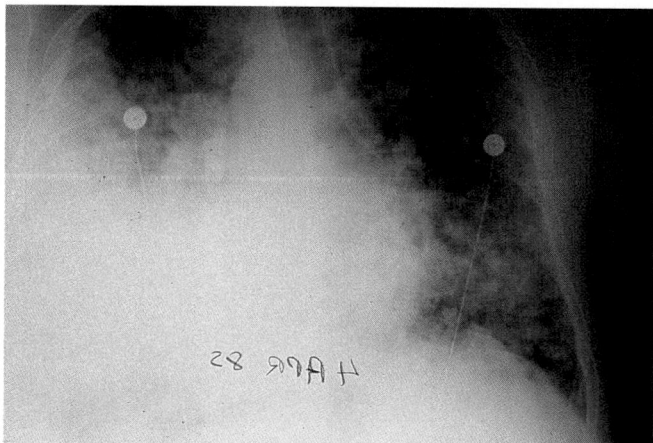

Figure 7–33. *Nocardia* pneumonia and pericarditis.
Chest x-ray—*Nocardia* pneumonia and pericarditis.

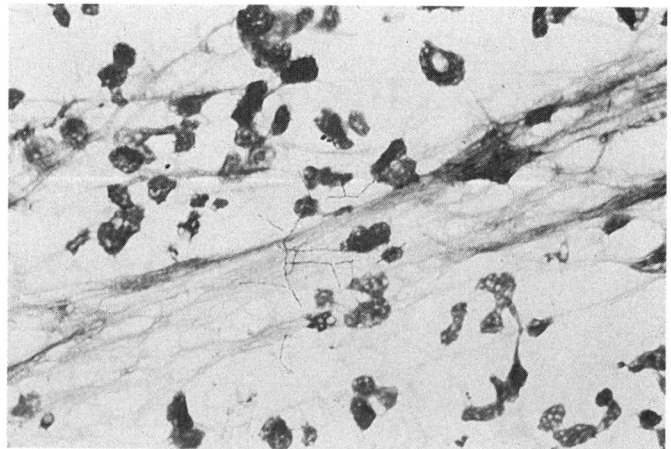

Figure 7–34. *Nocardia*.
AVB stain of *Nocardia* from the lung revealing branching acid-fast positive rods.

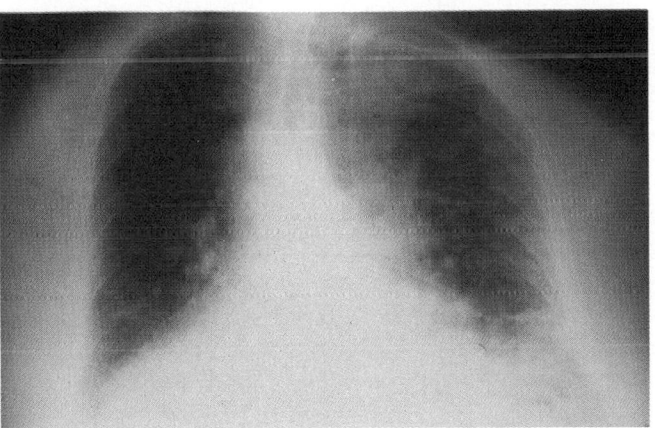

Figure 7–35. *Legionella pneumophila* pneumonia.
Chest x-ray–*Legionella pneumophila* pneumonia.

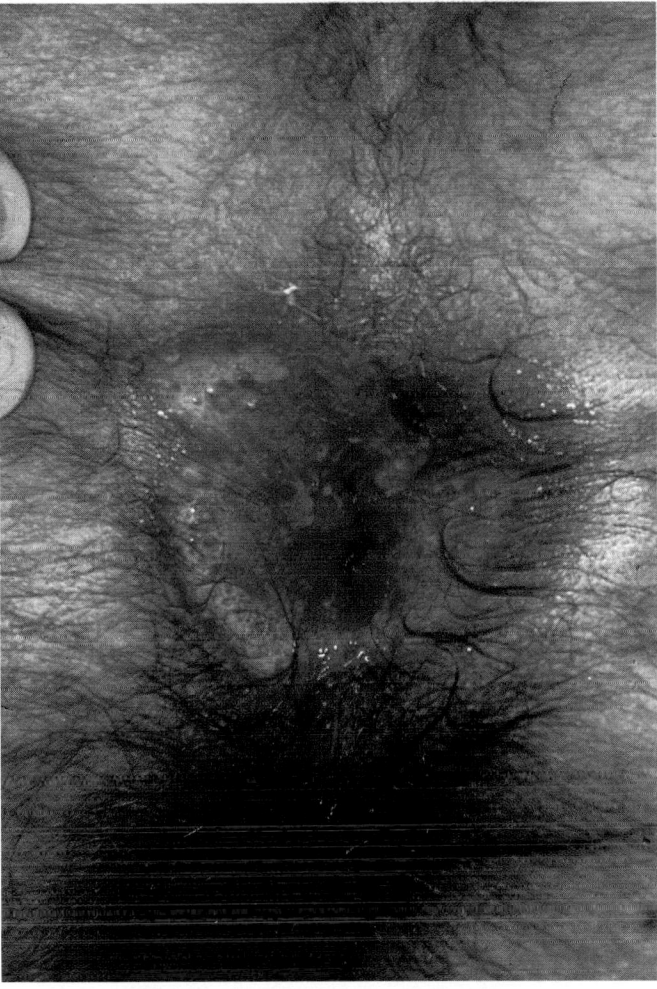

Figure 7–37. Herpes infection.
Chronic mucocutaneous perianal herpes infection. (From Still Picture Archives, Centers for Disease Control, Atlanta, Georgia.)

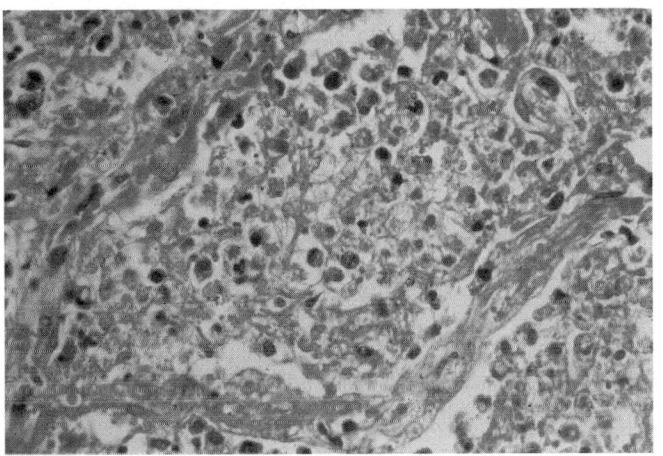

Figure 7–36. *Legionella* alveolitis.
Hematoxylin and eosin stain—*Legionella* alveolitis.

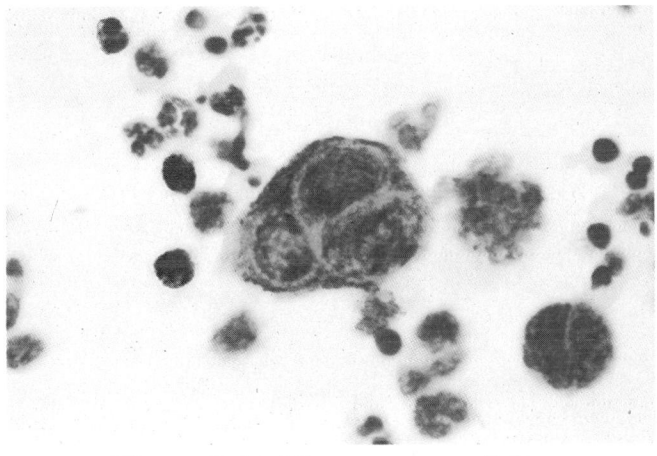

Figure 7–38. Herpes progenitalis.
Herpes progenitalis, multinucleated giant cell, penile lesion; Tzanck preparation.

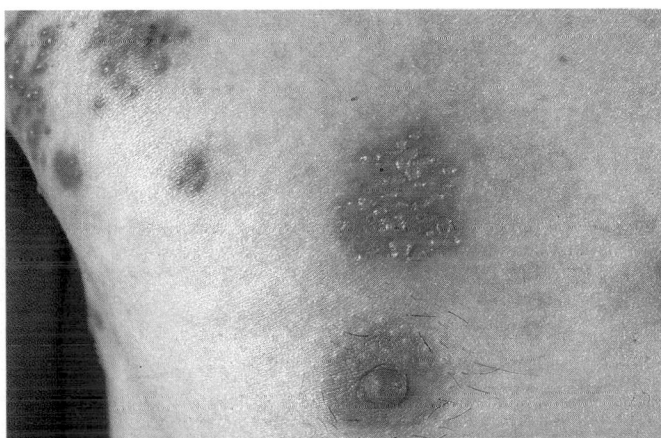

Figure 7–39. Varicella zoster.
Varicella zoster—reactivation as shingles.

Cytomegalovirus

Cytomegalovirus is a ubiquitous cause of infection in individuals with AIDS involving a wide variety of organ systems. Many of the higher risk groups for AIDS have particularly high seroprevalence for CMV, and the cellular immunity associated with AIDS allows the latent virus to reactivate and disseminate widely.[96] It is not known whether repeated exposures to the virus in gay and bisexual men result in hyperinfection with multiple strains and synergistic immunosuppression.[94]

Most individuals with AIDS have persistent CMV viremia. It is therefore often difficult to determine the role that CMV is playing in the pathogenesis of specific clinical syndromes. Individuals without exposure to HIV may have fever, malaise, and weight loss associated with primary CMV infection; however, coinfection with HIV and Epstein-Barr virus makes it difficult to assess the independent contribution of CMV in these syndromes in patients with AIDS and related disorders.

Visceral involvement with CMV may be demonstrated by histologic staining with a demonstration of inclusion bodies such as the classic "owl's eye" pattern (Figure 7–40). Culture alone often is not sufficient evidence because contamination with blood cells in patients who are viremic makes it difficult to assess the independent contribution of CMV.

Cytomegalovirus infection may result in a pneumonitis that is most often diagnosed at autopsy.[97] In addition, hemorrhagic gastrointestinal disease,[98] hepatitis, and chorioretinitis[99] may be associated with CMV infection (Figure 7–41). Hemorrhages and exudates found in the retina are more frequently due to cytomegalovirus than to *Tox-*

oplasma gondii in this population. Less common syndromes include CMV esophagitis, lymphadenitis, and adrenalitis.[100, 101]

Newer investigational drugs such as 9-[2-hydroxy-l-(hydroxymethyl)ethoxymethyl guananine] DHPG, an acyclovir derivative which appears to suppress viral replication, have been shown to be effective in the management of disseminated CMV infection, particularly chorioretinitis and colitis.[102, 103] In patients who are immunosuppressed because of renal transplants and develop CMV infection, diminution of the immunosuppressive drugs has resulted in resolution of CMV infection. Whether immunostimulatory treatment will work in individuals with AIDS remains to be seen.

Epstein-Barr Virus

Like CMV, Epstein-Barr virus can be isolated from multiple patients with AIDS and related disorders as well as people at increased risk for these syndromes.[94] The virus may result in fever, generalized lymphadenopathy, and malaise in individuals with or without exposure to HIV. It is, therefore, difficult to ascertain the independent role played by this virus in the pathogenesis of some of the disorders associated with AIDS. However, evidence of active Epstein-Barr virus resulting in B-cell proliferation has been suggested as a mechanism for the development of opportunistic lymphomas in individuals with AIDS. The diffuse lymphocytic interstitial pneumonitis described in the pediatric population with AIDS has been associated with active Epstein-Barr virus infection as well. Much more of the biology of the interaction of this virus with HIV remains to be clarified.

The multiplicity of organisms that may cause significant illness in in-

dividuals with AIDS have certain features in common, particularly their ubiquitous presence in nature, as well as the manner in which the immune system combats these organisms in immunocompetent hosts. Other organisms that require intact T-helper cell function have been described with increasing frequency in individuals with AIDS, such as strongyloidosis, histoplasmosis, and coccidioidomycosis.[35] It is possible, with increased observation of the epidemic, that new pathogens will be identified which contribute to the significant morbidity and mortality rates in individuals with AIDS and related disorders.

Helminthic Infections

Strongyloides stercoralis may persist in human hosts for decades asymptomatically and can reactivate when individuals become immunocompromised. Thus, persons with AIDS may develop disseminated disease without prior knowledge of infection, which may be manifested as diarrhea, abdominal pain, and intermittent pulmonary symptoms. Stool examination in the appropriate clinical context may be useful in establishing the diagnosis (Figure 7–42). Patients can be treated with thiabendazole. *Trichuris* (whipworm) infection may be seen in homosexually active males (Figure 7–43) and treated with mebendazole.

Conclusion

Persons with AIDS and HIV infection are subject to multiple types of viral, bacterial, protozoal, and helminthic infections because of immune deficits, as well as life-style practices. The astute clinician must be aware that multisystem disease may be due to the spread of an unusual pathogen, that common organisms may present in atypical ways, and that symptoms may be due to coinfection with multiple agents.

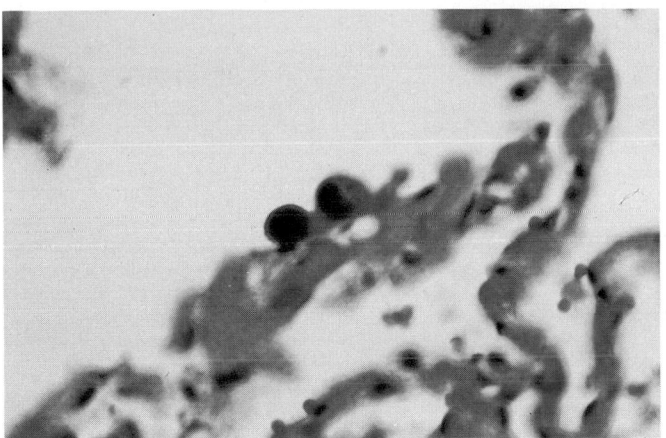

Figure 7–40. Cytomegalovirus.

Cytomegalovirus—intranuclear inclusions in cells in lung biopsy. (Courtesy of Jonathan W. M. Gold, MD, Associate Director, Special Microbiology Laboratory, Memorial Sloan-Kettering Cancer Center, New York.)

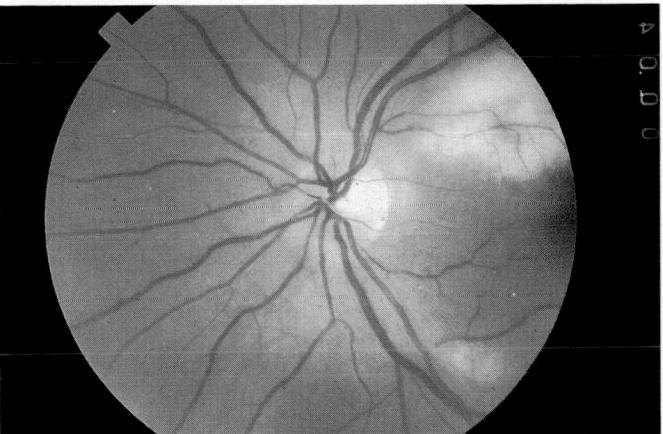

Figure 7–41. Cytomegalovirus retinitis.

Cytomegalovirus retinitis—hemorrhage and exudate.

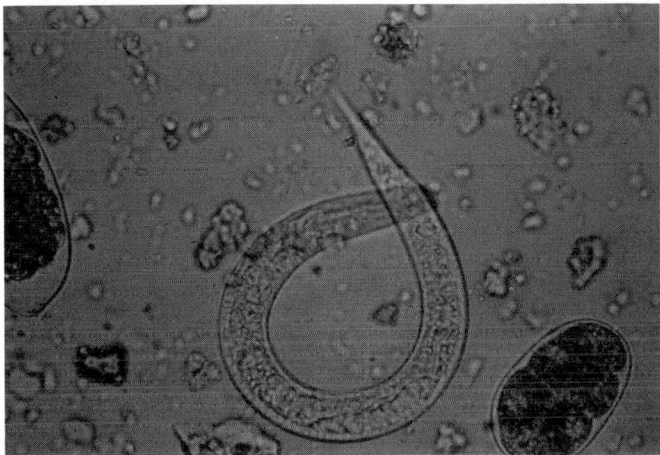

Figure 7–42. *Strongyloides stercoralis*.

Strongyloides stercoralis—rhabditiform larvae on stool specimen.

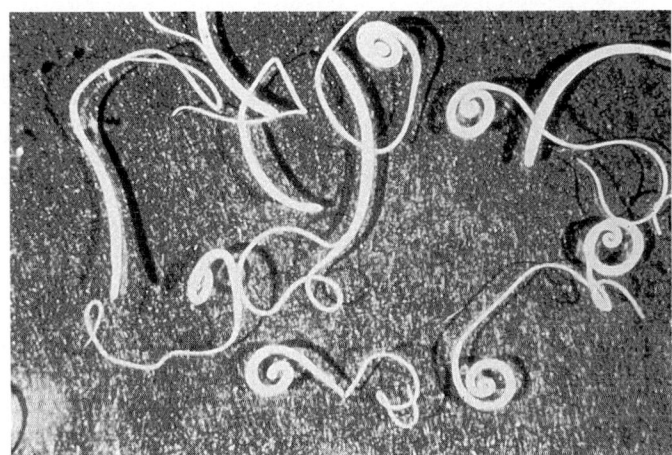

Figure 7–43. *Trichuris*.

Trichuris (whipworm) from stool specimen.

References

1. Barre-Sinoussi F, Chermann JC, Rety F, et al: Isolation of a T-lymphotropic retrovirus from a patient at risk for acquired immune deficiency syndrome (AIDS). Science 220:868, 1983.
2. Gallo RC, Salahuddin SZ, Popovic M, et al: Frequent detection and isolation of cytopathic retroviruses (HTLV-III) from patients with AIDS and at risk for AIDS. Science 224:500, 1984.
3. Bowen DL, Lane HC, Fouci AS: Immunologic features of AIDS. In DeVita VT Jr, Hellman S, Rosenberg SA (eds): AIDS: Etiology, Diagnosis, Treatment and Prevention. Philadelphia, J. B. Lippincott Company, pp. 89–109, 1985.
4. Fauci AS, Macher AM, Longo DL, et al: Acquired immunodeficiency syndrome: Epidemiologic, clinical, immunologic, and therapeutic considerations. Ann Intern Med 100:92–106, 1984.
5. Blaser MJ, Cohn DL: Opportunistic infections in patients with AIDS: Clues to the epidemiology of AIDS and the relative virulence of pathogens. Rev Infect Dis 8:21, 1986.
6. Kanki PJ, Alroy J, Essex M: Isolation of a T-lymphotropic retrovirus related to HTLV-III/LAV from wild-caught African green monkeys. Science 230:951–954, 1985.
7. Kanki PJ, Barin F, M'Boup S, Allan JS, Romet-Lemonne JL, Marlink R, et al: New human T-cell retrovirus related to simian T-lymphotropic virus type III (STLV-III$_{AGM}$). Science 232:238–243, 1986.
8. Letvin NL, Daniel MD, Sehgal PK, Desrosiers RC, Hunt LM, Waldron JJ, et al: Induction of AIDS-like disease in macaque monkeys with T-cell tropic retrovirus STLV-III. Science 230:71–73, 1985.
9. Sonigo P, Alizon M, Staskus K, Klatzman D, Cole S, Danos D, et al: Nucleotide sequence of the visna lentivirus: Relationship to the AIDS virus. Cell 42:369–382, 1985.
10. Weiss R, Teich N, Vermus H, Coffin J (eds): The Molecular Biology of Tumor Viruses: RNA Tumor Viruses. 2nd ed. Cold Spring Harbor, NY, Cold Spring Harbor Laboratory, 1985.
11. Ratner L, Haseltine W, Patarca R, Livak KJ, Starcich B, Josephs SF, et al: Complete nucleotide sequence of the AIDS virus, HTLV-III. Nature 313:277–284, 1985.
12. Sanchez-Pescador R, Power MD, Barr PJ, Steiner KS, Stempien MM, et al: Nucleotide sequence and expression of an AIDs-associated retrovirus (ARV-2). Science 227:484–492, 1985.
13. Wain-Hobson S, Sonigo P, Danos O, Cole S, Alizon M: Nucleotide sequence of the AIDS virus, LAV. Cell 40:9–17, 1985.
14. Meusing MA, Smith DH, Cabradilla CD, Benton CV, Lasky LA, Capon DJ: Nucleic acid structure and expression of the human AIDS/lymphadenopathy retrovirus. Nature 313:450–457, 1985.
15. Coffin JM: Genetic variation in AIDS viruses. Background paper. Washington, DC: Committe on a National Strategy for AIDS, 1987.
16. Dowbenko D, Bell J, Benton C, Groopman J, Nguyen H, Vetterlein D, et al: Bacterial expression of the AIDS retrovirus p24 GAG protein and its use as a diagnostic reagent. Proc Natl Acad Sci 82:7748–7752, 1985.
17. Sodroski JG, Rosen C, Haseltine WA: Trans-activating transcriptional activation of the long terminal repeat of human T-lymphotropic virus in infected cells. Science 225:381–385, 1984.
18. Sodroski JG, Goh WC, Rosen C, Tartar A, Portetella D, Burny A, et al: Replicative and cytopathic potential of HTLV-III/LAV with sor gene deletions. Science 231:1549–1553, 1986.
19. Allan JS, Coligan JE, Lee TH, McCane MF, Kanki PJ, Groopman JE, et al: A new HTLV-III/LAV encoded antigen detected by antibodies from AIDS patients. Science 230:810–813, 1985.
20. Lee TH, Coligan JE, Allan JS, McLane MF, Groopman JE, Essex M: A new HTLV-III/LAV protein encoded by a gene found in cytopathic retroviruses. Science 236:1546–1549, 1985.
21. Fisher AG, Feinberg MB, Josephs SF, Harper ME, Marselle IM, Broder S, et al: Infectious mutants of HTLV-III with changes in the 3' region and markedly reduced cytopathic effects. Science 233:655–659, 1986.
22. Harper ME, Marsell LM, Gallo RC, et al: Detection of HTLV-III-infected lymphocytes in lymph nodes and peripheral blood from AIDS patients by in situ hybridization. Proc Natl Acad Sci USA 83:772–776, 1986.
23. Salahuddin Z, Rose RM, Groopman JE, et al: Human alveolar macrophages: One of the possible reservoirs of HTLV-III. Blood 68:281–284, 1986.
24. Gartner S, Markovits P, Markovitz DM, Betts RF, Popovic M: Virus isolation from and identification of HTLV-III/LAV-producing cells in brain tissue from a patient with AIDS. JAMA 256:2365–2371, 1986.
25. Dalgleish AG, Beverly PCL, Clapham PR, Crawford DH, Greaves MF, Weiss RA: The CD4 (T4) antigen is an esential component antigen of the receptor for the AIDS retrovirus. Nature 312:763–767, 1984.
26. Klatzmann D, Barre-Sinoussi F, Nugeyre MT, et al: Selective tropism of lymphadenopathy associated virus (LAV) for helper-inducer T lymphocytes. Science 225:59–63, 1984.
27. Folks T, Powell DM, Lightfoote MM, Benn S, Martin MA, Fauci AS: Induction of HTLV-III/LAV from a nonvirus-producing T-cell line: Implications for latency. Science 231:600–602, 1986.
28. Zagury D, Bernard J, Leonard R, Cheynier R, Feldman M, Sarin PS, et al: Immune induction of T cell death in long term culture of HTLV-III infected T cells: A cytopathogenic model for AIDS T-cell depletion. Science 231:850–853, 1986.
29. Sodroski J, Goh WC, Rosen C, Campbell K, Haseltine WA: Role of HTLV-III/LAV envelope in syncytium formation and cytopathicity. Nature 322:470–474, 1986.
30. Bowen DL, Lane HC, Fauci AS: Immunopathogenesis of the acquired immunodeficiency syndrome. Ann Intern Med 103:704–709, 1985.
31. Lane HC, Depper JM, Greene WC, Whalen G, Waldmann TA, Fauci AS: Qualitative analysis of immune function in patients with the acquired immunodeficiency syndrome: Evidence for a selective defect in soluble antigen recognition. N Engl J Med 313:79–84, 1985.
32. Parks WP, Scott GB: An overview of pediatric AIDS: Approaches to diagnosis and outcome assessment. Background paper. Washington, DC, Committee on a National Strategy for AIDS, 1987.
33. Understanding of the disease and dimensions of the epidemic. In Baltimore D, Wolff SM (Co-chairs): Confronting AIDS, Directions for Public Health, Health Care, and Research. National Academy of Sciences, Washington, DC, 1986, pp 37–83.
34. Jaffe HW, Hardy AM, Meade Morgan W, Darrow WW: The acquired immunodeficiency syndrome in gay men. Ann Intern Med 103:662–664, 1985.
35. National Institute of Health: The impact of routine HTLV-III antibody testing of blood and plasma on public health. Draft report of a consensus conference. Bethesda, MD, July 7–9, 1986.
36. Sandstrom EG, Schooley RT, Ho DD, et al: Detection of human anti-HTLV-III antibodies using indirect immunofluorescences using fixed cells. Transfusion 25:308–312, 1985.
37. Mortimer PP, Parry JV, Mortimer JY: Which anti-HTLV-III/LAV assays for screening and confirmatory testing? Lancet 2:873–877, 1985.
38. Lange JMA, Coutinho RA, Krone WJA, Verdonck LF, Danner SA, van der Noordaa J, et al: Distinct IgG recognition patterns during progression of subclinical and clinical infection with LAV/HTLV-III. Br Med J 292:228–230, 1985.
39. Goudsmit J, de Wolf F, Paul DA, et al: Expression of human immunodeficiency virus antigen (HIV-Ag) in serum and cerebrospinal fluid during acute and chronic infection Lancet 2:177, 1986.
40. Margan J, Tate R, Farr AD, Urbaniak SJ: Potential source of errors in HTLV-III antibody testing (letter). Lancet 1:739–740, 1986.

41. Barr A, Dow BC, Arnott J, Crawford RS, Mitchell R: Anti-HTLV-III screening specificity and sensitivity (letter). Lancet 1:1032, 1986.

42. Saag MS, Britz J: Symptomatic blood donor with false positive HTLV-III Western Blot (letter). N Engl J Med 314:118, 1986.

43. Francis DP, Jaffe WH, Fultz PN, Getchell JP, McDougal JS, Feorino PM: The natural history of infection with the lymphadenopathy-associated virus human T-lymphotropic virus type III. Ann Intern Med 103:719–722, 1985.

44. Salahuddin SZ, Groopman JE, Markham PD, et al: HTLV-III in symptom-free seronegative persons. Lancet 2:1418–1420, 1984.

45. Mayer KH, Stoddard AM, McCusker J, Ayotte D, Ferriani R, Groopman JE: Human T-lymphotropic virus type III in high-risk, antibody-negative homosexual men. Ann Intern Med 104:194–196, 1986.

46. Cooper DA, Gold J, Maclean P, Donovan B, Finlayson R, Barnes TG, et al: Acute AIDS retrovirus infection: Definition of a clinical illness associated with seroconversion. Lancet 1:537–540, 1985.

47. Ho DD, Sarngadharan MG, Resnick L, et al: Primary human T-lymphotropic virus type III infection. Ann Intern Med 103:880–883, 1985.

48. Curran JW, Meade Morgan W, Hardy AM, Jaffe HW, Darrow WW, Dowdle WR: The epidemiology of AIDS: Current status and future prospects. Science 229:1352–1357, 1985.

49. Jaffe HW, Darrow WW, Echenberg DF, O'Malley PM, Getchel JP, Kalyanaraman VS, et al: The acquired immunodeficiency syndrome in a cohort of homosexual men. A six-year follow-up study. Ann Intern Med 103:210–214, 1985.

49a. Lifsen AR, Bodecker TW, Barnhart JL, et al: AIDS in the San Francisco City Clinic Cohort. Presented at the 27th Interscience Conference on Antimicrobial Agents and Chemotherapy. October 4–7, 1987, p. 95.

50. Redfield RR, Wright DC, Rhoades J, Burke DS: The natural history of HTLV-III/LAV infection. Abstracts of the Second International Conference on AIDS, Paris, June 23–25, 1986, p 128.

51. Mathur-Wagh U, Enlow RW, Spigland I, et al: Longitudinal study of persistent generalized lymphadenopathy in homosexual men: Relation to the acquired immunodeficiency syndrome. Lancet 1:1033–1038, 1984.

52. Abrams DI, Mess TP, Volberding P: Lymphadenopathy: Update of a 40-month prospective study. Presented at the International Conference on AIDS, Atlanta, GA, April 15, 1985.

53. Goedert JJ, Biggar RJ, Weiss SH, et al: Three year incidence of AIDS among HTLV-III infected risk group members: A comparison of five cohorts. Science 231:992–995, 1986.

54. Klein RS, Harris CA, Small CB, Moll B, Lesser M, Friedland GH: Oral candidiasis in high risk patients as the initial manifestation of the acquired immunodeficiency syndrome. N Engl J Med 311:354–358, 1984.

55. Hughes WT: Pneumocystis carinii pneumonia. N Engl J Med 297:1381, 1977.

56. Khadem M, Kalish SB, Goldsmith J, et al: Ophthalmologic findings in acquired immune deficiency syndrome (AIDS). Arch Ophthalmol 102:201, 1984.

57. Chalvardjian AM, Grawe LA: A new procedure for the identification of Pneumocystis carinii cysts in tissue sections and smears. J Clin Pathol 16:383, 1963.

58. Blumenfeld W, Wager E, Hadley WK: Use of the transbronchial biopsy for diagnosis of opportunistic pulmonary infections in acquired immunodeficiency syndrome (AIDS). Am J Clin Pathol 81:1, 1984.

59. Murray JF, Felton CP, Garay SM, et al: Pulmonary complications of the acquired immunodeficiency syndrome. Report of National Heart, Lung, and Blood Institute Workshop. N Engl J Med 310:1682, 1984.

60. Kovacs JA, Hiemenz JW, Macher AM, et al: Pneumocystis carinii pneumonia: A comparison between patients with the acquired immunodeficiency syndrome and patients with other immunodeficiencies. Ann Intern Med 100:663, 1984.

61. Coleman DL, Dodek PM, Luce JM, et al: Diagnosis utility of fiberoptic bronchoscopy in patients with Pneumocystis carinii pneumonia and the acquired immunodeficiency syndrome. Am Rev Respir Dis 128:795, 1983.

62. Broaddus C, Dake MD, Stulbarg MS, Blumenfeld W, Hadley K, Golden JA, et al: Bronchoalveolar lavage and transbronchial biopsy for the diagnosis of pulmonary infections in the acquired immunodeficiency syndrome. Ann Intern Med 102:747–752, 1985.

63. Bigby TD, Margolskee D, Curtis JL, Michael PF, Sheppard D, Hadley WK, et al: The usefulness of induced sputum in the diagnosis of Pneumocystis carinii pneumonia in patients with the acquired immunodeficiency syndrome. Am Rev Respir Dis 133:515–518, 1986.

64. Gordin FM, Simon GL, Wofsy CB, Mills J: Adverse reactions to trimethoprim-sulfamethoxazole in patients with AIDS. Ann Intern Med 100:495–499, 1984.

65. Haverkos HW: Assessment of therapy for Pneumocystis carinii pneumonia. Am J Med 76:501–508, 1984.

65a. Montgomery AB, Luce JM, Turner J, et al: Aerosolized pentamidine as sole therapy for Pneumocystis carinii pneumonia in patients with AIDS. Lancet 2:480, 1987.

66. Hughes WT, Smith BC: Efficiency of diaminodiphenylsulfone and other drugs in murine Pneumocystis carinii pneumonia. Antimicrob Agents Chemother 26:436, 1984.

67. Wong G, Gold JWM, Brown AE, et al: Central nervous system toxoplasmosis in homosexual men and parenteral drug abusers. Ann Intern Med 100:36, 1984.

68. Luft BJ, Brooks RG, Conley FK, et al: Toxoplasmosis encephalitis in patients with acquired immune deficiency syndrome. JAMA 252:913, 1984.

69. Whelan MA, Kricheff II, Handler M, et al: Acquired immunodeficiency syndrome: Cerebral computed tomographic manifestations. Radiology 149:477, 1983.

70. Current WL, Reese NC, Ernst JC, et al: Human cryptosporidiosis in immunocompetent and immunodeficient persons. N Engl J Med 308:1252, 1983.

71. Soave R, Danner RL, Honig CL, Ma P, Hart CC, Nash T, et al: Cryptosporidiosis in homosexual men. Ann Intern Med 100:504–511, 1984.

72. Margulis SJ, Honig CL, Soave R, Govoni AF, Mouradian JA, Jacobson IM: Biliary tract obstruction in the acquired immunodeficiency syndrome. Ann Intern Med 105:207–210, 1986.

73. Ma P, Soave R: Three-step stool examination with protracted watery diarrhea. J Infect Dis 147:824, 1983.

74. Portnoy D, Whiteside ME, Bukley E, et al: Treatment of intestinal cryptosporidiosis with spiramycin. Ann Intern Med 101:202, 1984.

75. Collier AC, Miller RA, Meyers JD: Cryptosporidiosis after marrow transplantation: Person-to-person transmission and treatment with spiramycin. Ann Intern Med 101:205–206, 1984.

76. Rolston K, Fainstein V, Mansell P, Sjoersdma A, Bodey GP: Alpha-difluoromethylornithine (DFMO) in the treatment of cryptosporidiosis in AIDS patients: Preliminary evaluation. Abstracts of the International Conference on AIDS, Atlanta, GA, April 14–17, 1985, p 77.

77. Westerman EL, Christensen RP: Chronic Isosporia belli infection treated with co-trimoxazole. Ann Intern Med 91:413–414, 1979.

78. Klein RS, Harris CA, Small CB, et al: Oral candidiasis in high risk patients as the initial manifestation of the acquired immunodeficiency syndrome. N Engl J Med 311:354, 1984.

79. Zuger A, Louie E, Holtzman RS, Simberkoff MS, Rahal JJ: Cryptococcal disease in patients with acquired immunodeficiency syndrome. Ann Intern Med 104:234–240, 1986.

80. Kovacs JA, Polis M, Macher AM, et al: Cryptococcus infections in patients with acquired immunodeficiency syndrome. Abstracts of the 24th ICAAC.

Washington, D.C., American Society for Microbiology, 1984.

81. Bennett JE, Dismukes WE, Duma RJ, et al: A comparison of amphotericin B alone and combined with flucytosine in the treatment of cryptococcal meningitis. N Engl J Med *301*:126–131, 1979.

82. Hawkins CC, Gold JWM, Whimbey E, Kiehn TE, Brannon P, Cammarata R, et al: *Mycobacterium avium* complex infections in patients with the acquired immunodeficiency syndrome. Ann Intern Med *105*:184–188, 1986.

83. Greene JB, Sidhu GS, Lewin S, et al: *Mycobacterium avium-intracellulare*: A cause of disseminated life-threatening infection in homosexuals and drug abusers. Ann Intern Med *97*:539, 1982.

84. Zakowski P, Fligiel S, Berlin GW, et al: Disseminated *Mycobacterium avium-intracellulare* in homosexual men dying of acquired immunodeficiency. JAMA *248*:2980, 1982.

85. Sohn CC, Schoroff RW, Kliewer KE, et al: Disseminated *Mycobacterium avium-intracellulare* infection in homosexual men with acquired cell-mediated immunodeficiency: A histologic and immunologic study of two cases. Am J Clin Pathol *79*:247, 1983.

86. Gillin JS, Urmacher C, West R, et al: Disseminated *Mycobacterium avium-intracellulare* infection in acquired immunodeficiency syndrome mimicking Whipple's disease. Gastroenterology *85*:1187, 1983.

87. Woodley CL, Kilburn JO: In vitro susceptibility of *Mycobacterium avium* complex and *Mycobacterium tuberculosis* strains to a spiropiperidyl rifamycin. Am Rev Respir Dis *126*:586, 1982.

88. Wu M, Kolonoski PT, Yadegar S, Inderlied CB, Young LS: In vitro suscep-tibility of *Mycobacterium avium* complex (MAC) to novel antimycobacterial drugs. Program and Abstracts of the 26th Interscience Conference on Antimicrobial Agents and Chemotherapy, New Orleans, LA, September 28–October 1, 1986, p 1102.

89. Pitchenik AE, Cole C, Russell BW, Fischl MA, Spira TJ, Snider DE: Tuberculosis, atypical mycobacteriosis and the acquired immunodeficiency syndrome among Haitian and non-Haitian patients in south Florida. Ann Intern Med *101*:641–645, 1984.

90. Glaser JB, Morton-Kute L, Berger SR, Weber J, Siegel FP, Lopez C, et al: Recurrent *Salmonella typhimurium* bacteremia associated with the acquired immunodeficiency syndrome. Ann Intern Med *102*:189–193, 1985.

91. Smith PD, Macher AM, Bookman MA, Poccia RV, Steis RG, Gill V, et al: *Salmonella typhimurium* enteritis and bacteremia in the acquired immunodeficiency syndrome. Ann Intern Med *102*:207–209, 1985.

92. Mayer KH, Hanson E: Recurrent salmonella infection with a single strain in the acquired immunodeficiency syndrome: Confirmation by plasmid fingerprinting. Diagn Microbiol Infect Dis *4*:71, 1986.

93. Siegel FP, Lopez C, Hammer GS, et al: Severe acquired immunodeficiency in male homosexuals manifested by chronic perianal ulcerative *herpes simplex* lesions. N Engl J Med *305*:1439, 1981.

94. Quinnan GV, Masur H, Rook AH, et al: Herpes virus infections in the acquired immunodeficiency syndrome. JAMA *252*:72, 1984.

95. Epstein E: Acyclovir for immunocompromised patients with herpes zoster. N Engl J Med *309*:1254, 1984.

96. Mintz L, Drew WL, Miner RC, et al: Cytomegalovirus infections in homosexual men. Ann Intern Med *99*:326, 1983.

97. Macher AM, Reichert CM, Straus SE, et al: Death in the AIDS patient: Role of cytomegalovirus. N Engl J Med *309*:1454, 1983.

98. Knapp AB, Horst DA, Eliopoulos G, et al: Widespread cytomegalovirus gastroenterocolitis in a patient with the acquired immunodeficiency syndrome. Gastroenterology *85*:1399, 1983.

99. Bachman DM, Rodrigues MM, Chu FC, et al: Culture-proven cytomegalovirus retinitis in a homosexual man with the acquired immunodeficiency syndrome. Ophthalmology *89*:797, 1982.

100. Laurence J: AIDS Report: CMV infections in AIDS patients. Infect Surg *5*:603–610, October 1986.

101. Tapper ML, Rotterdam HZ, Lerner CW, et al: Adrenal necrosis in the acquired immunodeficiency syndrome. Ann Intern Med *100*:239–241, 1984.

102. Masur H, Lane HC, Palestine A, et al: Effect of 9-(1,3-dihydroxy-2-propoxymethyl) guanine on serious cytomegalovirus disease in eight immunosuppressed homosexual men. Ann Intern Med *104*:41–44, 1986.

103. Koretz SH, Buhler WC, Brewin A, et al: Treatment of serious cytomegalovirus infection with 9-(1,3-dihydroxy-2-propoxymethyl) guanine in patients with AIDS and other immunodeficiencies. N Engl J Med *314*:801–805, 1986.

Index

Ear, Kaposi's sarcoma affecting, *19, 34*
Edema, *16, 23, 41*
Electrocautery, for Kaposi's sarcoma, 36
ELISA (enzyme-linked immunosorbent assay), 6, 129–130
Encephalitis-arthritis virus, in goats, 4
Encephalopathy, HIV-induced, 5
Endoplasmic reticulum, in epidemic Kaposi's sarcoma, 85, 86, *86,* 88, *88*
Entamoeba histolytica, 136, *137*
Enzyme-linked immunosorbent assay (ELISA), 6, 129–130
Eosinophilic pustular folliculitis, 118, *118–119*
Epidemiology, of AIDS, 3–4
   of HIV infection, 5–6
   of Kaposi's sarcoma variants, 44(t)
Epstein-Barr virus, 20, 31, 100, 101, 146
Equine anemia virus, 4
Erythema multiforme, 52, *59*
Erythematous plaques, of sarcoidosis, 69
Erythrocytes, extravasated, in dermatofibroma, *79*
   in Kaposi's sarcoma, *74, 75, 85, 86*
   in keloids, 78, *79*
Esophagitis, candidal, 108, 136, *137*
   herpetic, vs. candidal esophagitis, 144
Esophagus, epidemic Kaposi's sarcoma of, *39*
Etoposide, 36
Eye, epidemic Kaposi's sarcoma of, *33, 37*
Eyelashes, long, 120, *120*

Face, epidemic Kaposi's sarcoma of, *25, 27, 28, 41*
   herpes zoster infection of, *99*
   molluscum contagiosum infection of, *99*
   mycosis fungoides infection of, *65*
   sarcoidosis of, *68*
   seborrheic dermatitis-like eruption of, 113–114, *113*
Facial edema, *41*
Factor VIII preparation, 6
Fansidar, 133
Feet, Kaposi's sarcoma on, *15–18,* 29
   soles of, epidemic Kaposi's sarcoma on, *15, 17, 21, 25, 26*
      malignant melanoma on, *63*
      reticulum cell sarcoma on, *66*
      secondary syphilis on, *57, 105*
Fibroblasts, *85–87*
   vs. plasma cells, in epidemic Kaposi's sarcoma, *86, 86, 87*
Finger, Kaposi's sarcoma on, *18, 29*
Folliculitis, 102, *119*
   eosinophilic pustular, 118, *118–119*
   vs. mycobacterial infection, 106
Fordyce spots, 52
Foreskin, epidemic Kaposi's sarcoma on, *35*
Fungal infections, 2(t), 3(t)
   superficial, 108, *108–109*
   systemic, 110, *111*
Furuncles, 102

Gangrene, Kaposi's sarcoma and, *16*
Gastrointestinal lesions, Kaposi's sarcoma and, 30, *39*
   with perianal CMV ulcers, 96
Gene(s), *env,* of HIV, 5
   for retroviruses, 128
Genetic factors, of Kaposi's sarcoma, 46

Genital herpes, 144, *145*
Giardia lamblia, 136, *137*
Gingiva, epidemic Kaposi's sarcoma affecting, *38–39*
Glomus tumor, *67*
Granuloma, pyogenic, *62*
Granuloma annulare, 58, *59*
Granulomatous dermatitis, *61*
GRID, 2

Hair, absence of, 122, *123*
Haitian immigrants, 2
Halo, yellowish, in epidemic Kaposi's sarcoma, *28*
Hands, Kaposi's sarcoma on, *18, 22, 25*
   secondary syphilis on, *57*
Head and neck, angiosarcoma of, vs. epidemic Kaposi's sarcoma, *75–76, 76–77*
   epidemic Kaposi's sarcoma of, *41*
Health care workers, HIV infection in, 7
Helminthic infections, 2(t), 146, *147*
Hemangioma, *54, 55,* 120
Hemophiliacs, 2, 5, 31
Hemosiderin, *28, 52, 58, 72, 73*
Hepatitis B infection, 4, 7, 131
Herpes esophagitis, vs. candidal esophagitis, 136
Herpes simplex infection, 98, *99,* 144, *145*
   with CMV infection, *96, 97*
Herpes zoster infection, 98, *99,* 144, *145*
Heterosexuals, AIDS and, 6
   Kaposi's sarcoma and, 31, 33
Histoplasma capsulatum, 112, *117*
Histoplasmosis, 112, *112,* 140, *141*
HIV infection. See *Human immunodeficiency virus (HIV), infection with.*
Hives, 52
HLA-DR5, Kaposi's sarcoma and, 46
Homosexuals, 2, 4, 5, 31, 46
   hairy leukoplakia in, 100
   Kaposi's sarcoma in, 24, *25–26, 28–29,* 31, 36
   Pneumocystis carinii pneumonia in, 24
HTLV. See *Human T-cell lymphotropic virus (HTLV).*
Human immunodeficiency virus (HIV), 128, *129*
   entry into target helper T cells, 128
   genetic characteristics of, 5
   infection with, 2, 4
      antibody tests for, 6, 7
      antigenic variation of, 5
      asymptomatic, 131
      Centers for Disease Control classification system for, 131(t)
      clinical signs of, with seronegative results, *21–22*
      diagnostic tests for, 6, 129–130
      epidemiology and clinical spectrum of, 5–6
      future prospects for, 6–7
      immunology of, 47
      in Africa, vs. Europe and U.S., 6, 42
      in health care workers, 7
      latency period of, 5
      nervous system, 5, 129. See also *Central nervous system.*
      serum antibody to, endemic Kaposi's sarcoma and, 45
      spread of, 4, 6
      therapy and prevention of, 7–8

Human immunodeficiency virus (HIV) *(Continued)*
   infection with, therapy and prevention of, 7–8
   virology of, 4–7
Human immunodeficiency virus II (HIV-II), 4–5, 128
Human T-cell lymphotropic virus (HTLV), 4, 128
9-[(2-Hydroxy-l-(hydroxy-methyl)ethoxy-methyl guaninine] DHPG, for CMV infection, 146
Hypergammaglobulinemia, 129
Hyperkeratotic scales, with Kaposi's sarcoma, *17*
Hyperpigmentation, of basal cell carcinoma, *64*
   of Kaposi's sarcoma, 13, *16, 18, 26–28, 31–32, 37, 41*
   of lichen planus, *60*
   of pityriasis rosea, 58, *59*
   of purpuric lesions, *53*
   of sarcoidosis, *68*
   postinflammatory, *61*
Hypogammglobulinemia, 129

Immunodeficiency, 2, 4, 45, 128–129
   opportunistic infections indicative of, 127(t)
Immunologic basis, of AIDS-associated Kaposi's sarcoma, 24
   of HIV infection, 4–7
   of retroviral exposure, 127
Immunologic overload, 4
Immunosuppression, herpes zoster infection and, 98
   Kaposi's sarcoma and, 24
Impetigo, 102, *103*
Inclusions, cytomegalovirus, 146, *147*
   in biopsy material, 88, *88, 90, 91*
Infants. See also *Children.*
   born to HIV-infected mothers, 5
   lymphadenopathic Kaposi's sarcoma in, 42
Infection(s), associated with AIDS, 2(t), 3(t)
   modifiers of, 127
   bacterial 2(t), 3(t), 102, *103,* 140, *141–144*
   debilitation with, 129
   etiology of, 128
   fungal, 2(t), 3(t), 108, *108–109,* 110, *111*
   in Africa vs. U.S. and Europe, 42
   multiple, 4, *41, 43*
   nongenital viral, 2(t), 3(t)
   opportunistic, in AIDS patients, 125–150
      in epidemic Kaposi's sarcoma, 30
      indicative of immune defect, 127(t)
   pathogenesis of, 128–129
   prevalence of, in AIDS patients, 130(t)
   protozoan, 2(t), 3(t), 132–136, *132–136*
   repeated exposure to, HIV infection and, 46
Infectious diseases, signs of, *96–112.* See also specific diseases (e.g., *Cytomegalovirus infection; Molluscum contagiosum,* etc.)
Inflammatory lesions, vs. epidemic Kaposi's sarcoma, 58, *58–61*
Inguinal nodes, 22
Insect bites, 37, 117
Interferons, 36, 88
   recombinant leukocyte A, long eyelashes with, 120, *120*
International Committee on Taxonomy of Viruses, 4
Intestines, Kaposi's sarcoma of, endemic African, *23*
Isospora belli, 134